PCF1

PALLIATIVE CARE FORMULARY

Robert Twycross

Andrew Wilcock

Sarah Thorp

Radcliffe Medical Press

© 1998 Robert Twycross, Andrew Wilcock and Sarah Thorp

Radcliffe Medical Press Ltd
18 Marcham Road, Abingdon, Oxon OX14 1AA

Reprinted 1999

British Library Cataloguing in Publication Data

A catalogue record for this book is available from the British Library.

ISBN 1 85775 264 3

Typeset by Advance Typesetting Ltd, Oxon.
Printed and bound by Biddles Ltd, Guildford and King's Lynn.

PALLIATIVE CARE FORMULARY

Robert Twycross DM, FRCP, FRCR
Macmillan Clinical Reader in Palliative Medicine,
University of Oxford
Consultant Physician, Sir Michael Sobell House,
Churchill Hospital, Oxford
Director, WHO Collaborating Centre for Palliative Cancer Care,
Oxford

Andrew Wilcock DM, MRCP
Macmillan Senior Lecturer in Palliative Medicine and Medical Oncology,
University of Nottingham
Consultant Physician,
Hayward House Macmillan Specialist Palliative Care Unit,
Nottingham City Hospital NHS Trust,
Nottingham

Sarah Thorp MRPharmS, Dip Clin Pharm
Palliative Care Pharmacist,
Hayward House Macmillan Specialist Palliative Care Unit,
Nottingham City Hospital NHS Trust,
Nottingham

Contents

Preface

The NHS Executive Letter EL (96)85 on commissioning palliative care services stressed the need for continuity and consistency of care in all aspects of cancer services. In relation to palliative care, it stated that this would be assisted by a core drug formulary. Indeed, a core formulary, developed in consultation with specialist palliative care services and pharmacists, is a required standard for a Cancer Centre and its associated units. We hope that the Palliative Care Formulary will be seen as a significant step towards achieving this goal.

The PCF has evolved out of the Sobell House Department Formulary, hitherto revised annually. After 10 years, the time was ripe for major changes – including the opportunity of extending 'ownership' to Hayward House, Nottingham. It should be stressed that the PCF does not replace the British National Formulary or books on pain and symptom management; it is for use alongside them. We hope that the PCF will help clinicians steer their way successfully through the increasingly complex world of pharmacology and therapeutics.

Inside the back cover of the BNF there are several tear-out **yellow cards**. These are used to report suspected adverse drug reactions to the Medicines Control Agency (UK). Inside the back cover of the PCF there are several tear-out **red cards** and **green cards**. The red cards are for reporting syringe driver compatibilities and incompatibilities which are not listed in Section 14. The green cards are for making suggestions for additional drugs to be included in the next edition of the PCF. The ultimate success of the PCF depends in part on the use by readers of these cards.

There is obvious duplication between the contents of the PCF and *Symptom Management in Advanced Cancer* (Twycross 1997, Radcliffe Medical Press). In time, the overlap will be resolved and they will more clearly become companion volumes.

Acknowledgements are due to the BNF whose cover design is reflected in ours, and to the Neonatal Formulary whose format pointed us in the right direction. We are grateful to colleagues at Sobell House and Hayward House, and elsewhere, for their advice and support, particularly Jennifer Barraclough, John Chambers, Ray Corcoran, Vincent Crosby, Caroline Hare, Christine Hirsch, Andrew Hughes, Michael Minton, John Moyle, Lindsay Nearney, Sue Palmer and Meg Roberts. Thanks are also due to Margaret Scott (Hayward House) and Karen Allen (Sobell House) for their respective parts in preparing the typescript, and to Susan Brown for her invaluable contribution as copy editor.

Robert Twycross
Andrew Wilcock
Sarah Thorp
July 1998

Finding your way around the PCF

The sections generally follow the order in the BNF, but some have been omitted because they are irrelevant in palliative care. On the other hand, there is a section on syringe drivers. The appendices deal with themes which transcend the drug monographs, e.g. important drug interactions, the use of drugs for unlicensed purposes, and named patient supplies. The Index contains both the **recommended International Nonproprietary Names (rINNs)** and, where they differ, the more familiar (though outdated) **British Approved Names (BANs)**. You should take an early opportunity to familiarize yourself with the new rINNs (see p.xii). For a few drugs, both BAN and rINN will be used concurrently for 5 years. For the rest, the use of BANs will be illegal from the end of 1998.

Manufacturers' names are not included. For this, you should refer to the **BNF** or the **ABPI Compendium of Data Sheets and Summaries of Product Characteristics**. Drugs marked with an asterisk (*) should generally be used only by, or after consultation with, a specialist palliative care service. Drug prices are net prices based on those in the BNF Number 35 (March 1998).

Inevitably, the views expressed in the PCF reflect the experience and clinical practice of the authors. Many drugs featured in the PCF are recommended for unlicensed uses and routes, and at doses which exceed those in the manufacturers' **Data Sheets** and **Summaries of Product Characteristics** (see Appendix 7). While every effort has been made to indicate unlicensed uses with a dagger (†), the dividing line is not always clearcut. It is the reader's personal responsibility to decide how far to follow the recommendations in the PCF in such matters.

General guidance about the use of drugs in palliative care

Drugs are not the total answer for the relief of pain and other symptoms. For many symptoms, the concurrent use of nondrug measures is equally important, and sometimes more important. Further, drugs must always be used within the context of a systematic approach to symptom management, namely:

- evaluation
- explanation
- individualized treatment
- supervision
- attention to detail.

In palliative care, the axiom 'diagnosis before treatment' still holds true. Further, even when the cancer is responsible, a symptom may be caused in different ways, e.g. in lung cancer vomiting may be caused by hypercalcaemia or by raised intracranial pressure – to name but two out of many possible causes. Clearly, treatment will vary according to the cause.

Attention to detail includes **precision in taking a drug history**. Thus, if a patient says, 'I take morphine every 4 hours', the doctor should say, 'Tell me, when do you take your first dose?' 'And your second dose?' etc. When this is done, it often turns out that the patient is taking morphine q.d.s. rather than q4h, and possibly p.r.n. rather than prophylactically. On one occasion, 'every 4 hours' meant 0800, 1200, 1600, 2000h. It was not surprising, therefore, that this patient woke in excruciating pain at about 0300h – so much so that she dreaded going to bed at night.

Attention to detail also means **providing clear instructions for drug regimens**. 'Take as much as you like, as often as you like', is a recipe for anxiety and poor symptom relief. The drug regimen should be written out in full for the patient and his family to work from (Figures 1 & 2). This should be in an ordered and logical way, e.g. analgesics, anti-emetics, laxatives, followed by other drugs. Times to be taken, name of drugs, reason for use ('for pain', 'for bowels' etc.) and dose (x ml, y tablets) should all be stated. The patient should also be advised how to obtain further supplies, e.g. from the general practitioner.

When prescribing an additional drug, it is important to ask:

'What is the treatment goal?'
'How can it be monitored?'
'What is the risk of adverse effects?'
'What is the risk of drug interactions?'
'Is it possible to stop any of the current medications?'

'Good prescribing is a skill, and makes the difference between poor and excellent symptom control'.[1] It extends to considering size, shape and taste of tablets and solutions; and avoiding 'bastard' doses which force:

- patients to take more tablets than would be the case if doses were 'rounded up' to a more convenient tablet size. For example, it is better to prescribe m/r morphine 60mg (a single tablet) rather than 50mg (3 tablets: 30mg + 10mg + 10mg)
- nurses to spend more time refilling syringes for 24h infusions. For example, in the UK, pre-scribing diamorphine 100mg (a single ampoule) instead of 90mg (60mg ampoule + 30mg ampoule).

It is necessary to be equally thorough when re-evaluating a patient and supervising treatment. It is often difficult to predict the optimum dose of a symptom relief drug, particularly opioids,

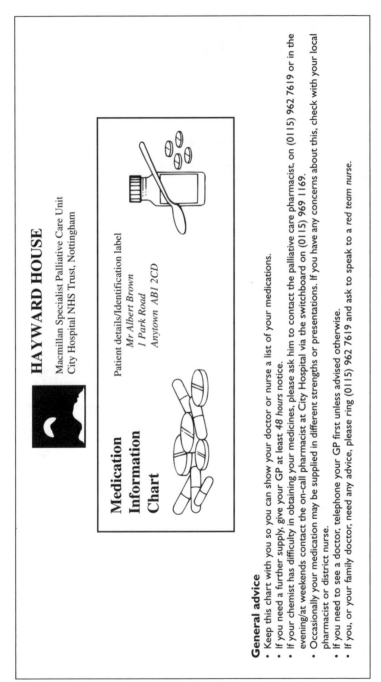

Figure 1 Side 1 of patient's Medication Information Chart.

| Regular medication | | Strength | Reason | When to take | | | | |
Description	(Trade name)			ON WAKING	LUNCH 2pm	TEA 6pm	BED TIME
MORPHINE SULPHATE MR Purple tablet	(MST)	30mg	PAIN RELIEF *take 12 hours apart*	1			1
DICLOFENAC Round brown tablet		50mg	BONE PAIN	1	1		1
SODIUM VALPROATE Lilac tablet	(Epilim)	200mg	NERVE PAIN				2
CODANTHRAMER Orange liquid		strong	FOR BOWELS			TWO 5ml spoons	
DOMPERIDONE Small white tablet	(Motilium)	10mg	STOP SICKNESS	2	2	2	2
As needed							
MORPHINE SOLUTION Clear liquid	(Oramorph)	10mg in 5ml	Breakthrough pain	Take ONE 5ml spoon every 2–4 hours if needed			
ASILONE Suspension White liquid			Indigestion	Take TWO 5ml spoonfuls FOUR times a day			

Completed by: S THORP   Nurse/Pharmacist   Checked by: M SMITH   On: 24-2-98

Figure 2 Side 2 of patient's Medication Information Chart.

laxatives and psychotropic drugs. Further, adverse effects put drug compliance in jeopardy. Arrangements must be made, therefore, for continuing supervision and adjustment of medication.

Finally, it may be necessary to compromise on complete relief in order to avoid unacceptable adverse effects. For example, antimuscarinic effects such as dry mouth or visual disturbance may limit dose escalation; and, with inoperable bowel obstruction, it may be better to aim to reduce the incidence of vomiting to once or twice a day rather than to seek to abolish it altogether.

1 Kaye P (1994) *A to Z of Hospices and Palliative Medicine*. EPL Publications, Northampton.

Drug names

For about 150 drugs marketed in the UK, the recommended International Nonproprietary Name (rINN) differs from the British Approved Name (BAN). In 1999, following a European Union Directive, the use of BANs will be discontinued and all drugs marketed in the UK will be known by their rINNs. For drugs where there is a high risk to health from possible confusion, there will be a 5-year transition period during which both the BAN and the rINN must be used (Table 1). In the case of a few drugs for which the INN is only 'proposed' (pINN) and not recommended (rINN), BANs will continue to be used.

Table 1 Main drugs for which both BAN and rINN must be used

BAN	rINN
Adrenaline	Epinephrine
Amethocaine	Tetracaine
Bendrofluazide	Bendroflumethiazide
Benzhexol	Trihexyphenidyl
Chlorpheniramine	Chlorphenamine
Dicyclomine	Dicycloverine
Dothiepin	Dosulepin
Frusemide	Furosemide
Mitozantrone	Mitoxantrone
Noradrenaline	Norepinephrine
Procaine penicillin	Procaine benzylpenicillin
Salcatonin	Calcitonin (salmon)
Trimeprazine	Alimemazine

For many drugs, the change is slight (e.g. danthron → dantron) but for others the rINN is very different (e.g. methotrimeprazine → levomepromazine). Certain general rules apply:

- 'ph' becomes 'f' (e.g. cephradine → cefradine)
- 'th' becomes 't' (e.g. indomethacin → indometacin)
- 'y' becomes 'i' (e.g. napsylate → napsilate).

Inevitably perhaps there are exceptions, e.g. amitriptyline which is unchanged. The main drugs affected are listed in Table 2.

Table 2 Main drugs affected by European Union Directive on rINN

BAN	rINN
Amylobarbitone	Amobarbital
Amoxycillin	Amoxicillin
Beclomethasone	Beclometasone
Bendrofluazide	Bendroflumethiazide
Benorylate	Benorilate
Benzathine penicillin	Benzathine benzylpenicillin
Benztropine	Benzatropine
Cephalexin (etc.)	Cefalexin (etc.)
Chlormethiazole	Clomethiazole
Cyclosporin	Ciclosporin
Danthron	Dantron
Dexamphetamine	Dexamfetamine
Dienoestrol	Dienestrol
Dimethicone	Dimeticone
Glycopyrronium	Glycopyrrolate
Guaiphenesin	Guaifenesin
Hexamine hippurate	Methenamine hippurate
Indomethacin	Indometacin
Lignocaine	Lidocaine
Methotrimeprazine	Levomepromazine
Oestradiol	Estradiol
Oxethazaine	Oxetacaine
Phenobarbitone	Phenobarbital
Sodium cromoglycate	Sodium cromoglicate
Stilboestrol	Diethylstilbestrol
Sulphasalazine	Sulfasalazine
Sulphathiazole	Sulfathiazole
Thyroxine	Levothyroxine
Vitamin A	Retinol

Outside Europe, it is important to note several differences between rINNs and USANs, i.e. the 'adopted' names used in the USA (Table 3). Note also that:

- diamorphine (available only in the UK) = di-acetylmorphine = heroin
- hyoscine = scopolamine
- liquid paraffin = mineral oil.

Table 3 Important differences between rINNs and USANs

rINN	USAN
Dimeticone[a]	Simethicone
Dextropropoxyphene	Propoxyphene
Paracetamol	Acetaminophen
Pethidine	Meperidine

a. in some countries, dimeticone is called (di)methylpolysiloxane.

List of abbreviations

General

BNF	British National Formulary
BP	British Pharmacopoeia
CSM	Committee on Safety of Medicines (UK)
IASP	International Association for the Study of Pain
IDIS	International Drug Information Service
MCA	Medicines Control Agency (UK)
PCU	palliative care unit
SPC	Summary of Product Characteristics
UK	United Kingdom
USA	United States of America
USP	United States Pharmacopoeia
WHO	World Health Organization

Medical

ADH	antidiuretic hormone (vasopressin)
β_2	beta 2 adrenergic (receptors)
CNS	central nervous system
COX	cyclo-oxygenase; alternative, prostaglandin synthase
COPD	chronic obstructive pulmonary disease
CSF	cerebrospinal fluid
CT	computed tomography
δ	delta opioid (receptors)
D_2	dopamine type 2 (receptors)
DIC	disseminated intravascular coagulation
ECG	electrocardiogram
FEV_1	forced expiratory volume in 1 second
FRC	functional residual capacity
FVC	forced vital capacity of lungs
H_1, H_2	histamine type 1, type 2 (receptors)
Ig	immunoglobulin
INR	International normalized ratio (prothrombin time)
κ	kappa opioid (receptors)
MAOI(s)	mono-amine oxidase inhibitor(s)
MRI	magnetic resonance imaging
MSU	mid-stream specimen of urine
μ	mu opioid (receptors)
NMDA	N-methyl D-aspartate
NSAID(s)	nonsteroidal anti-inflammatory drug(s)
$PaCO_2$	arterial partial pressure of carbon dioxide
PaO_2	arterial partial pressure of oxygen
PCA	patient-controlled analgesia
PG(s)	prostaglandin(s)
PPI(s)	proton pump inhibitor(s)
RIMA(s)	reversible inhibitor(s) of mono-amine oxidase type A
SSRI(s)	selective serotonin re-uptake inhibitor(s)
Tlco	transfer factor of the lung for carbon monoxide
UTI	urinary tract infection
VIP	vaso-active intestinal polypeptide

Drug administration

a.c.	ante cibum (before food)
amp	ampoule containing a single dose (cp. vial)
b.d.	bis die (twice daily); alternative, b.i.d.
CD	controlled drugs, i.e. subject to prescription requirements under the Misuse of Drugs Act (UK)
CIVI	continuous intravenous infusion
CSCI	continuous subcutaneous infusion
e/c	enteric-coated
ED	epidural
IM	intramuscular
IT	intrathecal
IV	intravenous
m/r	modified release; alternative, slow release, controlled release
NHS	not prescribable on NHS prescriptions
o.d.	omni die (daily, once a day)
o.m.	omni mane (in the morning)
o.n.	omni nocte (at bedtime)
OTC	over-the-counter (can be obtained without a prescription)
p.c.	post cibum (after food)
PO	per os, by mouth
POM	prescription only medicine
PR	per rectum
p.r.n.	pro re nata (as needed, when required)
PV	per vaginum
q.d.s.	quater die sumendus (four times a day); alternative, q.i.d.
q4h	quarta quaque hora (every 4 hours)
SC	subcutaneous
SL	sublingual
stat	immediately
t.d.s.	ter die sumendus (three times a day); alternative, t.i.d.
vial	sterile container with a rubber bung containing either a single or multiple doses (cp. amp)
WFI	water for injections

Units

cm	centimetre(s)
cps	cycles per sec
dl	decilitre(s)
g	gram(s)
Gy	Gray(s), a measure of radiation
h	hour(s)
Hg	mercury
IU	international unit(s)
kg	kilogram(s)
L	litre(s)
mcg	microgram(s); alternative, μg
mg	milligram(s)
ml	millilitre(s)
mm	millimetre(s)
mmol	millimole(s)
μg	microgram, alternative, mcg
min	minute(s)
mosmol	milliosmole(s)
nm	nanometre(s)
nmol	nanomole(s)

1: Drugs acting on the
GASTRO-INTESTINAL SYSTEM

Antacids
   Alginic acid
   Dimeticone
   Oxetacaine

Antimuscarinics
   Hyoscine butylbromide
   Propantheline

Prokinetics
   Cisapride

H_2-receptor antagonists

Misoprostol

Proton pump inhibitors (PPIs)

Loperamide

Laxatives
   Ispaghula husk
   Stimulant laxatives
   Docusate
   Lactulose
   Magnesium salts
   Rectal preparations (enemas)

Preparations for haemorrhoids

Pancreatin

ANTACIDS   BNF 1.1

Antacids taken by mouth to neutralize gastric acid include:
* sodium bicarbonate
* magnesium salts
* aluminium hydroxide
* hydrotalcite/aluminium magnesium carbonate
* calcium carbonate.

*Magnesium salts are laxative and can cause diarrhoea; **aluminium salts** constipate.* Most proprietary antacids contain a mixture of magnesium and aluminium salts so as to have a neutral impact on intestinal transit. With doses of 100–200ml/24h or more, the effect of magnesium salts increasingly overrides the constipating effect of aluminium.

The sodium content of some antacids may be detrimental in patients with hypertension or cardiac failure; **Gaviscon** liquid and **magnesium trisilicate mixture** both contain >6mmol/10ml compared with 0.1mmol/10ml in **Asilone**. Regular use of **sodium bicarbonate** may cause sodium loading and metabolic alkalosis. Regular use of **calcium carbonate** may cause hypercalcaemia, particularly if taken with sodium bicarbonate.

Aluminium hydroxide binds dietary phosphate. It is of benefit in patients with hyperphosphataemia in renal failure. Long-term complications of phosphate depletion and osteomalacia are not an issue in advanced cancer. **Hydrotalcite** binds bile salts and is of specific benefit in patients with bile salt reflux, e.g. after certain forms of gastroduodenal surgery. Note:
* *by reducing stomach acid, antacids may result in damage to enteric coatings designed to prevent dissolution in the stomach*
* apart from sodium bicarbonate, antacids delay gastric emptying and may thereby modify drug absorption

- some proprietary preparations contain peppermint oil which masks the chalky taste of the antacid and helps belching by decreasing the tone of the lower oesophageal sphincter
- most antacid tablets feel gritty when sucked; some patients dislike this
- some proprietary preparations are fruit-flavoured, e.g. Tums (chewable tablet) and Remegel (chewing gum)
- the cheapest preparations are **magnesium trisilicate BP** and **aluminium hydroxide gel BP** given alone or as a mixture.

Antacid preparations should generally be taken 1h p.c. This maximizes contact time with gastric acid (2–3h) and allows the antacid to coat the stomach in the absence of food; o.n. & p.r.n. doses can also be taken.

Some antacids contain additional substances for use in specific situations, e.g. **alginic acid** (see below), **dimeticone** (see p.3), **oxetacaine** (see p.3).

ALGINIC ACID   BNF 1.1.3

Class of drug: Alginate.

Indications: Acid reflux ('heartburn').

Pharmacology

Alginic acid prevents oesophageal reflux pain by forming an inert low-density raft on the top of the acidic stomach contents. Both acid and air bubbles are necessary to produce the raft. Alginic acid preparations may therefore be less effective if used with an H_2-receptor antagonist (reduces acid) and/or an antiflatulent (reduces air bubbles). **Gaviscon**, a proprietary alginic acid preparation, is a weak antacid; most of the antacid content adheres to the alginate raft. This neutralizes acid which seeps into the oesophagus around the raft but does nothing to correct the underlying causes, e.g. lax lower oesophageal sphincter, hyperacidity, delayed gastric emptying, obesity. Indeed, alginic acid preparations are no better than dimeticone-containing antacids in the treatment of acid reflux.[1] Alginic acid preparations have been largely superseded by a more radical pharmacological approach, i.e. acid suppression with H_2-receptor antagonists and PPIs.

Onset of action <5min.

Duration of action 1–2h.

Cautions

Gaviscon liquid contains Na^+ 6mmol/10ml and it should not be used in patients with fluid retention or heart failure.

Dose and use

Several preparations are available but none is recommended. For patients already taking Gaviscon and who are reluctant to change to Asilone (or other option), prescribe Gaviscon 1–2 tablets or Gaviscon liquid 10–20ml p.c. & o.n., and p.r.n.

Supply

Tablets peppermint or lemon flavour, contain 2mmol Na^+/tab, 60 = £2.25.

Liquid sugar-free peppermint or aniseed flavour, contains 3mmol Na^+/5ml, 500ml = £2.70.

---

1 Pokorny C et al. (1985) Comparison of an antacid/dimethicone mixture and an alginate/antacid mixture in the treatment of oesophagitis. *Gut.* **26**: A574.

DIMETICONE BNF 1.1.1 & 1.1.3

Class of drug: Antifoaming agent.

Indications: Acid dyspepsia (including acid reflux), gassy dyspepsia, [†]hiccup (if associated with gastric distension).

Pharmacology
Dimeticone (dimethylpolysiloxane) is an antifoaming agent present in several proprietary antacids, e.g. **Asilone**. By facilitating belching, dimeticone eases flatulence, distension and postprandial gastric discomfort. Dimeticone-containing antacids are as effective as Gaviscon in the treatment of acid reflux.[1] Asilone should be used in preference to Gaviscon because it is cheaper and contains almost no sodium.
Onset of action <5min.
Duration of action 1–2h.

Cautions
Although Asilone contains both aluminium and magnesium, if large amounts are used, e.g. 30–60ml q.d.s., the laxative effect of magnesium will override the constipating effect of aluminium.[2]

Dose and use
Asilone suspension is available on NHS prescription (tablets and liquid ~~NHS~~):
• starting dose 5ml p.r.n., or 5ml q.d.s. & p.r.n.
• if necessary, double dose to 10ml.

Supply
Suspension sugar-free **Asilone**, dried aluminium hydroxide 420mg, activated dimeticone 135mg, light magnesium oxide 70mg/5ml (low Na⁺), 500ml = £1.95; use within 28 days of opening.

---

1 Pokorny C *et al.* (1985) Comparison of an antacid/dimethicone mixture and an alginate/antacid mixture in the treatment of oesophagitis. *Gut.* **26**: A574.
2 Morrissey JF and Barreras RF (1974) Antacid therapy. *New England Journal of Medicine.* **290**: 550–554.

OXETACAINE BNF 1.1.1

Class of drug: Local anaesthetic.

Indications: Odynophagia (painful swallowing) caused by oesophagitis whatever its cause, including postradiation.

Pharmacology
Like lidocaine and bupivacaine, oxetacaine is a local anaesthetic of the amide type. It produces a reversible loss of sensation by preventing or diminishing the conduction of sensory nerve impulses near the site of its application. Because the mode of action decreases the permeability of the nerve cell membrane to sodium ions, local anaesthetics are said to have a membrane stabilizing effect. Oxetacaine is effective when applied topically, and is a constituent in some ointments and suppositories for the relief of pain from haemorrhoids.
Onset of action 5min.
Duration of action 2–3h.

[†] unlicensed use only.

Dose and use

For short-term symptomatic treatment while specific treatment of the underlying condition (hyperacidity, candidiasis) permits healing of the damaged mucosa:
• **Mucaine** suspension 5–10ml (without fluid) 15min a.c. & o.n., and p.r.n. before drinks.

Supply

Suspension sugar-free **Mucaine**, aluminium hydroxide mixture 4.75ml, magnesium hydroxide 100mg, oxetacaine 10mg/5ml, 200ml = 76p; use within 14 days of opening.

ANTIMUSCARINICS   BNF 1.2

The antimuscarinics – often called anticholinergics – comprise the natural belladonna alkaloids (**atropine** and **hyoscine**) together with synthetic and semisynthetic derivatives. The latter two are divided into tertiary amines (e.g. **dicycloverine**) and quaternary ammonium compounds (e.g. **hyoscine butylbromide** and **propantheline**). The quaternary ammonium compounds are less lipid-soluble than the natural alkaloids and do not cross the blood-brain barrier. They are also less well absorbed from the gut. Central atropine-like effects (e.g. delirium) are therefore not a problem but peripheral antimuscarinic effects are characteristic (Table 1.1).

Table 1.1   Peripheral antimuscarinic effects

Visual Mydriasis Loss of accommodation	} blurred vision	*Gastro-intestinal* Dry mouth Heartburn Constipation	
Cardiovascular Palpitations Extrasystoles Arrhythmias	} also related to norepinephrine (noradrenaline) potentiation and a quinidine-like action	*Urinary tract* Hesitancy of micturition Retention of urine	

Cautions

Antimuscarinics block the final common (cholinergic) pathway through which prokinetic drugs act; *the two types of drugs should not be prescribed concurrently*.[1] Antimuscarinics relax the lower oesophageal sphincter and, if possible, should be avoided in patients with symptomatic acid reflux. Antimuscarinics should be avoided in paralytic ileus. Glaucoma may be precipitated in those at risk, particularly the elderly.

---

1 Schuurkes JAJ et al. (1986) Stimulation of gastroduodenal motor activity: dopaminergic and cholinergic modulation. *Drug Development Research.* **8**: 233–241.

HYOSCINE BUTYLBROMIDE   BNF 1.2

Class of drug: Antimuscarinic antispasmodic and antisecretory.

Indications: Intestinal colic, [†]inoperable bowel obstruction, [†]sialorrhoea (drooling), [†]death rattle.

Contra-indications: Narrow-angle glaucoma (unless moribund).

† unlicensed use only.

Pharmacology

Hyoscine butylbromide has both smooth muscle relaxant (antispasmodic) and antisecretory properties. Unlike **hyoscine hydrobromide,** hyoscine butylbromide does not cross the blood-brain barrier and so does not have a central anti-emetic action or cause drowsiness. Because they are poorly absorbed, tablets of hyoscine butylbromide should be used only for mild–moderate bowel colic. In healthy volunteers, a bolus injection of 20mg has a maximum antisecretory duration of action of 2h;[1] the same dose by CSCI, however, is often effective for 24h in 'death rattle' (see p.76).

Oral bio-availability 8–10%.
Onset of action <10min SC/IM/IV; 1–2h PO.
Duration of action <2h in volunteers; probably longer in moribund patients.
Plasma halflife 5–6h.

Cautions

As for all antimuscarinic drugs (see p.225). Blocks the final common (cholinergic) pathway through which prokinetic drugs act.[2]

Dose and use

For patients with obstructive symptoms without colic, **metoclopramide** *should be tried before hyoscine butylbromide because the obstruction may well be more functional than mechanical* (see p.71). Hyoscine butylbromide is normally given SC (Table 1.2). For mild–moderate colic not associated with intestinal obstruction there may be a place for PO tablets. For sialorrhoea, an alternative oral antimuscarinic may be better and more convenient, e.g. **amitriptyline** (see p.64), **orphenadrine** (see p.82), **propantheline** (see p.6), **thioridazine** (see p.59).

Table 1.2   Dose recommendations for SC hyoscine butylbromide

Indication	Stat dose	Initial infusion rate/24h	Common range
Inoperable bowel obstruction with colic[3,4]	20mg	60mg	60–120mg[a]
Death rattle	20mg	20–40mg	20–40mg

a. maximum dose = 300mg/24h.

Supply

Tablets 10mg, 56 = £2.59.
Injection 20mg/ml, 1ml amp = 20p.

---

1 Herxheimer A and Haefeli L (1966) Human pharmacology of hyoscine butylbromide. *Lancet.* **ii:** 418–421.
2 Schuurkes JAJ et al. (1986) Stimulation of gastroduodenal motor activity: dopaminergic and cholinergic modulation. *Drug Development Research.* **8:** 233–241.
3 DeConno F et al. (1991) Continuous subcutaneous infusion of hyoscine butylbromide reduces secretions in patients with gastrointestinal obstruction. *Journal of Pain and Symptom Management.* **6:** 484–486.
4 Baines MJ (1997) ABC of palliative care: nausea and vomiting. *British Medical Journal.* **315:** 1148–1150.

---

† unlicensed use.

PROPANTHELINE   BNF 1.2

Class of drug: Antimuscarinic antispasmodic.

Indications: Intestinal smooth muscle spasm, urinary frequency, [†]paraneoplastic sweating.

Pharmacology
Propantheline is a typical antimuscarinic drug (see p.225). It doubles gastric emptying half-time[1] and slows gastro-intestinal transit generally, with variable effects on drug absorption (e.g. the *rate* of absorption of paracetamol is reduced). Propantheline is extensively metabolized in the small bowel before absorption. If taken with food, the effect of propantheline by mouth is almost abolished.[2]
Bio-availability 0–50%.
Onset of action 30–60min.
Duration of action 4–6h.
Plasma halflife 3–4h.

Cautions and adverse effects
As for all antimuscarinic drugs (see p.225).

Dose and use
Intestinal colic
- usual dose 15mg t.d.s. *1h a.c.* & 30mg o.n.
- maximum dose 30mg q.d.s.

Urinary frequency: same as for colic; generally superseded by **oxybutynin** (see p.150) and **amitriptyline** (see p.64).
Sweating: 15–30mg b.d.–t.d.s.; generally superseded by **thioridazine** (see p.59) and **propranolol** (see BNF 2.4).

Supply
Tablets 15mg, 100 = £4.56.

---

1 Hurwitz A *et al.* (1977) Prolongation of gastric emptying by oral propantheline. *Clinical Pharmacology and Therapeutics.* **22**: 206–210.
2 Ekenved G *et al.* (1977) Influence of food on the effect of propantheline and l-hyoscyamine on salivation. *Scandinavian Journal of Gastroenterology.* **12**: 963–966.

PROKINETICS   BNF 1.2

Prokinetics accelerate gastro-intestinal transit by a neurohumoral mechanism. The term is restricted to drugs which co-ordinate antroduodenal contractions and accelerate gastroduodenal transit (Table 1.3). This excludes other drugs which enhance intestinal transit such as bulk-forming agents and other laxatives, and drugs which cause diarrhoea by increasing gut secretions, e.g. misoprostol. Some drugs increase contractile motor activity but not in a co-ordinated fashion, and so do not reduce transit time e.g. bethanechol. Such drugs are promotility but not prokinetic. Erythromycin is the only readily available motilin agonist. Its action is limited mainly to the stomach; tolerance often develops after a few days.

† unlicensed use.

Table 1.3 Gastro-intestinal prokinetics[1]

Class	Examples	Main site of action
D_2-receptor antagonist	Domperidone	Stomach
	Metoclopramide	Stomach
$5HT_4$-receptor agonist	Metoclopramide	Stomach → jejunum
	Cisapride	Stomach → colon
Motilin agonist	Erythromycin	Stomach

Apart from erythromycin, prokinetics act by triggering a cholinergic system in the gut wall. This action is impeded by opioids (Figure 1.1). On the other hand, antimuscarinic drugs block the cholinergic receptors on the intestinal muscle fibres.[2] Thus, drugs with antimuscarinic properties will block the action of prokinetic drugs to a greater or lesser extent. *Prokinetic and antimuscarinic drugs should not be prescribed concurrently.* Domperidone and metoclopramide, however, will still exert an antagonistic effect at the dopamine receptors in the area postrema (see p.67).

Prokinetics are used in various conditions in palliative care (Table 1.4). D_2-receptor antagonists block the dopaminergic 'brake' on gastric emptying induced by stress, anxiety and nausea from any cause. In contrast, $5HT_4$-receptor agonists have a direct excitatory effect which in theory gives them an advantage over the D_2-receptor antagonists particularly for patients with gastric stasis or functional bowel obstruction. When used for dysmotility dyspepsia, however, metoclopramide is no more potent than domperidone in standard doses.[3,4] Cisapride is several times more potent; unlike metoclopramide and domperidone, it has no central effect.[5,6]

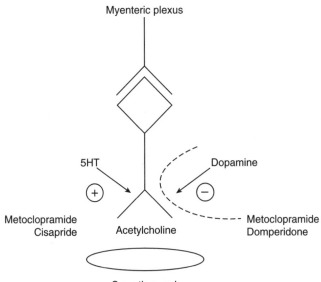

Figure 1.1 Schematic representation of drug effects on antroduodenal co-ordination via a postganglionic effect on the cholinergic nerves from the myenteric plexus.

⊕ stimulatory effect of 5HT triggered by metoclopramide and cisapride; ⊖ inhibitory effect of dopamine; − − − blockade of dopamine inhibition by metoclopramide and domperidone.

Table 1.4   Indications for prokinetics in palliative care

Gastro-oesophageal reflux	Functional bowel obstruction
Gastroparesis	cancer of head of pancreas
dysmotility dyspepsia	opioid-induced
opioid-induced	neoplastic
paraneoplastic visceral neuropathy	Constipation (cisapride only, see below)
	Irritable bowel syndrome (cisapride only, see below)

1 Debinski HS and Kamm MA (1994) New treatments for neuromuscular disorders of the gastrointestinal tract. *Gastrointestinal Journal Club.* **2**: 2–11.

2 Schuurkes JAJ et al. (1986) Stimulation of gastroduodenal motor activity: dopaminergic and cholinergic modulation. *Drug Development Research.* **8**: 233–241.

3 Loose FD (1979) Domperidone in chronic dyspepsia: a pilot open study and a multicentre general practice crossover comparison with metoclopramide and placebo. *Pharmatherapeutica.* **2**: 140–146.

4 Moriga M (1981) A multicentre double blind study of domperidone and metoclopramide in the symptomatic control of dyspepsia. In: Touse G (ed) *Progress with domperidone. A gastrokinetic and anti-emetic agent.* Royal Society of Medicine, London. pp 77–79.

5 McHugh S et al. (1992) Cisapride versus metoclopramide: an acute study in diabetic gastroparesis. *Digestive Diseases and Science.* **37**: 997–1001.

6 Fumagalli I and Hammer B (1994) Cisapride versus metoclopramide in the treatment of functional dyspepsia: a double-blind comparative trial. *Scandinavian Journal of Gastroenterology.* **29**: 33–37.

CISAPRIDE   BNF 1.2

Class of drug: Prokinetic, $5HT_4$-receptor agonist.

Indications: Dyspepsia or nausea associated with delayed gastric emptying unresponsive to metoclopramide (e.g. opioid-induced and paraneoplastic autonomic neuropathy), [†]nausea caused by venlafaxine and SSRIs,[1,2] [†]functional bowel obstruction, [†]constipation (as a 'co-laxative').

Contra-indications: Concurrent administration with oral or parenteral (but not topical) forms of imidazole antifungals (fluconazole, ketoconazole, itraconazole, miconazole), erythromycin and clarithromycin.

Pharmacology

Cisapride is a $5HT_4$-receptor agonist with a strong prokinetic action. It is 2–4 times more potent than metoclopramide.[3,4] It has a diffuse prokinetic effect ('panprokinetic' compared with 'gastrokinetic') and reverses opioid-induced delayed gastric emptying more completely. To explain the beneficial effect of cisapride in nausea caused by venlafaxine and SSRIs, it has been postulated that $5HT_4$-receptor activation reduces the release of 5HT from enterochromaffin cells.[5] At high plasma concentrations cisapride causes prolongation of the QT interval which predisposes to ventricular arrhythmias.

Oral bio-availability 50% (fasting), 65% (with food); PR <50% of PO.
Onset of action 0.5–1h.
Duration of action 12–16h.
Plasma halflife 10h.

[†] unlicensed use.

Cautions

> **Serious drug interactions:** rare cases of serious (occasionally fatal) cardiac arrhythmias, including ventricular arrhythmias and Torsade de Pointes associated with QT prolongation have been reported in patients taking cisapride in combination with **imidazole antifungals (fluconazole, ketoconazole, itraconazole, miconazole), erythromycin or clarithromycin**. The interaction relates to inhibition of one of the liver cytochrome P450 enzymes which results in an increase in plasma concentrations of cisapride (see Appendix 3, p.213). Most of those affected were receiving several other medications and had pre-existing cardiac disease or risk factors for arrhythmias. The original reports were of ketoconazole given in daily doses of 600–1200mg in patients with prostate cancer. Partly because it is given in smaller doses, fluconazole has less effect on the enzyme than ketoconazole. The likelihood of this interaction occurring with fluconazole 50–100mg o.d. is infinitesimal.[6]

The elderly, hepatic and renal impairment, cardiac disorders.

Adverse effects
Colic and diarrhoea, occasional headaches and lightheadedness. Liver function abnormalities (and possibly cholestasis) also reported.

Dose and use
Even though the BNF recommends 15–30min a.c. t.d.s. & o.n., administration b.d. is generally satisfactory:
- starting dose 10mg b.d.
- maximum dose 20mg b.d.

If causes colic or diarrhoea, halve the dose or give half the dose more frequently.

Supply
Tablets 10mg, 120 = £37.60.
Suspension 5mg/5ml, 500ml = £15.60.
Suppository 30mg (≈ 13mg by mouth) from IDIS on a named patient basis, 6 = £9.15.

---

1 Bergeron R and Blier P (1994) Cisapride for the treatment of nausea produced by selective serotonin reuptake inhibitors. *American Journal of Psychiatry.* **151**: 1084–1086.
2 Russel JL (1996) Relatively low doses of cisapride in the treatment of nausea in patients treated with venlafaxine for treatment of refractory depression. *Journal of Clinical Psychopharmacology.* **16**: 357.
3 McHugh S et al. (1992) Cisapride versus metoclopramide: an acute study in diabetic gastroparesis. *Digestive Diseases and Science.* **37**: 997–1001.
4 Fumagalli I and Hammer B (1994) Cisapride versus metoclopramide in the treatment of functional dyspepsia: a double-blind comparative trial. *Scandinavian Journal of Gastroenterology.* **29**: 33–37.
5 Gebauer A et al. (1993) Modulation by 5HT3 and 5HT4 receptors of the release of 5-hydroxytryptamine from the guinea-pig small intestine. *Naunyn-Schmiedeberg's Archives of Pharmacology.* **347**: 137–140.
6 Twycross RG (1997) *Symptom Management in Advanced Cancer.* Radcliffe Medical Press, Oxford.

H₂-RECEPTOR ANTAGONISTS   BNF 1.3.1

Class of drug: Ulcer-healing drugs.

Indications: Acid dyspepsia (including acid reflux), peptic ulceration.

Pharmacology
H_2-receptor antagonists reduce gastric acid output and reduce the volume of gastric secretions. **Ranitidine** is more effective if taken o.n. rather than with the evening meal.[1] In patients taking

NSAIDs, ranitidine is less effective than **PPIs** in healing gastroduodenal ulcers (63% v 80% at 8 weeks) and in preventing relapse (59% v 72% over 6 months).[2]
Bio-availability cimetidine 75%; ranitidine 50%.
Onset of action <1h.
Duration of action cimetidine 7h; ranitidine 8–12h.
Plasma halflife cimetidine 2h; ranitidine 2–3h.

Cautions

Serious drug interactions: **cimetidine** binds to microsomal cytochrome P450 and inhibits the metabolism of diazepam, methadone, phenytoin, theophylline and warfarin.

Hepatic impairment, renal impairment. **Cimetidine** causes a transient rise in the plasma concentrations of carbamazepine. Cumulation of **diazepam** and **methadone** can cause drowsiness and delirium.[3] Cimetidine, however, does not alter the metabolism of morphine in humans.[4] Famotidine, nizatidine and ranitidine do not share the drug metabolism inhibitory properties of cimetidine; ranitidine is recommended for use instead, even though it is more expensive (*see* Appendix 3, p.213).

Adverse effects

Dizziness, drowsiness or fatigue, and rash occur occasionally; rare reports of headache, liver dysfunction, and blood disorders. Cimetidine occasionally also causes gynaecomastia; rare reports of impotence and myalgia.

Dose and use

H_2-receptor antagonists have been largely superseded by PPIs (*see* p.12). The dose and duration of treatment is least with duodenal ulceration and most with reflux oesophagitis (Table 1.5). For any indication, the dose should be doubled if the initial response is poor. Parenteral formulations are available for IM and IV use if treatment is considered necessary in a patient with severe nausea and vomiting (*see* BNF 1.3.1).

Supply

Tablets cimetidine 400mg, 60 = £7.50; 800mg, 30 = £7.81.
Syrup cimetidine 200mg/5ml, 600ml = £28.49.
Tablets ranitidine 150mg, 60 = £26.89; 300mg, 30 = £26.45.
Tablets effervescent ranitidine 150mg (14.3mmol Na^+/tab), 60 = £27.88; 300mg (20.8mmol Na^+/tab), 30 = £27.42.
Syrup sugar-free ranitidine 75mg/5ml, 300ml = £22.32.

Table 1.5 Recommended dose regimens for H_2-receptor antagonists

Indication	Cimetidine	Ranitidine
Duodenal ulcer	400mg b.d. *or* 800mg o.n. for 4+ weeks	150mg b.d. *or* 300mg o.n. for 4–8 weeks
Gastric ulcer	400mg b.d. *or* 800mg o.n. for 6+ weeks	150mg b.d. *or* 300mg o.n. for 4–8 weeks
NSAID-associated ulcer	400mg b.d. *or* 800mg o.n. for 8+ weeks	150mg b.d. *or* 300mg o.n. for 8 weeks
Reflux oesophagitis	400mg q.d.s. *or* 800mg b.d. for 4-8 weeks	150mg b.d. *or* 300mg o.n. for 8–12 weeks
Reduction of degradation of pancreatin supplements	400mg t.d.s.-q.d.s. *1h a.c.*	[†]150mg t.d.s.–q.d.s. *1h a.c.*

† unlicensed use.

1 Johnston DA and Wormsley KG (1988) The effect of food on ranitidine-induced inhibition of nocturnal gastric secretion. *Alimentary Pharmacology and Therapeutics*. **2**: 507–511.
2 Yeomans ND et al. (1998) A comparison of omeprazole with ranitidine for ulcers associated with nonsteroidal anti-inflammatory drugs. *New England Journal of Medicine*. **338**: 719–726.
3 Sorkin E and Ogawa C (1983) Cimetidine potentiation of narcotic action. *Drug Intelligence and Clinical Pharmacy*. **17**: 60–61.
4 Mojaverian P et al. (1982) Cimetidine does not alter morphine disposition in man. *British Journal of Clinical Pharmacology*. **14**: 809–813.

MISOPROSTOL   BNF 1.3.4

Class of drug: Prostaglandin analogue.

Indications: Prevention or healing of NSAID-induced gastroduodenopathy.

Contra-indications: Pregnancy (misoprostol increases uterine tone).

Pharmacology
Misoprostol is a synthetic PG analogue with gastric antisecretory and protective properties which, after oral administration, is rapidly de-esterified to its free acid. It helps prevent NSAID-related gastroduodenal erosions and ulcers.[1,2] Misoprostol, however, is no more effective than a PPI in the treatment of NSAID-related gastroduodenal injury, and maintenance therapy with a PPI is associated with a lower relapse rate (61% v 48% misoprostol v 27% placebo).[3] Colic and diarrhoea may limit the use of misoprostol.
Bio-availability 90% (radio-labelled misoprostol given PO).
Onset of action <30min.
Duration of action 2–4h.
Plasma halflife 6min *in vitro*; 1–2h for free acid.

Cautions
Conditions where hypotension might precipitate severe complications (e.g. cerebrovascular disease, cardiovascular disease).

Adverse effects
Diarrhoea (may necessitate stopping treatment), colic, dyspepsia, flatulence, nausea and vomiting, abnormal vaginal bleeding (intermenstrual bleeding, menorrhagia, postmenopausal bleeding), rashes, dizziness.

Dose and use
NSAID-associated ulcers may be treated with an **H₂-receptor antagonist**, a **PPI** or **misoprostol**; the causal NSAID need not be discontinued during treatment.
Prophylaxis against NSAID-induced ulcers: 200µg b.d.–q.d.s. taken with the NSAID (see ketorolac, p.98).
NSAID-associated ulceration: 200µg t.d.s. with meals & o.n. or 400µg b.d. (breakfast and bedtime) for 4–8 weeks.[1] If causes diarrhoea, give 200µg t.d.s. & o.n. and avoid magnesium-containing antacids.

Supply
Tablets 200µg, 60 = £11.14.

1 Bardhan KD et al. (1993) The prevention and healing of acute NSAID-associated gastroduodenal mucosal damage by misoprostol. *British Journal of Rheumatology*. **32**: 990–995.
2 Silverstein FE et al. (1995) Misoprostol reduces serious gastrointestinal complications in patients with rheumatoid arthritis receiving nonsteroidal anti-inflammatory drugs. *Annals of Internal Medicine*. **123**: 241–249.

3 Hawkey CJ et al. (1998) Omeprazole compared with misoprostol for ulcers associated with nonsteroidal anti-inflammatory drugs. New England Journal of Medicine. **33**: 727–734.

PROTON PUMP INHIBITORS (PPIs)   BNF 1.3.5

Class of drug: Ulcer-healing drug.

Indications: Acid dyspepsia (including acid reflux), peptic ulceration.

Pharmacology

Because **lansoprazole**, **omeprazole** and **pantoprazole** are all rapidly degraded by acid, they are formulated as e/c granules or tablets. These dissolve in the duodenum where the drug is rapidly absorbed to be selectively taken up by gastric parietal cells and converted into active metabolites. These irreversibly inhibit the proton pump (H^+/K^+-ATPase) and thereby block gastric acid secretion. Elimination is predominantly by metabolism in the liver to inactive derivatives excreted mainly in the urine. The plasma halflives of PPIs are all <2h but, because they irreversibly inhibit the proton pump, the antisecretory activity continues for several days until new proton pumps are synthesized.

When treating peptic ulceration lansoprazole 30mg o.d. is as effective as omeprazole 40mg o.d. and is cheaper. Pantoprazole 40mg o.d. is as effective as omeprazole 20mg o.d.[1] Omeprazole, however, demonstrates a dose-response curve above the standard dose of 20mg o.d., whereas no further benefit is seen by increasing the dose of lansoprazole and pantoprazole above 30mg and 40mg o.d. respectively.[2,3] It is generally stated that the bio-availability of lansoprazole is reduced by food and that it should be given o.m. *1h before breakfast* (see Data Sheet). However, whether changes in the pharmacokinetic profile of lansoprazole affect its efficacy is debatable.[4–6] Certainly in one study, acid suppression was comparable after 7 days even though there was a significant difference on day 1.[7] Omeprazole 40mg o.d. is superior to lansoprazole 60mg o.d. and pantoprazole 80mg o.d. in the management of severe gastro-oesophageal reflux disease (oesophagitis and stricture).[8] For administration by nasogastric tube, the e/c granules of lansoprazole or omeprazole can be removed from the capsule and dissolved in sodium bicarbonate.

Bio-availability lansoprazole 80–90%; omeprazole 65%; pantoprazole 77%.
Onset of action <2h.
Duration of action >24h.
Plasma halflife lansoprazole 1–2h; omeprazole 0.5–1h; pantoprazole 1–2h.

Cautions

Serious adverse drug reactions: ocular damage, impaired hearing, angina, hypertension. Ocular damage has been reported either in humans or animals with all three available PPIs in the UK.[9] Most cases have been reported with IV omeprazole.[10] PPIs possibly cause vasoconstriction by blocking potassium-hydrogen ATPase. Because the retinal artery is an end-artery, anterior ischaemic optic neuropathy may result. If the PPI is stopped, visual acuity may improve. Several patients have become permanently blind, *in some instances after 3 days*. Impaired hearing and deafness have also been reported, again mostly with IV omeprazole. A similar mechanism may be responsible for the angina and hypertension included as adverse effects in the USA Data Sheet on omeprazole. (IV omeprazole is available only on a named patient basis.)

PPIs are metabolized by the cytochrome P450 family of liver enzymes. However, clinically important interactions are rare with all three drugs.[11,12] Omeprazole increases the bio-availability of digoxin by 10%. The SPC for omeprazole advises caution when using the drug in patients taking warfarin, phenytoin or diazepam, and the SPC for lansoprazole advises caution with oral contraceptives, warfarin, phenytoin and theophylline. No significant interactions between pantoprazole and other drugs have been identified[13] (see Appendix 3, p.213).

Adverse effects

Headache and diarrhoea occur in <3% of patients. PPIs may also cause dizziness, nausea, constipation, abdominal pain, pruritus and rashes. Occasional cases of acute interstitial nephritis have been reported, sometimes with eosinophilia ± a rash.[14]

Dose and use

PPIs are increasingly used in preference to H$_2$-receptor antagonists to treat hyperacidity. PPIs are used in combination with antibiotics for the eradication of *Helicobacter pylori* (see BNF 1.3), and for the treatment of NSAID-induced ulcers.

Lansoprazole

* 30mg o.m. for 4 weeks, followed by 15mg o.m. indefinitely
* some patients may need 30mg o.m. for 8 weeks.

A higher dose, i.e. 30mg b.d., is recommended only when lansoprazole is being used with antibiotics to eradicate *Helicobacter pylori*. The Data Sheet for lansoprazole states that administration should be o.m., a.c. in order to achieve 'optimal acid inhibition'. However, published data show that this precaution is unnecessary.[6,7] For patients with obstructive dysphagia and acid dyspepsia, or with severe gastritis and vomiting, the rectal route can be used.[15]

Omeprazole

* 20mg o.m.
* 40mg o.m. in reflux oesophagitis if poor response to standard dose.

For patients who require a liquid preparation and who are able to tolerate oral administration or who have feeding tubes of a sufficient diameter to allow the passage of lansoprazole or omeprazole granules without blockage, e.g. PEG tubes, administer the granules in an acidic drink, e.g. orange juice. This acidic solution ensures the integrity of the enteric coating, hence preventing degradation in the stomach. For patients with a small-bore nasogastric tube, a suspension of lansoprazole or omeprazole should be prepared (Box 1.A).

Box 1.A   Lansoprazole and omeprazole via a nasogastric tube

1   Prepare a suspension of lansoprazole 30mg or omeprazole 20mg:

  * empty the e/c granules from the capsule into a 20ml syringe
  * draw up 10ml of sodium bicarbonate 8.4% solution into the syringe
  * with the point of the syringe uncapped, leave for about 10min until a turbid suspension is formed.

2   Alkalinize the stomach contents with 10ml of sodium bicarbonate 8.4% and administer the suspension within 5min.

3   Rinse the syringe and nasogastric tube with 20ml of water.

Supply

Capsules enclosing e/c granules omeprazole 10mg, 28 = £19.95; 20mg, 28 = £30.13; 40mg, 28 = £60.24.

Capsules enclosing e/c granules lansoprazole 15mg, 28 = £18.95; 30mg, 28 = £29.69.

Tablets e/c pantoprazole 40mg, 28 = £29.76.

Suppositories lansoprazole or omeprazole can be made by mixing the contents of capsules with 1% arginine in Witepsol (a standard suppository base).[16]

---

1 Anonymous (1997) Pantoprazole – a third proton pump inhibitor. *Drug and Therapeutics Bulletin.* **35**: 93–94.

2 Dammann HG et al. (1993) The effects of lansoprazole, 30 or 60 mg daily on intragastric pH and on endocrine function in healthy volunteers. *Alimentary Pharmacology and Therapeutics.* **7**: 191–196.

3 Koop H *et al.* (1996) Intragastric pH and serum gastrin during administration of different doses of pantoprazole in healthy subjects. *European Journal of Gastroenterology and Hepatology.* **8**: 915–918.

4 Delhotal-Landes B *et al.* (1991) The effect of food and antacids on lansoprazole absorption and disposition. *European Journal of Drug Metabolism and Pharmacokinetics.* **3**: 315–320.

5 Andersson T *et al.* (1990) Bioavailability of omeprazole as enteric coated (EC) granules in conjunction with food on the first and seventh days of treatment. *Drug Investigations.* **2**: 184–188.

6 Moules I *et al.* (1993) Gastric acid inhibition by the proton pump inhibitor lansoprazole is unaffected by food. *British Journal of Clinical Research.* **4**: 153–161.

7 Brummer RJM *et al.* (1995) Acute and chronic effect of lansoprazole and omeprazole in relation to food intake. *Gut.* **37** (suppl 2): T127.

8 Jaspersen D *et al.* (1998) A comparison of omeprazole, lansoprazole and pantoprazole in the maintenance treatment of severe reflux oesophagitis. *Alimentary Pharmacology and Therapeutics.* **12**: 49–52.

9 Schonhofer PS *et al.* (1997) Ocular damage associated with proton pump inhibitors. *British Medical Journal.* **314**: 1805.

10 Schonhofer PS (1994) Intravenous omeprazole and blindness. *Lancet.* **343**: 665.

11 Andersson T (1996) Pharmacokinetics, metabolism and interactions of acid pump inhibitors. Focus on omeprazole, lansoprazole and pantoprazole. *Clinical Pharmacokinetics.* **31**: 9–28.

12 Tucker GT (1994) The interaction of proton pump inhibitors with cytochromes P450. *Alimentary Pharmacology and Therapeutics.* **8** (suppl 1): 33–38.

13 Steinijans WV *et al.* (1996) Lack of pantoprazole drug interactions in man: an updated review. *International Journal of Clinical Pharmacology and Therapeutics.* **34** (suppl 1): S31–S50.

14 Assouad M *et al.* (1994) Recurrent acute interstitial nephritis on rechallenge with omeprazole. *Lancet.* **344**: 549.

15 Zylicz Z *et al.* (1998) Rectal omeprazole in the treatment of reflux pain in esophageal cancer. *Journal of Pain and Symptom Management.* **15**: 144–145.

16 Choi M-S *et al.* (1996) Rectal absorption of omeprazole from suppository in humans. *Journal of Pharmaceutical Sciences.* **85**: 893–894.

LOPERAMIDE   BNF 1.4.2

Class of drug: Antimotility antidiarrhoeal.

Indications: Diarrhoea, ileostomy (to improve faecal consistency).

Pharmacology

Antimotility antidiarrhoeal drugs comprise the opioids and the non-analgesic opioid derivatives, **loperamide** and **diphenoxylate**. Loperamide is about 3 times more potent than diphenoxylate and 50 times more potent than codeine. It is longer acting and generally needs to be given only b.d. The following regimens are approximately equivalent:

    loperamide 2mg b.d.

    diphenoxylate 2.5mg q.d.s. (in co-phenotrope)

    codeine phosphate 60mg t.d.s.–q.d.s.

In AIDS-related diarrhoea, loperamide may need to be supplemented by morphine PO or diamorphine/morphine by CSCI to achieve control. Morphine and diamorphine have both peripheral and central constipating effects; because it is not absorbed, loperamide acts only peripherally.

Cautions

Ensure that the underlying cause of diarrhoea is not faecal impaction.

Adverse effects

Abdominal bloating, paralytic ileus, faecal impaction, overflow diarrhoea.

Dose and use
- for acute diarrhoea starting dose is generally 4mg
- then 2mg after each loose bowel action; usual maximum dose 16mg/24h
- occasionally doses up to 32mg/24h are needed; *this is twice the BNF recommended maximum dose.*

Supply
Capsules 2mg, 30 = £1.55.
Syrup 1mg/5ml, 100ml = £1.90.

LAXATIVES BNF 1.6

Constipation is common in advanced cancer, particularly in immobile patients with small appetites and those receiving constipating drugs such as opioids. Exercise and increased dietary fibre are rarely appropriate options. As a general rule, all patients prescribed morphine should also be prescribed a laxative. About 1/3 of patients also need rectal measures, either because of failed oral treatment or electively, e.g. in patients with paraplegia or bedbound debilitated elderly patients. There are several classes of laxatives (Table 1.6).

Table 1.6   Classification of commonly used laxatives

Bulk-forming agents	*Faecal softeners*
Ispaghula husk	Arachis (peanut) oil
	Docusate sodium
Stimulant laxatives	Glycerol
Bisacodyl	Liquid paraffin (mineral oil)
Dantron	
Senna	*Osmotic laxatives*
Sodium picosulphate	Lactulose
	Magnesium salts

In contrast to the BNF, **docusate sodium** is classed as a faecal softener and not a stimulant laxative because, at doses commonly used, it acts mainly by lowering surface tension, thereby enabling water to percolate into the substance of the faeces. A peristaltic stimulant action is generally apparent only at higher doses, e.g. 600mg/day or more.

Opioids cause constipation by enhancing ring contractions in the small and large intestines, thereby impeding peristalsis, and also by enhancing the absorption of fluid and electrolytes.[1] Colonic 'stimulant' laxatives reduce ring contractions and offer a logical approach to the correction of opioid-induced constipation. In the UK, a combination of a peristaltic stimulant and a faecal softener is generally prescribed.

1 Beubler E (1983) Opiates and intestinal transport: in vivo studies. In: Turnberg LA (ed) *Intestinal Secretion.* SKF Laboratories, Hertfordshire. pp 53–55.

ISPAGHULA HUSK BNF 1.6.1

Class of drug: Bulk-forming laxative.

Indications: Colostomy regulation, haemorrhoids, anal fissure, diverticular disease, irritable bowel syndrome (if unprocessed wheat bran unpalatable).

Contra-indications: Dysphagia, intestinal obstruction, colonic atony, faecal impaction.

Pharmacology

Ispaghula is derived from the husks of an Asian plant, *Plantago ovata*. It has very high water-binding capacity, is partly fermented in the colon, and increases bacterial cell mass. Like other bulk-forming laxatives, isphagula stimulates peristalsis by increasing faecal mass. Its water-binding capacity also helps to make loose faeces more formed in some patients with a colostomy.
Onset of action full effect obtained only after several days.
Duration of action best taken regularly to obtain a consistent ongoing effect; may continue to act for 2–3 days after the last dose.

Cautions

Adequate fluid intake should be maintained to avoid intestinal obstruction.

Adverse effects

Flatulence, abdominal distension, faecal impaction, intestinal obstruction.

Dose and use

Ispaghula swells in contact with fluid and needs to be drunk quickly before it absorbs water. Stir the granules or powder briskly in 150ml of water and swallow immediately; carbonated water can be used if preferred. Alternatively, the granules can be swallowed dry, or mixed with a vehicle such as jam, and followed by 100–200ml of water. Give 1 sachet o.m.–t.d.s., preferably after meals; not immediately before going to bed.

Supply

Granules Fybogel plain, orange or lemon flavour 3.5g/sachet (low Na+), 30 sachets = £2.12.
Powder Regulan orange or lemon-lime flavour 3.4g/sachet, 30 sachets = £2.12.

STIMULANT LAXATIVES   BNF 1.6.2

Indications: Prevention and treatment of constipation.

Contra-indications: Large bowel obstruction.

Pharmacology

Anthranoid laxatives such as **senna** are derived from plants. They are inactive glycosides which pass unabsorbed and unchanged through the small bowel and are hydrolyzed by bacterial glycosidases in the large bowel to yield active compounds. Thus, glycosides have no effect on the small bowel but become active in the large bowel. **Dantron**, a synthetic anthranoid, is not a glycoside and has a direct action on the small bowel as well as the large bowel.[1] Absorption of sennosides or any of their metabolites is small; whereas dantron is absorbed to some extent from the small bowel with subsequent significant urinary excretion. Active anthranoid compounds have both motor and secretory effects on the bowel. They act by stimulating first the submucosal (Meissner's) plexus and then the myenteric (Auerbach's) plexus. The motor effect precedes the secretory effect, and is the more important laxative action. There is a decrease in segmenting muscular activity and an increase in propulsive waves. Differences in bacterial flora may explain individual differences in responses to anthranoid laxatives.

Polyphenolics such as **bisacodyl** and **sodium picosulphate** have a similar laxative effect to the anthranoids. Bisacodyl and sodium picosulphate are hydrolyzed to the same active metabolite but the mode of hydrolysis differs.[2] Bisacodyl is hydrolyzed by intestinal enzymes and acts on both the small and large bowels. When applied to bowel mucosa, bisacodyl induces almost immediate powerful propulsive motor activity. In contrast, sodium picosulphate is hydrolyzed by colonic bacteria and its action is therefore confined to the large bowel. Its activity is more uncertain because it depends on bacterial flora. Bisacodyl tablets are enteric-coated, however, and this reduces the impact on the small bowel. **Phenolphthalein**, another polyphenolic laxative, is present in some proprietary laxatives. It undergoes enterohepatic circulation and can cause a drug rash; it is generally best avoided.

Onset of action
Bisacodyl tablets 10–12h; suppositories 20–60min.
Dantron 6–12h.
Senna 8–12h.
Sodium picosulphate 10–14h.

Cautions

Because very high doses in rodents revealed a potential carcinogenic risk,[3,4] UK licences for laxatives containing **dantron** are limited to constipation in geriatric practice, analgesic-induced constipation in terminally ill patients of all ages and constipation in cardiac failure and after coronary thrombosis.

Adverse effects

Intestinal colic, diarrhoea. Bisacodyl suppositories may cause local rectal inflammation. Dantron discolours urine, typically red but sometimes green or bluish. Prolonged contact with skin (e.g. in urinary or faecally incontinent patients) may cause a dantron burn – a red erythematous rash with a sharply demarcated border which, if ignored, may become excoriated.

Dose and use

The doses recommended here for opioid-induced constipation are higher (often much higher) than those featured in the BNF and the SPC. Because round-the-clock opioids constipate round-the-clock, b.d. or t.d.s. laxatives may well be necessary, rather than the traditional o.n. (or o.m.) dose.
Bisacodyl
• *by mouth,* 5–20mg o.n.–b.d.
• *by suppository,* 10–20mg o.d.
Dantron
Variable, according to preparation, individual need and patient acceptance (Box 1.B).

Box 1.B   Management of opioid-induced constipation

Note the patient's normal bowel habit and use of laxatives; record date of last bowel action.

Do a rectal examination if faecal impaction is suspected or if the patient reports diarrhoea or faecal incontinence (to exclude impaction with overflow).

For inpatients, record bowel activity daily.

Encourage fluids generally, and fruit juice and fruit specifically.

When an opioid is first prescribed, prescribe co-danthrusate 1 capsule o.n. prophylactically (or the equivalent as co-danthramer).

If already constipated, prescribe co-danthrusate 2 capsules o.n.

Adjust the dose every few days according to results, up to 3 capsules t.d.s.

If the patient prefers a liquid preparation, use co-danthrusate suspension (or equivalent dose of co-danthramer).

If necessary 'uncork' with suppositories, e.g. bisacodyl 10mg and glycerin 4g.

If suppositories are ineffective, administer a phosphate enema; possibly repeat the next day.

If the maximum dose of co-danthrusate is ineffective, reduce by half and add an osmotic laxative, e.g. lactulose 20–30ml b.d.

If co-danthrusate causes abdominal cramps divide the total daily dose into smaller, more frequent doses, e.g. change from co-danthrusate 2 capsules b.d. to 1 capsule q.d.s. or change to an osmotic laxative, e.g. lactulose 20–30ml o.d.–t.d.s.

Lactulose may be preferable to co-danthrusate in patients with a history of irritable bowel syndrome or of colic with other colonic stimulants, e.g. senna.

Sometimes it is appropriate to optimize a patient's existing bowel regimen, rather than change automatically to co-danthrusate.

Senna
- starting dose should be low, e.g. 15mg o.n.
- for patients receiving opioids, 15mg b.d. is generally apppropriate
- increase if necessary to 15–22.5mg t.d.s.

Sodium picosulphate
- 5–20ml o.n.–b.d.

Supply

Bisacodyl:
Tablets e/c 5mg, 20 = 24p.
Suppositories 10mg, 20 = £1.43.

Dantron:

Co-danthramer suspension 5ml =1 co-danthramer capsule.
Co-danthramer suspension 15ml ≈ 5ml **strong** co-danthramer suspension.
Strong co-danthramer suspension 5ml = 2 **strong** co-danthramer capsules.

Capsules co-danthramer 25/200 (dantron 25mg, poloxamer 188 200mg), 60 = £12.86.
Strong capsules co-danthramer 37.5/500 (dantron 37.5mg; poloxamer 188 500mg), 60 = £15.55.
Suspension co-danthramer 25/200 in 5ml (dantron 25mg, poloxamer 188 200mg/5ml), 300ml = £11.26.
Strong suspension co-danthramer 75/1000 in 5ml (dantron 75mg, poloxamer 188 1g/5ml), 300ml = £30.12.
Capsules co-danthrusate 50/60 (dantron 50mg, docusate sodium 60mg), 60 = £12.81.
Suspension co-danthrusate 50/60 (dantron 50mg, docusate sodium 60mg/5ml), 300ml = £9.60.

Senna:
Tablets total sennosides 7.5mg, 20 = 30p.
Granules total sennosides 15mg/5ml spoonful, 100g = £2.64.
Syrup total sennosides 7.5mg/5ml, 100ml = £1.98.

Sodium picosulphate:
Syrup 5mg/5ml, 100ml = £1.85.

The brand names NHS **Laxoberal** and **Dulco-lax Liquid** are used for sodium picosulphate elixir 5mg/5ml; the brand name **Dulco-lax** is also used for bisacodyl tablets and suppositories.

1 Lennard-Jones JE (1994) Clinical aspects of laxatives, enemas and suppositories. In: Kamm MA, Lennard-Jones JE (eds) *Constipation.* Wrightson Biomedical Publishing, Petersfield. pp 327–341.
2 Jauch R et al. (1975) Bis-(p-hydroxyphenyl)-pyridyl-2-methane: the common laxative principle of bisacodyl and sodium picosulfate. *Arzneimittel-Forschung Drug Research.* **25**: 1796–1800.
3 Mori H et al. (1985) Induction of intestinal tumours in rats by chrysazin. *British Journal of Cancer.* **52**: 781–783.
4 Mori H et al. (1986) Carcinogenicity of chrysazin in large intestine and liver of mice. *Japanese Journal of Cancer Research (Gann).* **77**: 871–876.

DOCUSATE   BNF 1.6.3

Indications: Constipation, [†]partial bowel obstruction.

Pharmacology
Although classified as a stimulant laxative in the BNF, docusate is principally an emulsifying and wetting agent and has a relatively weak effect on bowel transit. Other wetting agents include poloxamer 188 (in co-danthramer). Docusate lowers surface tension, thereby allowing water and fats to penetrate hard, dry faeces. It also stimulates fluid secretion by the small and large bowel.[1]

Cautions
Docusate enhances the absorption of liquid paraffin;[2] combined preparations of these substances are prohibited in some countries.

Adverse effects
Docusate solution may cause an unpleasant aftertaste or burning sensation, minimized by drinking plenty of water after taking the solution.

Dose and use
Docusate is used in combination with dantron in **co-danthrusate** as the laxative of choice for opioid-induced constipation (see p.15). Docusate is used alone for patients with persistent partial bowel obstruction. Dose varies according to individual need:
- usual starting dose 100mg b.d.
- usual maximum dose 200mg b.d.–t.d.s.; *the latter is higher than the manufacturer's maximum dose of 500mg/day.*

Supply
Capsules 100mg, 100 = £4.65.
Solution 50mg/5ml, 100ml = £2.48.
Docusate is also available as an enema (see p.21).

1 Moriarty KJ *et al.* (1985) Studies on the mechanism of action of dioctyl sodium sulphosuccinate in the human jejunum. *Gut.* **26**: 1008–1013.
2 Godfrey H (1971) Dangers of dioctyl sodium sulfosuccinate in mixtures. *Journal of the American Medical Association.* **215**: 643.

LACTULOSE   BNF 1.6.4

Indications: Constipation in patients who experience bowel colic with stimulant laxatives, or who fail to respond to a stimulant laxative alone; hepatic encephalopathy.

Contra-indications: Intestinal obstruction, galactosaemia.

Pharmacology
Lactulose is a synthetic disaccharide, a combination of galactose and fructose, which is not absorbed by the small bowel. It is a 'small bowel flusher', i.e. through an osmotic effect, lactulose deposits a large volume of fluid into the large bowel. Lactulose is fermented in the large bowel to acetic and lactic acids, hydrogen and carbon dioxide with an increase in faecal acidity, which also stimulate peristalsis. The low pH discourages the proliferation of ammonia-producing organisms, hence its use in hepatic encephalopathy. Lactulose does not affect the management of diabetes mellitus; 15ml contains 14 calories.
Onset of action up to 48h.

[†] unlicensed use.

Adverse effects

Abdominal bloating, discomfort and flatulence, intestinal colic.

Dose and use

Solution start with 15ml b.d. and adjust according to need. In hepatic encephalopathy, 30–50ml t.d.s., subsequently adjusted to produce 2–3 soft faecal evacuations per day.

Powder 10g b.d. adjusted according to need. In hepatic encephalopathy, 20–30ml t.d.s., subsequently adjusted to produce 2–3 soft faecal evacuations per day. The powder can be placed on the tongue and washed down with water or other liquid, or sprinkled on food, or mixed with water or other liquid before swallowing.

Supply

Solution 3.1–3.7g/5ml with other ketoses, 200ml = £1.05.
Powder 10g/sachet with other ketoses, 30 = £3.00.

MAGNESIUM SALTS   BNF 1.6.4

Indications: Constipation in patients who experience bowel colic with stimulant laxatives, or who fail to respond to a stimulant laxative alone.

Pharmacology

Magnesium and sulphate ions are poorly absorbed from the gut. Their action is mainly osmotic but other factors may be important, e.g. the release of cholecystokinin.[1,2] Magnesium ions also decrease absorption or increase secretion in the small bowel. Total faecal PGE_2 increases progressively as the dose of magnesium hydroxide is raised from 1.2 to 3.2g daily.[3] Increased PG in the gut lumen has been found with anthranoid laxatives and may have a role in their action.

Dose and use

Magnesium hydroxide mixture contains about 8% of hydrated magnesium oxide and the usual dose is 25–50ml. **Magnesium sulphate** is a more potent laxative which tends to produce a large volume of liquid stool. The compound is not popular with patients because it often leads to a sense of distension and the sudden passage of offensive liquid faeces which is socially inconvenient; it is very difficult to adjust the dose to produce a normal soft stool. The usual dose is 4–10g of crystals dissolved in warm water and taken with extra fluid.

Supply

Suspension magnesium hydroxide mixture BP (Cream of Magnesia) contains about 8% hydrated magnesium oxide; do not store in a cold place.

Powder magnesium sulphate (Epsom Salts) OTC; also **Andrews Liver Salts** (citric acid, magnesium sulphate, sodium bicarbonate) OTC (DHS).

Solution magnesium sulphate (Epsom Salts) 4–5g/10ml prepared extemporaneously.

---

1 Donowitz M (1991) Magnesium-induced diarrhea and new insights into the pathobiology of diarrhea. *New England Journal of Medicine.* **324**: 1059–1060.

2 Harvey RF and Read AE (1975) Mode of action of the saline purgatives. *American Heart Journal.* **89**: 810–813.

3 Donowitz M and Rood RP (1992) Magnesium hydroxide: new insights into the mechanism of its laxative effect and the potential involvement of prostaglandin E2. *Journal of Clinical Gastroenterology.* **14**: 20–26.

RECTAL PREPARATIONS (ENEMAS)   BNF 1.6.2 & 1.6.4

Indications: Constipation if oral laxatives and suppositories are ineffective.

Dose and use
There are 3 common types of laxative enema:
• osmotic
• lubricant
• faecal softener.
The osmotic laxative enemas comprise both small-volume preparations (micro-enemas) and large-volume preparations. Lubricant enemas contain oil and faecal softener enemas contain docusate. Osmotic micro-enemas are widely used when a laxative suppository is ineffective. Clinical experience suggests, however, that bisacodyl 20mg PR (2 standard suppositories) is often as effective as a micro-enema. A micro-enema may still be preferable because bisacodyl some-times causes colic and may cause faecal leakage after the initial evacuation.

Supply
Osmotic micro-enemas:
These all contain **sodium citrate**, **glycerol** and **sorbitol** and are supplied in 5ml single-dose disposable packs with nozzle:
Fleet 5ml = 45p.
Micolette 5ml = 32p.
Micralax 5ml = 45p.
Relaxit 5ml = 31p (only micro-enema licensed for children <3 years of age).
Standard osmotic enemas:
Fleet Ready-to-use Enema sodium acid phosphate 21.4g and sodium phosphate 9.4g/118ml, single-dose with standard tube = 46p.
Fletchers' Phosphate Enema sodium acid phosphate 12.8g and sodium phosphate 10.24g/128ml (corresponds to **Phosphates Enema Formula B**), 128ml with standard tube = 46p; with long rectal tube = 64p.
Lubricant enema:
Fletcher's Arachis (peanut) Oil Retention Enema in 130ml single-dose disposable pack = £1.07. *Do not use in patients with peanut allergy.*
Faecal softener enemas:
Fletcher's Enemette docusate sodium 90mg and glycerol 3.78g, 5ml unit = 32p.
Norgalax Micro-enema docusate sodium 120mg in 10g, 10g unit = 64p.

PREPARATIONS FOR HAEMORRHOIDS   BNF 1.7

Peri-anal pruritus (often associated with haemorrhoids), soreness and excoriation are best treated by the application of a bland ointment or cream. If associated with trauma caused by the evacuation of hard faeces, the constipation should be corrected (see p.15). Soothing preparations containing mild astringents such as **bismuth subgallate**, **zinc oxide** and **hamamelis** may give symptomatic relief in haemorrhoids. Many proprietary preparations also contain lubricants, vasoconstrictors and antiseptics.

Local anaesthetics relieve pruritus ani as well as pain associated with haemorrhoids. **Lidocaine** ointment can be used before defaecation to relieve pain associated with an anal fissure. Local anaesthetic ointments are absorbed through the rectal mucosa and could produce a systemic effect if applied excessively. They should be used for only a few days because, apart from lidocaine, they can cause contact dermatitis. **Corticosteroids** can be combined with local anaesthetics and astringents; suitable for short-term use after exclusion of infection, such as herpes simplex. Pain associated with spasm of the internal anal sphincter may be helped by topical **glyceryl trinitrate ointment** (see p.30).

Dose and use
Anusol
- apply ointment topically b.d. and after defaecation
- insert suppository after defaecation and o.n.

Scheriproct
- apply ointment b.d. for 5–7 days (t.d.s.–q.d.s. on first day if necessary), then o.d. for a few days after symptoms have cleared
- insert suppository after defaecation for 5–7 days (in severe cases initially b.d.–t.d.s.).

Supply
Anusol:
Cream bismuth oxide, perubalsam, zinc oxide, 23g = £1.63.
Ointment bismuth oxide, bismuth subgallate, perubalsam, zinc oxide, 23g = £1.63.
Suppositories same constituents as ointment, 12 = £1.54.

Scheriproct:
Ointment cinchocaine hydrochloride 0.5%, prednisolone hexanoate 0.19%, 30g = £4.41.
Suppositories cinchocaine hydrochloride 1mg, prednisolone hexanoate 1.3mg, 12 = £2.08.

PANCREATIN   BNF 1.9.4

Class of drug: Enzyme supplement.

Indications: *Symptomatic* steatorrhoea caused by biliary and/or pancreatic obstruction, e.g. cancer of the pancreas.

Pharmacology
Steatorrhoea (the presence of undigested faecal fat) often results in increased bowel frequency, typically with pale, bulky, offensive, frothy and greasy faeces which flush away only with difficulty; associated with abdominal distension, increased flatus, loss of weight, and mineral and vitamin deficiency (A, D, E and K).

Pancreatin is a standardized preparation of porcine lipase, protease and amylase. Pancreatin hydrolyzes fats to glycerol and fatty acids, degrades protein into amino acids, and converts starch into dextrin and sugars. Because they are inactivated by gastric acid, pancreatin preparations are best taken with food (or immediately before or after food). Gastric acid secretion may be reduced by giving cimetidine or ranitidine an hour beforehand (see p.9). Concurrent use of antacids further reduces gastric acidity. The newer e/c preparations (**Creon, Nutrizym GR, Pancrease**) deliver a higher enzyme concentration in the duodenum provided the granules are swallowed whole without chewing.

Cautions
Fibrotic strictures of the colon have developed in children aged 2–13 years with cystic fibrosis who have used certain high-strength preparations of pancreatin, e.g. **Nutrizym 22** and **Pancreatin HL**. Fibrosing colonopathy has not been reported in adults or in patients without cystic fibrosis. **Creon 25 000** has not been implicated.

Adverse effects
Nausea, vomiting and abdominal discomfort. Peri-anal irritation with larger doses.

Dose and use
There are several different proprietary preparations of pancreatin; Creon capsules are the preparations of first choice. Capsules are taken whole or their contents added to fluid or soft food and swallowed without chewing:
- Creon, initially give 1–2 capsules with each meal
- Creon 25 000, initially give 1 capsule with each meal.

The dose is adjusted upwards according to size, number, and consistency of stools, so that the patient thrives; extra allowance may be needed if snacks are taken between meals. If a pancreatin preparation continues to seem ineffective, prescribe a **PPI** or **H$_2$-receptor antagonist**.

Supply

Capsule strength denotes lipase unit content.

Capsules enclosing e/c granules **Creon 10 000**, 100 = £16.66.
Capsules enclosing e/c pellets **Creon 25 000**, 100 = £39.

2: Drugs used in
CARDIOVASCULAR DISEASES

Furosemide (Frusemide)

Spironolactone

*Flecainide

*Mexiletine

*Clonidine

Glyceryl trinitrate

Nifedipine

Dalteparin

Etamsylate

Tranexamic acid

FUROSEMIDE (FRUSEMIDE)   BNF 2.2.2

Class of drug: Loop diuretic.

Indications: Sodium and fluid retention, malignant ascites (normally with spironolactone *see* below).

Contra-indications: Hepatic encephalopathy, anuric renal failure.

Pharmacology

Furosemide inhibits sodium (and hence water) resorption from the ascending limb of the loop of Henle in the renal tubule. It also increases urinary excretion of K^+, H^+, Cl^+ and Mg^{2+}. Alone it has little effect on malignant ascites, even when used in daily doses of 100–200mg PO.[1,2] However, furosemide 100mg CIVI over 24h can have a marked short-term effect with a decrease in girth of up to 10cm and only a modest diuresis (<3L in 24h), suggesting part of the impact is fluid redistribution within the body.[2] Even so, its use in malignant ascites is best limited to when treatment alone with **spironolactone**, an aldosterone antagonist, is insufficient.
Oral bio-availability 60–70%.
Onset of action <1h.
Duration of action <6h.
Plasma halflife 30–120min.

Cautions

Increased risk of hypokalaemia with corticosteroids, β_2-adrenoceptor stimulants, amphotericin and carbenoxolone; increased risk of hyponatraemia with carbamazepine and aminoglutethimide; increased risk of hypotension with ACE inhibitors and tricyclic antidepressants.

Adverse effects

Nausea and gastro-intestinal disturbances, hypokalaemia (may precipitate encephalopathy in hepatic failure), hyponatraemia, hyperglycaemia (worsening diabetic control), hyperuricaemia (precipitating gout), urinary retention (in prostatic hypertrophy), hypotension, rashes, photosensitivity, bone marrow depression, tinnitus, deafness.

---

* specialist use only.

Dose and use
- starting dose 40mg o.m.
- usual maintenance dose 20mg o.m.; usual maximum dose 80mg o.m.

Supply
Tablets 20mg, 20 = 31p; 40mg, 20 = 22p.
Solution 5mg/5ml, 150ml = £1.10; 20mg, 40mg and 50mg/5ml from Rosemont as a special order (see Appendix 8).

---

1 Fogel MR et al. (1981) Diuresis in the ascitic patient: a randomised controlled trial of three regimens. *Journal of Clinical Gastroenterology.* **3** (suppl 1): 73–80.
2 Amiel SA et al. (1984) Intravenous infusion of frusemide as treatment for ascites in malignant disease. *British Medical Journal.* **288**: 1041.

SPIRONOLACTONE   BNF 2.2.3

Class of drug: Potassium-sparing diuretic; aldosterone antagonist.

Indications: Sodium and fluid retention, malignant ascites.

Contra-indications: Hyperkalaemia, hyponatraemia.

Pharmacology
Spironolactone is a potassium-sparing diuretic which inhibits the action of aldosterone on distal tubules. Hyperaldosteronism is a common concomitant of malignant ascites.[1] Treatment with even very large PO doses of a loop diuretic (e.g. furosemide (frusemide) ⩾200mg) generally fails to relieve ascites.[2] On the other hand, spironolactone in a median daily dose of 300mg is successful in about 2/3 of patients.[1,2]
Bio-availability 90%.
Onset of action peak effect at 7h; maximum response after 2–3 days.
Duration of action 24h.
Plasma halflife 80min.

Cautions

Serious drug interactions: risk of hyperkalaemia with potassium-sparing diuretics and ACE inhibitors.

Elderly, hepatic impairment, renal impairment. Risk of hyperkalaemia, particularly if prescribed concurrently with an NSAID. Effect reduced by aspirin and possibly other NSAIDs. Spironolactone enhances the effect of digoxin.

Adverse effects
Nausea and vomiting, impotence, gynaecomastia, menstrual irregularities, lethargy, headache, delirium, rashes, hyperkalaemia, hyponatraemia, hepatotoxicity, osteomalacia and blood disorders.

Dose and use
- monitor body weight and renal function
- starting dose 100–200mg o.m.
- increase dose by 100mg every 3–7 days to achieve a weight loss of 0.5–1kg/day
- usual maintenance dose 300mg daily; usual maximum dose 400mg daily.[1,2]
If not achieving the desired weight loss with spironolactone 300–400mg daily, consider the addition of furosemide 40mg o.m. Elimination of ascites may take 10–28 days.

Supply
Tablets 100mg, 20 = £2.33.
Capsules 100mg, 20 = £5.40.
Suspension 50mg/5ml and 100mg/5ml from Rosemont as a special order (see Appendix 8).

---

1 Greenway B et al. (1982) Control of malignant ascites with spironolactone. British Journal of Surgery. **69**: 441–442.
2 Fogel MR et al. (1981) Diuresis in the ascitic patient: a randomised controlled trial of three regimens. Journal of Clinical Gastroenterology. **3** (suppl 1): 73–80.

*FLECAINIDE   BNF 2.3

Class of drug: Class 1C anti-arrhythmic.

Indications: [†]Neuropathic pain.

Contra-indications: Recent myocardial infarction, heart disease requiring medication, abnormal ECG.

Pharmacology
Flecainide is a chemical congener of lidocaine (lignocaine). It is a membrane stabilizer, i.e. it inhibits sodium ion channels in nerve membranes, thereby decreasing excitability and slowing conduction velocity. Flecainide is licensed for use primarily in the treatment of ventricular arrhythmias but is used at some PCUs as the adjuvant analgesic of choice for nerve injury pain (as an alternative to **mexiletine**, see p.28); more often it is used as third-line treatment after failure with a combination of an **antidepressant** and an **anticonvulsant**. Benefit is seen in about 2/3 of patients.[1–4] Other third-line treatments include **methadone** (see p.120), **ketamine** (see p.175) and **spinal analgesia**.
When used as prophylaxis against arrhythmias after myocardial infarction, flecainide was associated with an increased incidence of sudden death.[5] In consequence, when used as an anti-arrhythmic, the manufacturer recommends that treatment is started in hospital. At some PCUs, however, flecainide for neuropathic pain is started on an outpatient basis without an ECG provided the patient is in normal rhythm, is not in cardiac failure and has no history of myocardial infarction.
Onset of action 65min (range 31–110min) as an anti-arrhythmic.
Duration of action 15–23h as an anti-arrhythmic.
Plasma halflife 14h.

Cautions
Hepatic and renal impairment. Risk of myocardial depression increased by β-blockers, calcium-channel blockers and hypokalaemia: risk of arrhythmia if used with a pro-arrhythmic drug (e.g. tricyclic antidepressants). Plasma concentration increased by amiodarone, fluoxetine, quinine, cimetidine; decreased by phenytoin, phenobarbital and carbamazepine.

Adverse effects
Dizziness, visual disturbances (corneal deposits), cardiac arrhythmias or block, nausea, vomiting, photosensitivity, abnormal liver function tests, ataxia, peripheral neuropathy, pulmonary fibrosis, pneumonitis, psychosis, delirium.[3,4,6]

Dose and use
Generally, tricyclic antidepressants should be stopped at least 48h before starting flecainide. Initial doses are comparable to those used in cardiology:
• starting dose 50mg b.d.
• usual dose 100mg b.d.; maximum 200mg b.d.

Supply
Tablets 50mg, 60 = £16.28; 100mg, 60 = £23.26.

---

1 Dunlop R et al. (1988) Analgesic effects of oral flecainide. Lancet. 1: 420–421.
2 Sinnot C et al. (1991) Flecainide in cancer nerve pain. Lancet. 337: 1347.
3 Chong et al. (1997) Pilot study evaluating local anesthetics administered systemically for treatment of pain in patients with advanced cancer. Journal of Pain and Symptom Management. 13: 112–117.
4 Broadley K (1998) Personal communication.
5 Cardiac arrhythmia suppression trial (CAST) (1989) Investigators' preliminary report: effect of encainide and flecainide on mortality in a randomized trial of arrhythmia suppression after myocardial infarction. New England Journal of Medicine. 321: 406–412.
6 Bennett MI (1997) Paranoid psychosis due to flecainide toxicity in malignant neuropathic pain. Pain. 70: 93–94.

*MEXILETINE BNF 2.3

Class of drug: Class 1B anti-arrhythmic.

Indications: [†]Neuropathic pain.

Contra-indications: Heart disease requiring medication, abnormal ECG.

Pharmacology

Mexiletine is a chemical congener of lidocaine (lignocaine). It is a membrane stabilizer, i.e. it inhibits sodium ion channels in nerve membranes, thereby decreasing excitability and slowing conduction velocity. Mexiletine is used primarily in the treatment of ventricular arrhythmias. Mexiletine is also of proven value in pain caused by nerve injury.[1,2] Some PCUs use mexiletine as the adjuvant analgesic of choice for nerve injury pain; more often it is used as third-line treatment after failure with a combination of an **antidepressant** and an **anticonvulsant**. Benefit is seen in about 2/3 of patients.[3] Other third-line treatments include **methadone** (see p.120), **ketamine** (see p.175) and **spinal analgesia**.
Bio-availability 80–88%.
Onset of action 1–3h.
Duration of action 6–8h.
Plasma halflife 6–12h.

Cautions

Hepatic impairment. Opioid analgesics and antimuscarinics delay absorption. Risk of myocardial depression with other anti-arrhythmics ($\rightarrow$ hypotension); risk of arrhythmia if used with a pro-arrhythmic drug (e.g. tricyclic antidepressants). Effect reduced by drugs causing hypokalaemia (e.g. loop and thiazide diuretics). Plasma concentration of mexiletine increased by amitriptyline but decreased by phenytoin and rifampicin. Mexiletine increases the plasma concentration of theophylline (see Appendix 3, p.213).

Adverse effects

Nausea, vomiting, constipation, bradycardia, hypotension, cardiac arrhythmias, drowsiness, tremor, delirium, convulsions, altered mood, psychosis, dysarthria, ataxia, paraesthesia, nystagmus, jaundice, hepatitis and blood disorders.

Dose and use

Generally, tricyclic antidepressants should be stopped at least 48h before starting mexiletine. Compared with use in cardiology, the initial dose of mexiletine is low:
• starting dose 50mg t.d.s.
• increase dose by 50mg t.d.s. every 3–7 days to a maximum of 10mg/kg/day.
In the event of troublesome adverse effects, give a smaller dose more frequently p.c. to delay absorption, thereby reducing the maximum plasma concentration.

At one centre, mexiletine is given in high doses (400mg PO stat, 200mg q6h) *with amitriptyline* to patients with *poststroke central pain* which has failed to respond to antidepressant mono-therapy.[4] This is done on an inpatient basis following cardiological review; combined treatment definitely *not* recommended in debilitated cancer patients.

Supply
Capsules 50mg, 100 = £4.95; 200mg, 100 = £11.87.

---

1 Dejgard A et al. (1988) Mexiletine for treatment of chronic painful diabetic neuropathy. *Lancet.* i: 9–11.
2 Chabal C et al. (1992) The use of oral mexiletine for the treatment of pain after peripheral nerve injury. *Anaesthesiology.* **76**: 513–517.
3 Chong et al. (1997) Pilot study evaluating local anesthetics administered systemically for treatment of pain in patients with advanced cancer. *Journal of Pain and Symptom Management.* **13**: 112–117.
4 Bowsher D (1995) The management of central post-stroke pain. *Postgraduate Medical Journal.* **71**: 598–604.

*CLONIDINE   BNF 2.5.2

Class of drug: α-adrenergic agonist.

Indications: [†]Pain poorly responsive to spinal morphine and bupivacaine.

Pharmacology
Clonidine is a mixed α_1- and α_2-adrenergic agonist (mainly α_2). It reduces the responsiveness of peripheral blood vessels to vasoconstrictor and vasodilator substances, and to sympathetic nerve stimulation.[1] Clonidine can cause a reduction in venous return and mild bradycardia, resulting in a reduced cardiac output. It is licensed for use as migraine prophylaxis and as an antihypertensive. Clonidine attenuates the opioid withdrawal syndrome, indicating an interaction with the opioid system. Reproducible pain relief in some patients with neuropathic pain has been observed, par-ticularly when given spinally.[2–5] Significant plasma concentrations are present after epidural administration (reflected clinically by a hypotensive effect) and it is debatable whether clonidine has a 'selective' spinal effect.[6] The analgesic effect of clonidine can be reversed by α-adrenergic antagonists but not by naloxone.[5] It is probable that clonidine analgesia is mediated by an agonist effect at α_2-adrenergic receptors or imidazoline receptors resulting in:
- peripheral and/or central suppression of sympathetic transmitter release[5,7,8]
- presynaptic inhibition of nociceptive afferents[9]
- postsynaptic inhibition of spinal cord neurones[10,11]
- facilitation of brain stem pain modulating systems.[12]

Spinal doses above 300µg/24h generally do not yield additional benefit.[13] Clonidine can also be given by mouth, as a transdermal patch,[4,8] and by SC infusion. Exceptionally, patients have received up to 1.5mg CSCI (10 × 150µg amp) with increasing effect.[13]
Bio-availability 75–100%.
Onset of action 30–60min PO.
Duration of action 8h PO.
Plasma halflife 6–24h.

Cautions
After stopping long-term treatment: agitation, rebound hypertension.

Adverse effects
Hypotension (after bolus injection), sedation and dry mouth (initially), dizziness, headache, euphoria, nocturnal restlessness, nausea, constipation, rash, impotence (rare), depression (long-term use).

Dose and use

Clonidine is used infrequently and is generally given spinally with diamorphine/morphine ± bupivacaine. A typical regimen for ED use would be:
- a test bolus dose of 50–150µg in 5ml saline injected over 5min
- if relief obtained, 150–300µg/24h by infusion.

It is also used IT.

Supply
Injection 150µg, 1 amp = 29p.

---

1 Hieble JP and Ruffolo RR (1991) Therapeutic applications of agents interacting with alpha-adrenoceptors. In: Ruffolo RR (ed) *Alpha-adrenoceptors: molecular biology, biochemistry and pharmacology.* **vol 8**. Karger, Basel. pp 180–220.

2 Glynn C et al. (1988) A double-blind comparison between epidural morphine and epidural clonidine in patients with chronic noncancer pain. *Pain.* **34**: 123–128.

3 Max MB et al. (1988) Association of pain relief with drug side effects in postherpetic neuralgia: a single-dose study of clonidine, codeine, ibuprofen, and placebo. *Clinical Pharmacology and Therapeutics.* **43**: 363–371.

4 Zeigler D et al. (1992) Transdermal clonidine versus placebo in painful diabetic neuropathy. *Pain.* **48**: 403–408.

5 Quan DB et al. (1993) Clonidine in pain management. *Annals of Pharmacotherapy.* **27**: 313–315.

6 Wells JCD and Hardy PAJ (1987) Epidural clonidine. *Lancet.* **i**: 108.

7 Langer SZ et al. (1980) Recent developments in noradrenergic neurotransmission and its relevance to the mechanism of action of certain antihypertensive agents. *Hypertension.* **2**: 372–382.

8 Davis KD et al. (1991) Topical application of clonidine relieves hyperalgesia in patients with sympathetically maintained pain. *Pain.* **47**: 309–318.

9 Calvillo O and Ghignone M (1986) Presynaptic effect of clonidine on unmyelinated afferent fibers in the spinal cord of the cat. *Neuroscience Letters.* **64**: 335–339.

10 Yaksh TL (1985) Pharmacology of spinal adrenergic systems which modulate spinal nociceptive processing. *Pharmacology, Biochemistry and Behaviour.* **22**: 845–858.

11 Michel MC and Insel PA (1989) Are there multiple imidazoline binding sites? *TIPS.* **10**: 342–344.

12 Sagen J and Proudfit H (1985) Evidence for pain modulation by pre- and postsynaptic noradrenergic receptors in the medulla oblongata. *Brain Research.* **331**: 285–293.

13 Glynn C (1997) Personal communication.

GLYCERYL TRINITRATE — BNF 2.6

Class of drug: Nitrate.

Indications: †Severe smooth muscle spasm pain (particularly of the oesophagus, rectum and anus), biliary and renal colic.

Contra-indications: Hypotension, aortic or mitral stenosis, cardiac tamponade, constrictive pericarditis, marked anaemia, cerebral haemorrhage, narrow-angle glaucoma.

Pharmacology

Glyceryl trinitrate reduces the amount of intracellular calcium available for muscle contraction. It is rapidly absorbed through the buccal mucosa but inactivated by the gastro-intestinal mucosa. Many patients on long-acting or transdermal nitrates develop tolerance; i.e. experience a reduced therapeutic effect. Tolerance is generally prevented if nitrate levels are allowed to fall for 4–8h in every 24h (a 'nitrate holiday').

---

† unlicensed use.

Sublingual bio-availability 60–75%.
Onset of action 1–3min.
Duration of action 20–30min.
Plasma halflife 1–4min.

Cautions

Severe hepatic or renal impairment; hypothyroidism, malnutrition or hypothermia; recent diagnosis of myocardial infarction. Exacerbates the hypotensive effect of other drugs. Drugs causing a dry mouth may reduce the effect of sublingual nitrates.

Adverse effects

Headache, flushing, dizziness, postural hypotension, tachycardia.

Dose and use

- starting dose 500µg SL, maximum 1mg
- instruct the patient to swallow or spit out tablet once pain relief obtained
- warn of possible adverse effects; these generally settle with repeated use.

Repeat as needed when spasm/colic is transient and intermittent. For persistent spasm consider:
- glyceryl trinitrate skin patches
- orally active nitrates, e.g. **isosorbide mononitrate**
- ointment 0.2% for pain due to anal fissure.[1]

If ineffective or poorly tolerated, consider the use of other smooth muscle relaxants e.g. **nifedipine** (see below), **hyoscine butylbromide** (see p.4). In contrast to exercise-induced angina pectoris, it may not be possible for patients with persistent pain to have a 'nitrate holiday'. If tolerance develops it will be necessary to increase the dose to restore efficacy.

Supply

Tablets SL 500µg, 100 = 75p; because of degradation, unused tablets should be discarded after 8 weeks.
Ointment 0.2% from Queen's Medical Centre Pharmacy, Nottingham, 20g = £8.77.

---

1 Lund JN and Scholefield JH (1997) A randomised, prospective, placebo-controlled trial of glyceryl trinitrate ointment in treatment of anal fissure. *Lancet.* **349**: 11–14.

NIFEDIPINE   BNF 2.6

Class of drug: Calcium-channel blocker.

Indications: [†]Severe smooth muscle spasm pain (particularly of the oesophagus, rectum and anus[1–3]), [†]intractable hiccup.[4,5]

Contra-indications: Cardiogenic shock, severe aortic stenosis.

Pharmacology

Calcium-channel blockers inhibit the influx of calcium into cells, thereby modifying cell function, e.g. smooth muscle contraction and nerve cell transmission of messages.[6] They have an antinociceptive effect and augment opioid antinociception. Nifedipine may help hiccup by relieving oesophageal spasm or by interference with neural pathways involved in hiccup.[4,5]
Bio-availability 50–60%.
Onset of action 20min.
Duration of action 6h.
Plasma halflife 3–4h.

[†] unlicensed use.   31

Cautions

Serious drug interactions: augments the hypotensive and negative inotropic effects of other drugs.

Hepatic impairment, may impair glucose tolerance. Plasma concentration increased by grapefruit juice and cimetidine; reduced by rifampicin, carbamazepine, phenobarbital and phenytoin. Nifedipine increases plasma concentrations of cyclosporin, digoxin, phenytoin and theophylline; reduces plasma concentrations of quinidine; inhibits the inotropic effect of theophylline on muscle.

Adverse effects

Headache, flushing, dizziness, lethargy, tachycardia, palpitations, gravitational oedema, rash, nausea, urinary frequency, eye pain, gum hyperplasia, depression.

Dose and use

- starting dose 10mg PO/SL stat
- followed by 10–20mg t.d.s. with or after food, or m/r 20mg b.d.
- usual maximum dose 60–80mg/day.

Up to 160mg/day have been used for intractable hiccup with concurrent fludrocortisone 0.5–1mg to overcome orthostatic hypotension.[5]

Supply

Capsules 10mg, 20 = £1.80.
Tablets m/r 20mg, 20 = £3.08–£4.57.

---

1 Cargill G *et al.* (1982) Nifedipine for the relief of oesophageal chest pain. *New England Journal of Medicine.* **307**: 187–188.
2 McLoughlin R and McQuillan R (1997) Using nifedipine to treat tenesmus. *Palliative Medicine.* **11**: 419–420.
3 Celik AF *et al.* (1995) Hereditary proctalgia fugax and constipation: report of a second family. *Gut.* **36**: 581–584.
4 Lipps DC *et al.* (1990) Nifedipine for intractable hiccups. *Neurology.* **40**(3 Pt 1): 531–532.
5 Bringham B and Bolin T (1992) High dose nifedipine and fludrocortisone for intractable hiccups. *Medical Journal of Australia.* **157**: 70.
6 Castell DO (1985) Calcium channel blocking agents for gastrointestinal disorders. *American Journal of Cardiology.* **55**: 210B–213B.

DALTEPARIN BNF 2.8

Class of drug: Low molecular weight heparin (LMWH).

Indications: Deep vein thrombosis, prevention and treatment, [†]thrombophlebitis migrans, [†]disseminated intravascular coagulation (DIC).

Contra-indications: Patients at risk of haemorrhage, (e.g. bleeding diathesis, thrombocytopenia *except disseminated intravascular coagulation*), peptic ulcer, recent cerebral haemorrhage and severe liver disease, subacute bacterial endocarditis.

Pharmacology

Dalteparin acts within minutes by potentiating the inhibitory effect of antithrombin III on Factor Xa and thrombin. It has a relatively higher ability to potentiate Factor Xa inhibition than to prolong plasma clotting time (APTT) which cannot be used to guide dosage. Anti-factor Xa can be

† unlicensed use.

measured if necessary but routine monitoring is not required because the dose is determined by the patient's weight. Other advantages over standard heparin include a better safety profile (it has less effect on platelet function and thus primary haemostasis) and a longer duration of action which allows administration o.d.

Heparin is the treatment of choice for chronic DIC, which commonly presents as recurrent thromboses in both superficial and deep venous systems. It does not respond to warfarin. Even when haemorrhagic manifestations (e.g. ecchymoses and haematomas) are the predominant manifestations, the correct treatment is still heparin because the original trigger for DIC is clot formation. Tranexamic acid (an antifibrinolytic drug) should not be used because it would increase the risk of end-organ damage from microvascular thromboses.

Bio-availability 87% SC.
Onset of action 3min IV, 2–4h SC.
Duration of action 10–24h SC.
Plasma halflife 2h SC, 3.5–4 h IV.

Cautions

Serious drug interactions: enhanced anticoagulant effect with anticoagulant/antiplatelet drugs, e.g. NSAIDS; reduced anticoagulant effect with antihistamines, cardiac glycosides, tetracycline, ascorbic acid.

Renal failure, uncontrolled hypertension, retinopathy.

Adverse effects

Local skin reactions at the injection site (erythema, induration, pruritus) or, rarely, systemic reactions (urticaria, angioedema, anaphylaxis). Abnormal liver function tests have been reported.

Both standard heparin and LMWH can cause thrombocytopenia (platelet count below 100×10^9/l). *Immune-mediated thrombocytopenia* typically develops after 5–10 days and is associated with heparin-dependent IgG antibodies and risk of severe venous and arterial thromboses.[1] Immune-mediated thrombocytopenia occurs in <3% of patients treated with standard heparin irrespective of dose. In one trial, heparin-dependent antibodies developed less frequently with LMWH than with standard heparin (2.2% v 7.8%).[2] Ideally, any patient receiving heparin should have a full blood count done on day 4–6 of treatment, possibly repeated a few days later. LMWH must be stopped immediately if thrombocytopenia is found and alternative anticoagulant therapy given. The heparinoid, **danaparoid**, is a suitable choice as cross-reactivity is rare (see BNF 2.8.1).

Dose and use

Inject SC, preferably into the abdomen or lateral thigh; introduce the total length of the needle vertically into the thickest part of a skin fold produced by squeezing the skin between the thumb and forefinger.

Surgical thromboprophylaxis
• give 2500 units 1–2h before and 8–12h after the operation, then 5000 units daily thereafter until mobile
• double the dose in high-risk patients.

Thrombophlebitis migrans
• generally responds rapidly to a small dose, i.e. 2500–5000 units SC daily
• titrate dose if necessary to maximum allowed according to weight (see below).

Deep vein thrombosis
• confirm diagnosis radiologically (ultrasound or venogram)
• give 200 units/kg SC o.d., up to a maximum of 18 000 units
• use 100 units/kg SC b.d. if patients are considered to be at a greater risk of bleeding.

Because of haemorrhagic complications in nearly 50% of patients when using warfarin in advanced cancer (possibly related to drug interactions and hepatic dysfunction), dalteparin can be used alone for 4–8 weeks.[3]

Disseminated intravascular coagulation (DIC)

* confirm the diagnosis:
    thrombocytopenia (platelet count <150 000 × 10^9/L in 95% of cases)
    decreased plasma fibrinogen concentration
    elevated plasma D-dimer concentration – a fibrin degradation product (85% of cases)
    prolonged prothrombin time and/or partial thromboplastin time.[4]

A normal plasma fibrinogen concentration (200–250mg/100ml) is also suspicious because fibrinogen levels are generally raised in cancer (e.g. 450–500mg/100ml) unless there is extensive hepatic disease. Infection and cancer both may be associated with an increased platelet count which likewise may mask an evolving thrombocytopenia.

* give dalteparin o.d. as for deep vein thrombosis
* *do not use warfarin because ineffective.*

Overdose

In emergencies, 1mg of **protamine sulphate** inhibits 100 units of dalteparin; maximum dose 50mg by slow IV injection.

Supply

Injection single dose syringe 12 500 units/ml, 0.2ml (2500 units) = £1.95; 25 000 units/ml, 0.2ml (5000 units) = £2.96.
Injection vial 25 000 units/ml, 4ml = £50.95.

1 Anonymous (1998) Low molecular weight heparins for venous thromboembolism. *Drug and Therapeutics Bulletin.* **36**: 25–29.

2 Warkentin TE *et al.* (1995) Heparin-induced thrombocytopenia in patients treated with low-molecular-weight heparin or unfractionated heparin. *New England Journal of Medicine.* **332**: 1330–1335.

3 Johnson MJ and Sherry K (1997) How do palliative physicians manage venous thrombo-embolism? *Palliative Medicine.* **11**: 462–468.

4 Spero JA *et al.* (1980) Disseminated intravascular coagulation: findings in 346 patients. *Thrombosis and Haemostasis.* **43**: 28–33.

ETAMSYLATE   BNF 2.11

Class of drug: Haemostatic agent.

Indications: [†]Surface bleeding from ulcerating tumours, nasal cavity and other organs (bladder, uterus, rectum, stomach and lungs).

Pharmacology

Etamsylate is thought to act by increasing capillary vascular wall resistance and platelet adhesiveness in the presence of a vascular lesion, by inhibiting the biosynthesis and actions of those PGs which cause platelet disaggregation, vasodilation and increased capillary permeability; it does not have a vasoconstricting action. Etamsylate does not affect normal coagulation; administration is without effect on prothrombin time, fibrinolysis, platelet count or function. Etamsylate is licensed for use in menorrhagia. It can be used in conjunction with tranexamic acid (see p.35). Etamsylate is absorbed slowly but completely from the gastro-intestinal tract and excreted in the urine mainly unchanged.
Onset of action no data.
Duration of action no data.
Plasma halflife 5–17h PO; 1.7–2.5h IM; 1.8–2h IV.

Adverse effects

Headache, rash, nausea (when taken on an empty stomach).

† unlicensed use.

Dose and use
500mg q.d.s., either indefinitely or for 1 week after cessation of bleeding; if causes nausea, take p.c.

Supply
Tablets 500mg, 20 = £4.43.

TRANEXAMIC ACID   BNF 2.11

Class of drug: Antifibrinolytic agent.

Indications: [†]Surface bleeding from ulcerating tumours, nasal cavity and other organs (bladder, uterus, rectum, stomach and lungs).

Contra-indications: Thrombo-embolic disease, DIC.

Pharmacology
Tranexamic acid inhibits the breakdown of fibrin clots. It acts primarily by competitively blocking the binding of plasminogen and plasmin; direct inhibition of plasmin occurs to a limited extent. Tranexamic acid is excreted in the urine mainly as unchanged drug. In DIC, even when haemorrhagic manifestations (e.g. ecchymoses and haematomas) are the predominant manifestations, tranexamic acid should not be used because clot formation is the trigger for further intravascular coagulation and platelet consumption – and an increased risk of end-organ damage from microvascular thromboses.
Bio-availability 30–50%.
Onset of action no data.
Duration of action no data.
Plasma halflife 2h.

Cautions

Serious drug interactions: increased risk of thrombosis with other thrombogenic drugs.

In renal failure, excretion is retarded with resultant cumulation. In patients with haematuria, there is risk of ureteric obstruction and retention.

Adverse effects
Nausea, vomiting, diarrhoea, disturbance of colour vision (withdraw treatment).

Dose and use
- 1.5g stat and 1g t.d.s.
- maximum dose 1.5g q.d.s.
- discontinue or reduce to 500mg t.d.s. 1 week after cessation of bleeding.
- restart if bleeding occurs.[1]

Supply
Tablets 500mg, 20 = £4.99.
Syrup 500mg/5ml, 300ml = £15.60.

---

1 Dean A and Tuffin P (1997) Fibrinolytic inhibitors for cancer-associated bleeding problems. *Journal of Pain and Symptom Management.* **13**: 20–24.

[†] unlicensed use.

3: Drugs used in
RESPIRATORY DISEASES

Bronchodilators
  Ipratropium
  Salbutamol
  Theophylline

Inhaled corticosteroids

Oxygen

Cough suppressants

Aromatic inhalations

Carbocisteine

BRONCHODILATORS   BNF 3.1

Selective β_2-adrenoceptor stimulants (e.g. **salbutamol, terbutaline**) are the safest and most effective bronchodilators for patients with airflow obstruction. British Thoracic Society guidelines for their use in patients with asthma and COPD are available (Boxes 3.A–3.C).[1,2] Ideally, a patient should be evaluated before and after a test dose of a bronchodilator or a corticosteroid to confirm benefit, and the results documented in the patient's notes (Box 3.D).

Patients with mild–moderate asthma should use the minimum dose of short-acting β_2-stimulants to control their symptoms, e.g. salbutamol p.r.n. In more severe asthma a long-acting β_2-stimulant, e.g. **salmeterol**, is prescribed in addition to inhaled corticosteroid (step 3 and above).

Inhalation delivers the drug directly to the bronchi and enables a smaller dose to work more quickly and with fewer systemic adverse effects. Inhaler technique should be carefully explained and checked periodically. The patient should be instructed to inhale slowly and then to hold their breath for 10 seconds if possible. If inhaler technique does not improve with training, a spacer should be used to improve drug delivery. Breath-actuated aerosol inhalers and turbohalers are other options.

In patients with lung cancer, concurrent COPD can be a major cause of breathlessness but may be unrecognized and so go untreated. Breathlessness can be improved in most patients with lung cancer and COPD by a combination of a β_2-stimulant and an antimuscarinic.[3] Administration by aerosol inhaler through a spacer is as effective as a nebulizer.[3] A summary of the use of nebulized drugs in palliative care is given in Appendix 9, p.241.

1 British Thoracic Society and others (1997) The BTS guidelines on asthma management. *Thorax.* **52** (suppl 1): S1–S21.
2 British Thoracic Society and others (1997) BTS guidelines for the management of chronic obstructive pulmonary disease. *Thorax.* **52** (suppl 5): S1–S28.
3 Congelton J and Meurs MF (1995) The incidence of airflow obstruction in bronchial carcinoma, its relation to breathlessness and response to bronchodilator therapy. *Respiratory Medicine.* **89**: 291–296.

Box 3.A Management of chronic asthma in adults[1]

Start at the step most appropriate to the initial severity. *A corticosteroid should be prescribed for a nonresponsive acute exacerbation, e.g. prednisolone 30–60mg o.m.*

Step 1: occasional relief bronchodilators
Inhaled short-acting β_2-stimulant p.r.n.
Move to step 2 if needed more than o.d. or if symptoms at night.

Step 2: regular inhaled preventer therapy
Regular standard dose of inhaled corticosteroid (beclometasone dipropionate or budesonide 100–400µg b.d. *or* fluticasone propionate 50–200µg b.d.)
+ inhaled short-acting β_2-stimulant p.r.n.
High-dose inhaled corticosteroid may be required to gain initial relief; some people benefit from doubling the dose for a short period during an exacerbation.

Step 3: high-dose inhaled corticosteroids *or* standard-dose inhaled corticosteroids + long-acting inhaled β_2-stimulant
Regular high-dose inhaled corticosteroids (beclometasone dipropionate or budesonide 800–2000µg daily *or* fluticasone 400–1000µg daily; given in 2–4 doses via a large-volume spacer), *or*
Regular standard-dose inhaled corticosteroids + regular long-acting inhaled β_2-stimulant (salmeterol 50µg b.d., eformoterol 12µg b.d.)
+ inhaled short-acting β_2-stimulant p.r.n.
The few who have problems (i.e. sore throat, hoarse voice) with high-dose inhaled corticosteroids should change to standard-dose inhaled corticosteroid with long-acting β_2-stimulant (as above) or regular oral m/r theophylline or try regular cromoglicate or nedocromil.

Step 4: high-dose inhaled corticosteroids + regular bronchodilators
Regular high-dose inhaled corticosteroids
+ sequential therapeutic trial of one or more of:
    inhaled long-acting β_2-stimulant
    oral m/r theophylline
    inhaled antimuscarinic
    oral m/r β_2-stimulant
    high-dose inhaled bronchodilators
    inhaled sodium cromoglicate or nedocromil
+ inhaled short-acting β_2-stimulant p.r.n.

Step 5: regular corticosteroid tablets
Regular prednisolone tablets (the minimum dose that controls symptoms o.m.)
+ regular high-dose inhaled corticosteroid
+ one or more long-acting bronchodilators (see step 4)
+ inhaled short-acting β_2-stimulant p.r.n.
Refer to asthma clinic.

Stepping down
Review treatment every 3–6 months; if good control has been achieved for 1–3 months, it may be possible to go down one or more steps. If treatment started recently at step 4 or 5 (or contains corticosteroid tablets) reduction should be considered after a shorter interval.

Box 3.B   Severe acute asthma

Characterized by persistent breathlessness despite usual bronchodilators, exhaustion, tachycardia (>110/min) and a low peak expiratory flow rate ($<50\%$ of best). It requires urgent treatment by experienced physicians with:
* oxygen
* corticosteroids (hydrocortisone 200mg IV *or* prednisolone 30–60mg PO)
* salbutamol 5mg or terbutaline 10mg by nebulizer (repeat as necessary).

If little response, consider:
* ipratropium bromide 500μg by nebulizer
* aminophylline 250mg by slow IV injection (*only if patient not already on oral theophylline*)
* change route of administration of β_2-stimulant to SC/IV.

If continued decline, consider:
* intermittent positive pressure ventilation.

Box 3.C   Bronchodilator therapy in COPD[2]

At all stages patients must be taught how and when to use their treatments. The use of medication which may cause bronchoconstriction (e.g. β-blockers) should be avoided.

Mild COPD
FEV_1 60–79% of predicted value; FEV_1/FVC and other indices of expiratory flow mildly reduced:
* asymptomatic $\rightarrow$ no drug treatment
* symptomatic $\rightarrow$ a trial of an inhaled β_2-stimulant *or* an antimuscarinic taken p.r.n. using an appropriate inhaler device, stop if ineffective.

Moderate COPD
FEV_1 40–59% of predicted value, often with increased FRC and reduced Tlco.
Some patients are hypoxaemic but not hypercapnic:
* regular inhaled bronchodilators as above.

Treatment depends on the severity of symptoms and their effect on lifestyle; most patients need only a single drug but a few require combined treatment.
Oral bronchodilators are generally not necessary.

Severe COPD
FEV_1 <40% of predicted value with marked overinflation; Tlco variable but often low. Hypoxaemia usual, hypercapnia in some:
* combined treatment with a β_2-stimulant and an antimuscarinic bronchodilator
* theophyllines can be tried but must be monitored for adverse effects.

Some patients request 'stronger' therapy. The dose-response curve is limited, however, by the maximum bronchodilation available. High-dose treatment including nebulized drugs should be prescribed only after a formal assessment.

Box 3.D Bronchodilator and corticosteroid reversibility testing[2]

These tests are done when a patient is clinically stable in order to:
- detect patients whose FEV_1 increases substantially, i.e. are asthmatic

- establish the post-bronchodilator FEV_1 (the best predictor of long-term outcome).
The patient should not have taken inhaled short-acting bronchodilators in the previous 6h, long-acting ones in the previous 12h, or m/r theophylline in the preceding 24h.

Response
Measure FEV_1:
- before and 15min after 2.5–5mg nebulized salbutamol *or* 5–10mg terbutaline

- before and after 500µg nebulized ipratropium bromide

- before and after both in combination

or

- before and after a course of oral prednisolone (e.g. 30mg o.m. for 2 weeks) or inhaled corticosteroid (e.g. beclometasone 500µg b.d. for 6 weeks).

Interpretation
- an increase in FEV_1 that is both greater than 200ml and a 15% increase over the pre-bronchodilator value is the definition of reversibility

- a negative FEV_1 response does not preclude benefit from bronchodilators in terms of improved walking distance or a reduction in the perception of breathlessness.

IPRATROPIUM   BNF 3.1.2

Class of drug: Quarternary ammonium antimuscarinic bronchodilator.

Indications: Reversible airways obstruction, particularly in COPD.

Pharmacology
Antimuscarinic drugs are as effective as β_2-stimulants in patients with COPD with some studies suggesting a greater and more prolonged bronchodilator response.[1,2] The combination of an antimuscarinic with a β_2-stimulant should be tried only when individually they have failed to give adequate relief.
Bio-availability 10–20% of the dose reaches the lower airways.
Onset of action maximum effect 30–60min.
Duration of action 3–6h.
Plasma halflife 2.3–3.8h

Cautions
Glaucoma, prostatic hypertrophy.

Adverse effects
Narrow-angle glaucoma, dry mouth. Rarely urinary retention, constipation and paradoxical bronchoconstriction.

Dose and use
In most patients, bronchodilation can be maintained with administration t.d.s.
Aerosol inhalation
- 20–40µg (1–2 puffs) t.d.s.–q.d.s. p.r.n.
- 20–40µg (1–2 puffs) before exercise in exercise-induced bronchoconstriction.

Nebulizer solution
• 250–500µg q.d.s. p.r.n.

Supply
Aerosol inhalation 20µg /metered inhalation, 200 dose unit = £4.21.
Nebulizer solution 0.025% 250µg/ml, 20 × 1ml (250µg) = £6.14; 20 × 2ml (500µg) = £7.20.

1 Tashkin DP *et al.* (1986) Comparison of the anticholinergic bronchodilator ipratropium bromide with metaproterenol in chronic obstructive pulmonary disease: a multicentre study. *American Journal of Medicine.* **81** (suppl 5a): 61–65.
2 Combivent inhalation aerosol study group (1994) In chronic obstructive pulmonary disease a combination of ipratropium and albuterol is more effective than either agent alone. *Chest.* **105**: 1411–1419.

SALBUTAMOL   BNF 3.1.1

Class of drug: β_2-adrenoceptor agonist (sympathomimetic).

Indications: Asthma and other conditions associated with reversible airways obstruction.

Pharmacology
Salbutamol has predominantly a β_2-stimulant bronchodilator effect, i.e. it does not have a major impact on the heart. It is safer than less selective β-adrenoceptor agonists, e.g. orciprenaline and epinephrine (adrenaline) although some patients develop prolongation of the QT interval.
Bio-availability 10–20% of the dose reaches the lower airways.
Onset of action 5min inhaled; 3–5min nebulized.
Duration of action 4–6h inhaled and nebulized.
Plasma halflife 4–6h inhaled and nebulized.

Cautions

Serious drug interactions: increased risk of hypokalaemia with corticosteroids, diuretics, theophylline.

Hyperthyroidism, myocardial insufficiency, hypertension, diabetes mellitus (risk of keto-acidosis if given by CIVI).

Adverse effects
Tremor, palpitations, muscle cramps. In higher doses: tachycardia (occasionally arrhythmias), tenseness, headaches, peripheral vasodilatation, hypokalaemia, allergic reactions.

Dose and use
Aerosol inhalation
• 100–200µg (1–2 puffs) t.d.s.–q.d.s. p.r.n.
• 200µg (2 puffs) before exercise in exercise-induced bronchoconstriction.
Nebulizer solution
• 2.5–5mg up to q.d.s., occasionally q4h.

Supply
Aerosol inhalation 100µg/metered inhalation, 200 dose unit = £1.80.
Nebulizer solution 0.1% 1mg/ml, 20 × 2.5ml (2.5mg) = £3.06; *0.2%* 2mg/ml, 20 × 2.5ml (5mg) = £6.14.

Inhaler devices
Haleraid to aid operation by patients with impaired strength in hands, available for 120- and 200-dose inhalers = £1.38.

Nebuhaler large-volume spacer device, for terbutaline and budesonide = £4.28.
Volumatic large-volume spacer device, for salbutamol, salmeterol, ipratropium, beclomethasone, fluticasone = £2.75.

THEOPHYLLINE   BNF 3.1.3

Class of drug: Methylxanthine.

Indications: Reversible airways obstruction, severe acute asthma (see Box 3.B).

Pharmacology
Theophylline shares the actions of the other xanthine alkaloids (e.g. caffeine) on the CNS, myocardium, kidney and smooth muscle. It has a relatively weak CNS effect but a more powerful relaxant effect on bronchial smooth muscle. It probably acts by inhibiting cyclic nucleotide phosphodiesterase. This leads to an accumulation of cyclic AMP/GMP which prevents the use of intracellular calcium for muscle contraction. In addition, an immunomodulator effect on cells important in airway inflammation has been demonstrated at plasma concentrations as low as $5\mu g/ml$.[1,2] Other effects include an improvement in respiratory muscle strength, the release of catecholamines from the adrenal medulla, inhibition of catechol-O-methyl transferase and blockade of adenosine receptors – all of which may play a part in the beneficial effect of theophylline.

Theophylline is given by injection as **aminophylline**, a mixture of theophylline with ethylenediamine; it is 20 times more soluble than theophylline alone. Aminophylline must be given by *very slow* IV injection; it is too irritant for IM use and is a potent gastric irritant PO. Theophylline is metabolized by the liver. Its therapeutic index is narrow and some patients experience adverse effects even in the therapeutic range. Plasma concentrations of theophylline are influenced by infection, hypoxia, smoking, various drugs, hepatic impairment and heart failure; all these can make the use of theophylline difficult.

Steady-state theophylline levels are attained within 3–4 days of adjusting the dose of a m/r preparation. Blood for theophylline levels should be taken 6–8h after the last dose. *It is not possible to ensure bio-equivalence between different m/r theophylline products and they should not be interchanged; the Royal Pharmaceutical Society requires a prescription to specify the brand name of the product.*
Bio-availability ≥90% (m/r = 80% of ordinary tablet).
Onset of action (?) 40–60min PO (immunomodulation ≤3 weeks).
Duration of action (?) 3–6h PO (immunomodulation = several days).
Plasma halflife 7–9h.

Cautions

Serious drug interactions: plasma concentrations of theophylline are increased by allopurinol, cimetidine, ciprofloxacin, clarithromycin, diltiazem, erythromycin, fluconazole, fluvoxamine, norfloxacin, thiabendazole, verapamil, viloxazine and oral contraceptives. Plasma concentrations are decreased in smokers, heavy drinkers and by barbiturates, carbamazepine, isoprenaline, phenytoin, rifampicin and sulphinpyrazone. May potentiate hypokalaemia associated with β_2-stimulants, corticosteroids, diuretics and hypoxia. See also Appendix 3, p.213.

Elderly, cardiac disease, hypertension, hyperthyroidism, peptic ulcer, liver failure, pyrexia.

Adverse effects
Dyspepsia, nausea, headache, CNS stimulation (less with m/r preparations). Arrythmias and convulsions (IV use).

Dose and use

Generally, a m/r preparation is preferable (e.g. Uniphyllin-Continus):
* usual starting dose 200mg b.d.; increase after 1 week
* in the elderly or patients weighing <70kg, the usual maintenance dose is 300mg b.d.
* in younger heavier patients, the usual maintenance dose is 400mg b.d.
* in patients whose symptoms manifest diurnal fluctuation, a larger evening or morning dose is appropriate to ensure maximum therapeutic benefit when symptoms are most severe
* the recommended therapeutic range is 10–20µg/ml.

In view of the beneficial immunomodulator effect of theophylline in patients with asthma at relatively low plasma concentrations,[2,3] dose adjustments should be made according to clinical response rather than necessarily trying to achieve the recommended therapeutic range.

Give by injection in severe acute asthma if the patient is not already taking oral theophylline:
* aminophylline 250–500mg (maximum 5mg/kg) IV *over 20min*
* continue as 500µg/kg/h CIVI; adjust dose according to theophylline levels.

Patients already receiving theophylline PO should not receive theophylline IV unless plasma theophylline concentrations can be monitored so as to guide dosing.

Supply

Tablets m/r **theophylline (Uniphyllin-Continus)** 200mg, 56 = £4.05; 300mg, 56 = £6.17; 400mg, 56 = £7.32.
Injection **aminophylline** 25mg/ml, 10ml amp = 61p.

---

1 Sullivan P *et al.* (1994) Anti-inflammatory effects of low-dose oral theophylline in atopic asthma. *Lancet.* **343**: 1006–1008.
2 Kidney J *et al.* (1995) Immunomodulation by theophylline in asthma: demonstration by withdrawal of therapy. *American Journal of Respiratory and Critical Care Medicine.* **151**: 1907–1914.
3 Evans DJ *et al.* (1997) A comparison of low-dose inhaled budesonide plus theophylline and high-dose inhaled budesonide for moderate asthma. *New England Journal of Medicine.* **337**: 1412–1418.

INHALED CORTICOSTEROIDS BNF 3.2

Indications: Reversible airways obstruction, [†]stridor, [†]lymphangitis carcinomatosa, [†]radiation pneumonitis, [†]cough after insertion of a bronchial stent (*see* Appendix 9, p.225).

Pharmacology

Corticosteroids reduce the inflammatory response by lowering peripheral lymphocyte levels and inhibiting phospholipase A_2, the enzyme which releases arachidonic acid (the precursor of PGs and leukotrienes) from cell membrane phospholipid. Inhaled corticosteroids reduce bronchial mucosa inflammation and are indicated in asthma (*see* Boxes 3.A & 3.B). Symptoms may take 3–7 days to improve. In patients with COPD, long-term use should be restricted to those who demonstrate objective improvement after a trial of corticosteroid therapy (*see* Box 3.D). The only evidence to support the other uses of inhaled or nebulized corticosteroids listed above is clinical experience.

Bio-availability 10–20% of the dose reaches the lower airways.
Onset of action up to 7 days.
Duration of action no data.
Plasma halflife beclometasone 10min, active metabolite 1–2h.

Cautions

Active or quiescent tuberculosis.

Adverse effects

Oropharyngeal candidiasis, sore throat, hoarse voice, paradoxical bronchospasm, hypersensitivity reactions (e.g. rashes). At higher doses, (e.g. beclomethasone >1500µg/day) adrenal suppression and osteoporosis.

---

† unlicensed use.

Dose and use
Aerosol inhalation
- check the patient's inhaler technique
- use a spacer device if:
   poor inhaler technique
   patient is on a high dose (e.g. beclometasone >1000µg/day)
   patient develops a hoarse voice or sore throat
- take the corticosteroid 5min *after* a β_2-stimulant if being used concurrently
- instruct patient to rinse mouth after use
- usual starting dose beclometasone 200µg b.d.
- titrate dose against symptoms; usual maximum dose beclometasone 2000µg/day in divided doses.

Nebulizer solution
- budesonide 1–2mg b.d.; occasionally more.

Patients should be given a **steroid card** with doses associated with adrenal suppression (*see* Box 7.D, p.139).

Supply
Aerosol inhalation beclometasone 100µg/metered inhalation, 200-dose unit = £8.24; 200µg/metered inhalation, 200-dose unit = £19.61; 250µg/metered inhalation, 200-dose unit = £18.02.

Aerosol inhalation budesonide 200µg/metered inhalation, 200-dose unit = £19.00.

Turbohaler budesonide 100µg/inhalation, 200-dose unit = £18.50; 200µg/inhalation, 100-dose unit = £18.50.

Nebulizer solution budesonide 250µg/ml, 20 × 2ml (500µg) = £32.00; 500µg/ml, 20 × 2ml (1mg) = £44.64.

OXYGEN   BNF 3.6

Indications: Breathlessness on exertion (intermittent use); breathlessness at rest (continuous use).

Pharmacology
Oxygen is prescribed for breathless patients to increase alveolar oxygen tension and decrease the work of breathing necessary to maintain a given arterial tension. The concentration given varies with the underlying condition. Inappropriate prescription can have serious or fatal effects. Ideally, domiciliary oxygen should be prescribed only after careful evaluation, preferably by a respiratory specialist. Some patients obtain as much benefit from piped air delivered by nasal prongs.[1] This suggests that a sensation of airflow is an important determinant of benefit.[2–5] Patients should be encouraged to test the benefit of a cool draught (open window or fan) before being offered oxygen. In mildly hypoxic patients, the benefit from oxygen is independent of the degree of arterial oxygen desaturation.[1] In severely hypoxic patients (oxygen saturation <90%), oxygen is generally better than air.[6]

Helium 80%–oxygen 20% mixture is less dense and viscous than room air.[7] Its use helps to reduce the respiratory work required to overcome upper airway obstruction. It can be used as a temporary measure while more definitive therapy is arranged.

Cautions
Patients with hypercapnic ventilatory failure who are dependent upon hypoxia for their respiratory drive. Patients should be advised of the fire risks of oxygen therapy:
- no smoking in the vicinity of the cylinder
- no naked flames, including candles, matches and gas cookers
- keep cylinders away from sources of heat, e.g. radiators and direct sunlight.

Adverse effects

An oxygen mask may be claustrophobic for some; use of nasal prongs can cause dryness and soreness of the nasal mucosa.

Dose and use

Oxygen therapy should be available for severely hypoxic patients – most of whom will be breathless at rest and/or on minimal exertion. In those less hypoxic the role of oxygen is more difficult to determine as there is great variation in response to oxygen which cannot be predicted by the level of oxygen saturation at rest or the degree of desaturation on exercise. A trial of oxygen therapy can be given via nasal prongs for 10–15min. Although initial oxygen saturation is a poor predictor of who will benefit subjectively, a pulse oximeter will help identify those patients whose oxygen saturation is objectively improved by oxygen therapy. If on review the patient has persisted in using the oxygen and has found it useful it can be continued; if the patient has any doubts about its efficacy then it should be discontinued.

Short-term/intermittent

High concentration oxygen (60%) is given for pneumonia, pulmonary embolism and fibrosing alveolitis. In these situations a low arterial oxygen (PaO_2) is usually associated with normal or low levels of carbon dioxide ($PaCO_2$). High concentrations of oxygen are also given in acute asthma when $PaCO_2$ levels are usually subnormal but can rise rapidly with deterioration; if these patients fail to improve with treatment, ventilation needs to be considered urgently.

Low concentration oxygen (≤28%) is reserved for patients with ventilatory failure related to COPD and other causes. The aim is to improve breathlessness caused by hypoxaemia without worsening pre-existing CO_2 retention.

Long-term/continuous

Long-term oxygen (≥15h/day) may prolong survival in patients with severe COPD and cor pulmonale (FEV_1 <1.5L, PaO_2 <7.3kPa ± hypercapnia). Blood gas tensions should be measured to ensure that the set flow is achieving a PaO_2 of >8kPa without an unacceptable rise in $PaCO_2$. It is more economical to use a concentrator if oxygen is given >8h/day.

Supply

Oxygen cylinders 1360L (domiciliary use) and 3400L (hospital use) supplied by pharmacy contractors; flow settings medium (2L/min) or high (4L/min). Patients are supplied with either constant or variable performance masks. Constant supply masks such as the Intersurgical 010 28% (97p) or Ventimask MK IV 28% (£1.36) provide an almost constant supply of 28% oxygen over a wide range of oxygen supply (generally 4L/min) irrespective of the patient's breathing pattern. The variable performance masks include the Intersurgical 005 mask (78p) and the Venticaire masks (65p); the concentration of oxygen supplied to the patient varies with the rate of flow of oxygen (2L/min is recommended and provides 24% oxygen) and with the patient's breathing pattern.

Portable oxygen cylinders (NHS), supplied by Medigas or BOC, PD oxygen cylinder (300L capacity) allows 2h of use at 2L/min.

Oxygen concentrators are prescribed by GPs specifying the flow rate (2–4L/min) and the recommended h/day. If necessary, two concentrators can be linked by tubing and T-piece to deliver higher flow rates (4–8L/min). The GP should contact the supplier (see BNF 3.6) who will arrange to deliver the concentrator and collect the FP10 from the patient. Suppliers include: De Vilbiss, Omnicare and Oxygen Therapy. An installation fee is charged to the Health Authority (about £90) plus a monthly rental and service charge (about £35) and an additional fee if a back-up cylinder is required (about £4). The price for private purchase is about £1000 (+ VAT). Patients may be re-imbursed for the electricity costs.

1 Booth S et al. (1996) Does oxygen help dyspnea in patients with cancer? American Journal of Respiratory Critical Care Medicine. **153**: 1515–1518.
2 Schwartzstein RM et al. (1987) Cold facial stimulation reduces breathlessness induced in normal subjects. American Review of Respiratory Diseases. **136**: 58–61.
3 Burgess KR and Whitelaw WA (1988) Effects of nasal cold receptors on pattern of breathing. Journal of Applied Physiology. **64**: 371–376.
4 Freedman S (1988) Cold facial stimulation reduces breathlessness induced in normal subjects. American Review of Respiratory Diseases. **137**: 492–493.

5 Kerr D (1989) A bedside fan for terminal dyspnea. *American Journal of Hospice Care.* **89**: 22.
6 Bruera E *et al.* (1993) Effects of oxygen on dyspnoea in hypoxaemic terminal cancer patients. *Lancet.* **342**: 13–14.
7 Boorstein JM *et al.* (1989) Using helium-oxygen mixtures in the emergency management of acute upper airway obstruction. *Annals of Emergency Medicine.* **18**: 688–690.

COUGH SUPPRESSANTS   BNF 3.9

Indications: Dry cough which is distressing to the patient, nocturnal wet cough which is disturbing sleep, wet cough in a patient too weak to expectorate properly.

General information
Cough is a physiological reflex which clears the central airways of foreign material and secretions and expectoration should generally be encouraged. It becomes pathological when it is dry and disrupts sleep, rest, eating or social functioning. It may lead to muscular strain and discomfort, rib or vertebral fracture, syncope, headache or retinal haemorrhage. The primary aim is to identify and treat the cause of the distressing cough but, when this is not possible or is inappropriate, a cough suppressant should be used (Figure 3.1).[1]

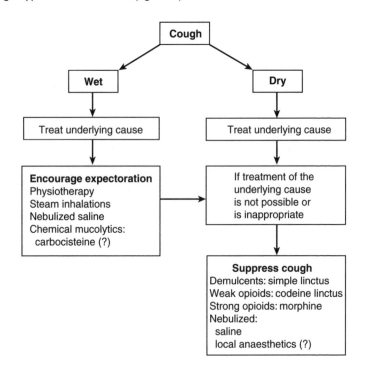

Figure 3.1 Management strategy for cough.

Dose and use
Demulcents: contain soothing substances such as syrup or glycerol. The high sugar content stimulates the production of saliva and soothes the oropharynx. The associated swallowing may also interfere with the cough reflex. The effect is short-lived and there is no evidence that

compound preparations are better than **simple linctus BP** (5ml t.d.s.–q.d.s.). Thus, if simple linctus is ineffective, there is little point in trying compound preparations.

Opioids: act primarily by suppressing the cough reflex centre in the brain stem.

Codeine, pholcodine and **dextromethorphan** are common ingredients in compound cough preparations. Dextromethorphan is a synthetic opioid derivative but does not act through opioid receptors. The effective dose of codeine or dextromethorphan is greater than the dose typically recommended by manufacturers of compound preparations.[2] The benefit of compound preparations may reside mainly in the sugar content. If **codeine** linctus 5–10ml (15–30mg) t.d.s.–q.d.s. is ineffective, a strong opioid such as morphine should be used. If a patient is already receiving a strong opioid for pain relief it is nonsense to prescribe codeine as well. **Morphine solution** can be used instead of codeine linctus, initially 2.5–5mg q.d.s.–q4h, or when codeine linctus fails to relieve, 5–10mg q.d.s.–q4h. The dose is titrated up as necessary or until unacceptable adverse effects occur. For patients already receiving strong opioids, if an 'as needed' dose relieves the cough, continue to use in this way or increase the regular morphine dose. If no benefit is obtained from a p.r.n. dose of morphine, there is little point in further regular dose increments. Some patients with cough but no pain benefit from a bedtime dose of morphine to prevent cough disturbing sleep.

Nebulized local anaesthetics: of limited value because of the unpleasant taste, oropharyngeal numbness, risk of bronchoconstriction and short duration of action (10–30min). The use of nebulized local anaesthetics in patients with cough caused by cancer has not been evaluated and cannot be routinely recommended. There are case reports of patients with chronic lung disease, sarcoid or cancer, however, when a single treatment with nebulized **lidocaine** 400mg has relieved cough for periods of 1–8 weeks.[3–5] They should be considered only when other avenues have failed, including nebulized saline. Suggested doses are 2% lidocaine (5ml) or 0.25% **bupivacaine** (5ml) q8h-q6h.

Supply
Linctus **simple linctus BP**, 100ml = 17p.
Linctus **codeine** 15mg/5ml, 100ml = 31p.
Diabetic linctus **codeine** 15mg/5ml, 100 ml = 68p.
Solution **morphine** 10mg/5ml, 100ml = £2.31.

1 Wilcock A (1998) The management of respiratory symptoms. In: Carter Y, Faull C and Woof R (eds) *The Handbook of Palliative Care*. Blackwell Scientific, London. pp 157–176.
2 Fuller RW and Jackson DM (1990) Physiology and treatment of cough. *Thorax.* **45**: 425–430.
3 Howard P *et al.* (1977) Lignocaine aerosol and persistent cough. *British Journal of Chest Diseases.* **71**: 19–24.
4 Saunders RV and Kirkpatrick MB (1984) Prolonged suppression of cough after inhalation of lidocaine in a patient with sarcoid. *Journal of the American Medical Association.* **252**(17): 2456–2457.
5 Stewart CJ and Coady TJ (1977) Suppression of intractable cough. *British Medical Journal.* **1**: 1660–1661.

AROMATIC INHALATIONS   BNF 3.8

Class of drug: Demulcent.

Indications: Wet cough (to aid expectoration).

Dose and use
Add 5ml to 500ml ('one teaspoon to a pint') of hot (not boiling) water and inhale vapour.

Supply
Tincture **benzoin compound BP (Friars' Balsam)** balsamic acids 4.5%, 100ml = 73p.
Inhalation **menthol and eucalyptus BP 1980**, 100ml = 53p.

CARBOCISTEINE   BNF 3.7

Class of drug: Mucolytic.

Indications: Reduction of sputum viscosity.

Contra-indications: Active peptic ulceration.

Pharmacology
Carbocisteine reduces the viscosity of bronchial secretions and facilitates expectoration. It alters the physical and chemical characteristics of the mucin components of sputum to a more 'normal' pattern (by reducing fructose and sulphate content and increasing the proportion of sialomucins). There is no clinical trial evidence to support the routine use of carbocisteine. However, some individual patients benefit from its use and a therapeutic trial may be justified if all other approaches have failed.
Bio-availability high.
Onset of action no data.
Duration of action no data.
Plasma halflife 1.3h.

Cautions
Rare reports of rashes and gastro-intestinal bleeding.

Adverse effects
Occasional gastro-intestinal irritation.

Dose and use
* starting dose 750mg t.d.s.
* reduce to 750mg b.d. once satisfactory response obtained.

Supply
Capsules 375mg, 30 = £4.48 (NHS).
Liquid 250mg/5ml, 300ml = £6.28 (NHS).
Available on NHS prescription for children in specific circumstances (see BNF 3.7).

4: Drugs acting on the
CENTRAL NERVOUS SYSTEM

Psychotropics

Benzodiazepines
　Diazepam
　Midazolam

Antipsychotics (neuroleptics)
　Haloperidol
　Levomepromazine (methotrimeprazine)
　Thioridazine

Antidepressants
　Amitriptyline
　Sertraline

Anti-emetics
　Metoclopramide
　Domperidone
　Cyclizine
　$5HT_3$-receptor antagonists

Hyoscine

Anticonvulsants

Orphenadrine

PSYCHOTROPICS   BNF 4.2

Psychotropic drugs are primarily used to alter a patient's psychological state. They can be classified as:
• anxiolytic sedatives
• antipsychotics (neuroleptics)
• antidepressants
• psychostimulants
• psychodysleptics (hallucinogens).

Generally, smaller doses should be used in debilitated patients with advanced cancer than in physically fit patients, particularly if they are already receiving morphine or another psychotropic drug. After an initial test dose, the dose can be increased fairly quickly to the modal dose or until troublesome adverse effects appear. Close supervision is essential, particularly during the first few days. There may be a need for either a reduction in dose because of drug cumulation or a further increase because of a lack of efficacy. A few patients respond paradoxically when prescribed psychotropic drugs, e.g. diazepam (become more distressed) or amitriptyline (become wakeful and restless at night). Other patients derive little benefit from a benzodiazepine, e.g. diazepam, but are helped by an antipsychotic, e.g. haloperidol.

Psychostimulants have little place in palliative care despite their ability to enhance post-operative analgesia. Cannabinoids are the only psychodysleptic drugs which are used in palliative care; they are used occasionally in the management of:
• nausea and vomiting[1]
• dyspnoea[2]
• spasticity in multiple sclerosis.[3]

Psychostimulants and psychodysleptics are not included in the PCF.

1 Mannix KA (1997) Palliation of nausea and vomiting. In: Doyle D, Hanks GWC, MacDonald N (eds) *Oxford Textbook of Palliative Medicine. (2nd edn)* Oxford University Press, Oxford. pp 489–499.
2 Ahmedzai S (1997) Palliation of respiratory symptoms. In: Doyle D, Hanks GWC, MacDonald N (eds) *Oxford Textbook of Palliative Medicine. (2nd edn)* Oxford University Press, Oxford. pp 583–616.
3 Martyn CN et al. (1995) Nabilone in the treatment of multiple sclerosis. *Lancet.* **345**: 579.

BENZODIAZEPINES   BNF 4.1, 4.8.3, 10.2.2 & 15.1.4.1

Benzodiazepines are a group of anxiolytic sedative drugs of differing potency (Table 4.1) with muscle relaxant and anticonvulsant properties (Table 4.2). Although the relationship is nonlinear, the plasma halflives of a benzodiazepine and its pharmacologically active metabolites reflect its duration of action (Figure 4.1); those with long halflives can be taken o.d., preferably o.n. The main adverse effects of benzodiazepines are dose-dependent drowsiness, impaired psychomotor skills and hypotonia (manifesting as unsteadiness). Benzodiazepines with long halflives cumulate when given repeatedly and adverse effects may manifest only after several days, or even later. Because benzodiazepines can cause physical and psychological dependence, the CSM discourages long-term use in the general population (Box 4.A). Benzodiazepines, however, are essential drugs in palliative care (Box 4.B).

Table 4.1   Approximate equivalent anxiolytic–sedative doses[1]

Drug	Dose
Lorazepam	500µg
Diazepam	5mg
Nitrazepam	5mg
Temazepam	10mg
Chlordiazepoxide	15mg
Oxazepam	15mg

Table 4.2   Pharmacological properties of selected benzodiazepines[2]

Drug name	Anxiolytic	Night sedative	Muscle relaxant	Anticonvulsant
Diazepam	+++	++	+++	+++
Lorazepam	+++	++	+	+
Clonazepam	+	+++	+	+++
Nitrazepam	++	+++	+	++
Oxazepam	+++	+	0	0
Temazepam	+	0[a]	0	0

Pharmacological activity: 0 = minimal effect; + = slight; ++ = moderate; +++ = marked.

a. the failure to demonstrate significant night sedative effect with temazepam emphasizes a limitation of the study, namely the restriction to one dose in volunteers.

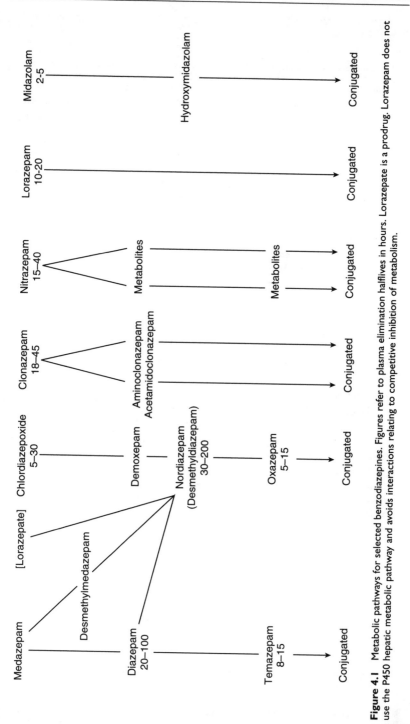

Figure 4.1 Metabolic pathways for selected benzodiazepines. Figures refer to plasma elimination halflives in hours. Lorazepate is a prodrug. Lorazepam does not use the P450 hepatic metabolic pathway and avoids interactions relating to competitive inhibition of metabolism.

Box 4.A   CSM advice

1   Benzodiazepines are indicated for short-term relief of anxiety (2–4 weeks only) that is severe, disabling or subjecting the individual to unacceptable distress, occurring alone or in association with insomnia or short-term psychosomatic organic or psychotic illness.

2   The use of benzodiazepines to treat short-term mild anxiety is inappropriate and unsuitable.

3   Benzodiazepines should be used to treat insomnia only when it is severe, disabling, or subjecting the individual to extreme distress.

Box 4.B   Benzodiazepines in palliative care

Night sedation

Short-acting drugs

- **midazolam** is not available in tablet form in the UK (halflife = 2–5h)
- **zopiclone** and **zolpidem** are alternatives available in the UK (halflives = 2–5h); they are not benzodiazepines, but act on the same receptors.

Intermediate-acting drug

- **temazepam** 10–40mg PO o.n., occasionally 60mg, is widely used (halflife = 8–15h).

Long-acting drug

- **flunitrazepam**, although marketed as a night sedative (0.5–2mg), has a plasma halflife of 16–35h; it is therefore *not* recommended as a night sedative in palliative care.

Some patients with insomnia respond better to an antipsychotic drug or a tricyclic antidepressant.

Anxiolytic

Intermediate-acting drugs

- **oxazepam** 10–15mg PO b.d.–t.d.s. (halflife = 5–15h).
- **lorazepam** 1–2mg PO b.d.–t.d.s. (halflife = 10–20h).

Lorazepam tablets are used SL at some centres for episodes of acute severe distress (e.g. respiratory panic attacks). For regular use, given its halflife, o.n. or b.d. administration should suffice.

Long-acting drug

- **diazepam** 2–20mg PO o.n. (halflife = 20–100h).

The BNF recommends t.d.s. administration but the long halflife means that o.n. will generally be as effective – and easier for the patient.

Muscle relaxant

- **diazepam** 2–10mg PO o.n., occasionally more
- **baclofen** is a useful nonbenzodiazepine alternative, particularly if diazepam is too sedative and if anxiety is not an associated problem (see p.162).

Anticonvulsant

Short-acting drug

- **midazolam** 10mg SC/IV stat, 30–60mg/24h CSCI and 10mg p.r.n.

Long-acting drugs

- **diazepam** 10mg PO, PR, IV stat, o.n.–b.d. & p.r.n.
- **clonazepam** 0.5–1mg PO o.n., rising by 0.5mg every 3–5 days up to 2–4mg, occasionally more; doses above 2mg can be divided, e.g. 2mg o.n. and the rest o.m.

Lower doses are generally satisfactory when treating multifocal myoclonus in moribund patients, e.g. **midazolam** 5mg stat and 10mg/24h CSCI.

1 Anonymous (1998) Hypnotics and anxiolytics. *British National Formulary No. 35*. BMA and RPS of Great Britain, London. p 154.

2 Ansseau M *et al.* (1984) Methodology required to show clinical differences between benzodiazepines. *Current Medical Research and Opinion*. 8 (suppl 4): 108–113.

DIAZEPAM BNF 4.1.2, 4.8.3, 10.2.2 & 15.1.4.1

Class of drug: Benzodiazepine.

Indications: Anxiety, insomnia, muscle tension/spasm, multifocal myoclonus, epilepsy.

Pharmacology

Diazepam is a typical benzodiazepine with GABA-potentiating actions in the CNS, notably spinal cord, hippocampus, cerebellum and cerebrum; at all these sites, diazepam reduces neuronal activity. Diazepam is rapidly absorbed with peak plasma concentrations at about 1h after PO administration. Standard parenteral preparations are oil-based and absorption from muscle after IM injection is slower and more variable than after PO and PR administration. Diazepam has a long plasma halflife and several active metabolites, one of which has a plasma halflife of up to 200h in the elderly. Because of marked interindividual variation, the effects of a constant dose will vary greatly. Doses for individual patients are determined empirically.

Oral bio-availability ≈100%.

Onset of action 15min PO.

Duration of action variable from 3–4h to 3–4 days, or longer.

Plasma halflife 20–100h; active metabolite nordiazepam (desmethyldiazepam) 30–200h.

Cautions

Cumulation of active metabolites may necessitate a dose reduction after several days. If given IV can cause hypotension and transient apnoea. *See* Appendix 3, p.213.

Adverse effects

Daytime drowsiness, muscle flaccidity, unsteadiness. When given IV, the oil-based solution may cause painful thrombophlebitis.

Dose and use

Typical doses for diazepam are shown in Table 4.3. The initial dose will depend on the patient's age, general condition, previous use of diazepam and other benzodiazepines, the intensity of distress, and the urgency of relief.

Table 4.3 Dose recommendations for diazepam

Indication	Stat and p.r.n. doses	Initial daily dose	Common range
Anxiety[a]	2–10mg PO	2–10mg PO o.n.	2–20mg PO
Muscle tension/spasm[b] Multifocal myoclonus	5mg PO	5mg PO o.n.	2–10mg PO
Anticonvulsant[c]	10mg PR/IV	10–20mg	10–30mg

a. given as an adjunct to nondrug approaches, e.g. relaxation therapy and massage

b. if localized, consider injection of a trigger point with local anaesthetic or acupuncture

c. acute use but in the moribund can be used as a convenient substitute for long-term oral anti-epileptic therapy (see also midazolam, p.54).

B.d.–t.d.s. dosing is sometimes indicated in an agitated moribund patient to reduce the number of hours awake. Rectal diazepam is useful in a crisis or if the patient is moribund:
- suppositories 10mg
- rectal solution 5–10mg in 2.5ml
- parenteral formulation administered with a cannula.

If IV administration is necessary, use diazepam oil-in-water emulsion (**Diazemuls**) if possible or substitute **midazolam** (see below). Patients occasionally react paradoxically, i.e. become more distressed; if this happens, **haloperidol** or **levomepromazine (methotrimeprazine)** should be given instead.

Supply
Tablets, 2mg, 20 = 7p; 5mg, 20 = 8p; 10mg, 20 = 15p.
Solution 2mg/5ml, 100ml = £2.16.
Injection (oil-based solution) 5mg/ml, 2ml amp = 25p.
Injection (oil-in-water emulsion) 5mg/ml, 2ml amp = 76p.
Suppositories 10mg, 1 = £1.09.
Rectal tubes (rectal solution) 5mg/2.5ml tube = £1.27; 10mg/2.5ml tube = £1.62.

MIDAZOLAM   BNF 15.1.4.1

Class of drug: Benzodiazepine.

Indications: Anaesthetic induction agent, sedative for minor procedures, multifocal myoclonus, epilepsy, [†]sedative for terminal agitation,[1,2] [†]intractable hiccup.[3]

Pharmacology
In single doses for sedation, midazolam is 3 times more potent than diazepam; as an anticonvulsant, it is twice as potent. With multiple doses, diazepam will gain in potency because of its prolonged plasma halflife, i.e. 20–100h versus 2–5h for midazolam (but about 10h when given by infusion). The main advantage of midazolam is that it is water-soluble and is miscible with most of the drugs commonly given by CSCI. It is also better for IV injection because it does not cause thrombophlebitis.
Bio-availability >90% IM; 30–70% PO.
Onset of action 5–10min SC; 2–3min IV.
Duration of action 15min to several hours.
Plasma halflife 2–5h.

Cautions
If given IV can cause hypotension and transient apnoea. Enhanced effect if given concurrently with diltiazem, erythromycin, fluconazole (possibly), itraconazole, ketoconazole. See also Appendix 3, p.213.

Adverse effects
Drowsiness.

Dose and use
Typical doses for midazolam are shown in Table 4.4. In terminal agitation, if the patient does not settle on 30mg/24h, an antipsychotic (e.g. **haloperidol**) should be introduced before further increasing the dose of midazolam. Its use for intractable hiccup is limited to patients in whom persistent distressing hiccup is contributing to terminal restlessness at a time when sedation is acceptable to aid symptom relief.

[†] unlicensed use.

Table 4.4 Dose recommendations for SC midazolam

Indication	Stat and p.r.n. doses	Initial infusion rate/24h	Common range
Muscle tension/spasm Multifocal myoclonus	5mg	10mg	10–30mg
Terminal agitation Intractable hiccup	5–10mg[a]	30mg	30–60mg[b]
Anticonvulsant	10mg	30mg	30–60mg

a. for hiccup, give initial stat dose IV
b. reported upper dose range 120mg for hiccup; 240mg for agitation.

Supply
Injection 5mg/ml, 2ml amp = 85p.

1 Bottomley DM and Hanks GW (1990) Subcutaneous midazolam infusion in palliative care. *Journal of Pain and Symptom Management.* **5**: 259–261.
2 McNamara P et al. (1991) Use of midazolam in palliative care. *Palliative Medicine.* **5**: 244–249.
3 Wilcock A and Twycross RG (1996) Midazolam for intractable hiccup. *Journal of Pain and Symptom Management.* **11**: 1–3.

ANTIPSYCHOTICS (NEUROLEPTICS)   BNF 4.2.1

Antipsychotics comprise mainly **phenothiazines** and **butyrophenones**. They are principally D_2-receptor antagonists; phenothiazines also antagonize muscarinic, α-adrenergic and H_1-receptors. Antipsychotics can cause extrapyramidal effects (see Appendix 5, p.227). **Haloperidol** is the antipsychotic of choice in palliative care. It is used as much for its anti-emetic properties as for antipsychotic purposes.

Antipsychotics have been used as part of an analgesic 'cocktail'. In chronic pain, however, the combination of an antipsychotic with an antidepressant is no more effective than treatment with an antidepressant alone,[1] and in combination with morphine causes more sedation without more pain relief.[2] Antipsychotics are of benefit, however, in selected highly anxious patients overwhelmed by persisting pain and insomnia.[3] Benefit may also be seen in patients whose pain escalates with the onset of delirium (acute confusion) and who derive no benefit from increased doses of opioids.[4] **Levomepromazine** (**methotrimeprazine**) is the only phenothiazine with specific analgesic properties.[5]

Phenothiazines are classified according to chemical structure (Table 4.5). The pharmacology of phenothiazines is complex because they interact with numerous transmitter systems in both the CNS and the periphery. The antipsychotic effect is mediated through D_2-receptor blockade in the mesolimbic and cortical areas. D_2-receptor blockade also has an inhibitory effect on the area postrema (chemoreceptor trigger zone), stimulates prolactin release, and reduces growth hormone levels. Extrapyramidal effects may occur as a result of D_2-receptor blockade in the basal ganglia (globus pallidus and corpus striatum). Phenothiazines bind to α-adrenoceptors to varying extents and cause postural hypotension; they also bind to H_1-receptors and cause sedation. Some phenothiazines are less sedative than others, and **trifluoperazine** may be stimulating. Akathisia, an extrapyramidal effect, may be misinterpreted as cerebral stimulation or deterioration of an underlying psychosis. Phenothiazines have differing antimuscarinic activity, which may be marked (e.g. **thioridazine**). Antiparkinsonian drugs with antimuscarinic properties (e.g. **orphenadrine, procyclidine**) are used to treat extrapyramidal effects but their antimuscarinic effects will be additive to those of the antipsychotic drug itself. In these circumstances, the antiparkinsonian drug could precipitate a toxic confusional psychosis and so complicate the underlying psychosis.

Table 4.5 Classification of phenothiazines

Ethylamino derivatives	*Piperidine derivatives*
Promethazine	Thioridazine
Propylamino derivatives	*Piperazine derivatives*[a]
Alimemazine	Fluphenazine
Chlorpromazine	Perphenazine
Levomepromazine	Prochlorperazine
(methotrimeprazine)	Thiethylperazine
Promazine	Trifluoperazine

a. possess a halogenated R_I side chain.

Given their respective plasma halflives, most phenothiazines need be given b.d.–t.d.s. at most; sometimes just o.n. (Table 4.6). Injections are generally IM because SC is too irritant. Prochlorperazine, however, is sometimes given by intermittent SC injection.

Table 4.6 Comparative features of selected antipsychotic drugs

Drug	Oral bio-availability (%)	Plasma halflife (h)	Equivalent oral dose (mg)[6]
Haloperidol[7]	60	12–36	2–3
Fluphenazine[8]	3	15	1–2
Trifluoperazine[9]	?	8–12	5
Prochlorperazine[10]	15	8[18][a]	?
Thioridazine[11]	60	6–40	100
Chlorpromazine[12,13]	10–25	7–15	100
Levomepromazine[14] (methotrimeprazine)	40	16–30	25–50

a. chronic administration.

1 Getto CJ et al. (1987) Antidepressants and chronic nonmalignant pain: a review. *Journal of Pain and Symptom Management.* **2**: 9–18.

2 Houde RW (1966) On assaying analgesics in man. In: Knighton RS, Dumke PR (eds) *Pain.* Little Brown, Boston. pp 183–196.

3 Maltebie A and Cavenar J (1977) Haloperidol and analgesia: case reports. *Military Medicine.* **142**: 946–948.

4 Coyle N et al. (1994) Delirium as a contributing factor to 'crescendo' pain: three case reports. *Journal of Pain and Symptom Management.* **9**: 44–47.

5 Bonica JJ and Halpern LM (1972) Analgesics. In: Modell W (ed) *Drugs of Choice 1972–1973.* CV Mosby, St Louis. pp 185–217.

6 Foster P (1989) Neuroleptic equivalence. *Pharmaceutical Journal.* September 30: 431–432.

7 Data Sheet: haloperidol (1996) *ABPI Compendium of Data Sheet and Summaries of Product Characteristics 1996–1997.* Datapharm Publications, London. pp 449–450.

8 Koytchev R et al. (1996) Absolute bioavailability of oral immediate and slow release fluphenazine in healthy volunteers. *European Journal of Clinical Pharmacology.* **51**: 183–187.

9 Smith Kline Beecham Pharmaceuticals (1997). Personal communication.

10 Dahl SG and Strandjord RE (1997) Pharmacokinetics of chlorpromazine after single and chronic dosage. *Clinical Pharmacology and Therapeutics.* **21**: 437–445.

11 Reynolds JEF (1996) Thioridazine. In: *Martindale. The Extra Pharmacopoeia. (31st edn)* Royal Pharmaceutical Society, London. pp 738–739.

12 Yeung PKF et al. (1993) Pharmacokinetics of chlorpromazine and key metabolites. *European Journal of Clinical Pharmacology.* **45**: 563–569.

13 Koytchev R et al. (1994) Absolute bioavailability of chlorpromazine, promazine and promethazine. *Arzneimittel-Forschung.* **44**: 121–125.

14 Dahl SG (1975) Pharmacokinetics of methotrimeprazine after single and multiple doses. *Clinical Pharmacology and Therapeutics.* **19**: 435–442.

HALOPERIDOL   BNF 4.2.1

Class of drug: Butyrophenone.

Indications: Nausea and vomiting, psychotic symptoms, agitated delirium (including disturbed nights in the elderly), [†]intractable hiccup.

Pharmacology

Haloperidol is well absorbed by mouth and after SC injection; peak plasma concentrations are reached in about 30–40min. Steady-state plasma concentrations do not vary greatly between patients after injection, but after PO administration vary up to 30-fold. The metabolism of haloperidol is not as complex as that of the phenothiazines but, even so, there are many metabolites. It is not possible to relate clinical response to plasma haloperidol concentrations. Haloperidol in solution is odourless, colourless and tasteless, and has been administered clandestinely in various extreme situations, e.g. to captors in sieges involving hostages. As a potent D_2-receptor antagonist, it is theoretically possible that haloperidol has a prokinetic effect comparable to domperidone, and might therefore correct gastric stasis induced by stress, anxiety or nausea from any cause (see p.6). Haloperidol demonstrates 10-fold greater affinity at dopamine receptors than domperidone.[1] Compared with chlorpromazine, haloperidol is a more potent anti-emetic. It has less effect on the cardiovascular system, has less antimuscarinic effects and is less sedative. It causes more extrapyramidal effects (more likely at daily doses of >5mg). Because these do not occur predictably, an antiparkinsonian drug should not be prescribed prophylactically.
Oral bio-availability 60–70%.
Onset of action 10–15min SC, >1h PO.
Duration of action up to 24h, sometimes longer.
Plasma halflife 13–35h.

Cautions

Parkinson's disease. Potentiation of CNS depression caused by other CNS depressants e.g. anxiolytics, alcohol. Increased risk of extrapyramidal effects and possible neurotoxicity with lithium. Plasma concentration of haloperidol is approximately halved by concurrent use of carbamazepine.

Adverse effects

Extrapyramidal effects (including tardive dyskinesia), hypothermia, sedation, antimuscarinic effects (occasional or mild), hypotension, tachycardia, arrhythmias, endocrine effects, blood disorders, alteration in liver function, neuroleptic malignant syndrome.

Dose and use

Anti-emetic (for chemical/toxic causes of vomiting)
- starting dose 1.5mg stat & o.n. (standard for morphine-induced vomiting)
- usual dose 3–5mg o.n.; maximum dose 10–20mg o.n. (or in divided dosage).

If 10mg o.n. or 5mg b.d. is ineffective, it is generally advisable to substitute **levomepromazine (methotrimeprazine)** for haloperidol (see p.58).

Antipsychotic–anxiolytic
- 1.5–3mg stat & o.n. in the elderly
- 5mg stat & o.n. in the younger patients or if poor response in the elderly
- 10–30mg o.n. (or in divided dosage) if poor response.

Although haloperidol exacerbates Parkinson's disease, a small daily dose (i.e. 1–1.5mg) may not cause noticeable deterioration.

[†] unlicensed use.

Supply
Liquid 1mg/ml, 100ml = £7.65; 2mg/ml, 100ml = £5.08.
Capsules 0.5mg, 20 = 65p.
Tablets 1.5mg, 20 = 92p; 5mg, 20 = £2.64; 10mg, 20 = £5.00; 20mg, 20 = £9.10.
Injection 5mg/ml, 1ml amp = 33p.

---

1 Sanger GJ (1993) The pharmacology of anti-emetic agents. In: Andrews PLR and Sanger GJ (eds) *Emesis in anti-cancer therapy: mechanisms and treatment.* Chapman & Hall, London. pp 179–210.

LEVOMEPROMAZINE (METHOTRIMEPRAZINE) BNF 4.2.1

Class of drug: Anti-emetic, phenothiazine antipsychotic.

Indications: Nausea and vomiting, insomnia, terminal agitation, intractable pain.

Pharmacology
Levomepromazine is a broad-spectrum anti-emetic which is widely used as a second- or third-line drug in patients who fail to respond to more specific drugs (*see* p.67). Like chlorpromazine, it is a potent D_2- and α_1-receptor antagonist; unlike chlorpromazine, levomepromazine also manifests potent $5HT_2$-receptor antagonism. This probably accounts for both its greater anti-emetic efficacy and its analgesic effect.[1] Levomepromazine, however, is more sedative and more likely to cause postural hypotension.
Bio-availability 40%.
Onset of action 30min.
Duration of action 12–24h.
Plasma halflife 15–30h.

Cautions
Parkinsonism, postural hypotension, antihypertensive medication, epilepsy, hypothyroidism, myasthenia gravis.

Adverse effects
Sedation (particularly with SC dose of $\geqslant$25mg/24h), dose-dependent postural hypotension. *See* also pp 225 & 227.

Dose and use
Anti-emetic
• starting dose 6.25mg PO o.d.–b.d., 2.5–6.25mg SC/24h
• usual dose 12.5–25mg PO o.n., 6.25–12.5mg SC/24h; higher doses often limited by sedation.
Terminal agitation ± delirium
• stat dose 25mg SC and 50–75mg/24h CSCI
• titrate dose according to response; usual maximum dose 300mg/24h, occasionally more.[2,3]
Analgesic
May be of benefit in a very distressed patient with severe pain unresponsive to other measures:
• stat dose 25mg PO/SC and o.n.
• titrate dose according to response; usual maximum daily dose 100mg SC/200mg PO.

Supply
Tablets 25mg, 20 = £3.00.
Injection 25mg/ml, 1ml amp = £1.75.

1 Twycross RG et al. (1997) The use of low dose levomepromazine (methotrimeprazine) in the management of nausea and vomiting. Progress in Palliative Care. 5 (2): 49–53.
2 Johnson I and Patterson S (1992) Drugs used in combination in the syringe driver: a survey of hospice practice. Palliative Medicine. 6: 125–130.
3 Regnard CFB and Tempest S (1998) A guide to symptom relief in advanced disease. (4th edn) Hochland & Hochland.

THIORIDAZINE   BNF 4.2.1

Class of drug: Phenothiazine antipsychotic.

Indications: Need for a more sedative antipsychotic than haloperidol, [†]cancer-related sweating.[1]

Contra-indications: Parkinson's disease.

Pharmacology
Thioridazine is equipotent with chlorpromazine as an antipsychotic.[2] Compared with chlorpromazine, thioridazine is less anti-emetic, causes less postural hypotension and extrapyramidal effects, but has more antimuscarinic effects.[3]
Oral bio-availability 60%.
Onset of action 30–60min.
Duration of action 12–24h.
Plasma halflife 6–40h; active metabolite mesoridazine.

Cautions
Parkinsonism. Potentiation of CNS depression when taken with other CNS depressants e.g. anxiolytics, alcohol. Increased risk of extrapyramidal effects and possible neurotoxicity with lithium (see also Appendix 3, p.213).

Adverse effects
See pp 55, 225 & 227. Electrolyte disturbance (e.g. as a result of severe diarrhoea) makes thioridazine more cardiotoxic.[4]

Dose and use
Antipsychotic
• usual starting dose 25mg stat & b.d.
• titrate according to response; usual maximum dose 100–200mg o.n. (or in divided dosage).
Night sedative
• usual starting dose 25–50mg o.n.
• titrate according to response; usual maximum dose 100–200mg o.n.
Sweating
Thioridazine is one option for cancer-related sweating (Box 4.C).
• usual starting dose 10mg o.n.
• usual effective dose 10–25mg o.n.; usual maximum dose 50mg o.n.

Supply
Tablets 10mg, 20 = 22p; 25mg, 20 = 31p; 50mg, 20 = 60p; 100mg, 20 = £1.14.
Suspension 25mg/5ml, 500ml = £2.98; 100mg/5ml, 500ml = £10.89.

1 Regnard C (1996) Use of low dose thioridazine to control sweating in advanced cancer. Palliative Medicine. 10: 78–79.
2 Foster P (1989) Neuroleptic equivalence. Pharmaceutical Journal. September 30: 431–432.

[†] unlicensed use.

Box 4.C   Drugs to relieve cancer-related sweating

If the sweating is associated with fever, prescribe an antipyretic (and an antibiotic if appropriate):

- **paracetamol** 500–1000mg
- NSAID, e.g. **ibuprofen** 200–400mg or locally preferred alternative.

Naproxen 250–500mg b.d. may be the NSAID of choice for paraneoplastic sweating associated with a remittent temperature;[5] this view, however, has been challenged.[6] NSAIDs are probably more effective than paracetamol and corticosteroids in this situation.

If sweating is not associated with fever or fails to respond to a NSAID, one of the following drugs may be helpful:

- **thioridazine** 10–50mg o.n.
- tricylic antidepressant, e.g. **amitriptyline** 25–50mg o.n.   antimuscarinic
- **propantheline** 15–30mg b.d.–t.d.s.
- **propranolol** 10–20mg b.d.–t.d.s.

Thioridazine is effective in 90% of patients,[1] but sedation may occur with doses >10mg.

---

3 Axelsson R and Martensson E (1976) Serum concentration and elimination from serum of thioridazine in psychiatric patients. *Current Therapeutic Research.* **19**: 242–265.

4 Denvir MA *et al.* (1998) Thioridazine, diarrhoea and torsades de pointe. *Journal of the Royal Society of Medicine.* **91**: 145–147.

5 Tsavaris N *et al.* (1990) A randomised trial of the effect of three non-steroidal anti-inflammatory agents in ameliorating cancer induced fever. *Journal of Internal Medicine.* **228**: 451–455.

6 Johnson M (1996) Neoplastic fever. *Palliative Medicine.* **10**: 217–224.

ANTIDEPRESSANTS   BNF 4.3

There are many subtle differences between the actions of different antidepressants (Table 4.7). It is important to study the Data Sheets and the BNF when developing a prescribing policy for antidepressants in palliative care. Tricyclic drugs have a range of actions, including:

- blockade of re-uptake by presynaptic terminals of:
  serotonin (5-hydroxytryptamine, 5HT)   responsible for antidepressant
  norepinephrine (noradrenaline)   and analgesic effects.
- receptor blockade:
  muscarinic, responsible for benefit in urgency and bladder spasms
  H_1-histaminergic, responsible for sedation   tend to be
  α_1-adrenergic, responsible for postural hypotension   correlated.

Tricyclic antidepressants are used for [†]pain relief (particularly neuropathic pain) and for [†]bladder spasms as well as for depression. The situation in relation to SSRIs and pain relief, however, is less clear. In randomized controlled trials in diabetic neuropathy and postherpetic neuralgia, fluoxetine and zimelidine were no better than placebo.[1–3] On the other hand, paroxetine and sertraline relieve diabetic neuropathic pain.[4,5] Relief correlates with plasma drug concentrations; a paroxetine plasma concentration above 150nmol provides relief similar to that obtained with imipramine and with fewer adverse effects.[4] Even so, a meta-analysis of 39 controlled trials concluded that mixed serotonin and norepinephrine (noradrenaline) re-uptake inhibitors are more effective.[6] SSRIs are of value in some patients with pruritus.[7]

     [†] unlicensed use.

Table 4.7 Pharmacological properties of some antidepressant drugs[a]

Drug name	Plasma elimination half-life (h) [active metabolite]	Norepinephrine (noradrenaline) re-uptake inhibition	Serotonin (5HT) re-uptake inhibition	Antimuscarinic effects	Sedative effects	Postural hypotension
Tricyclic and related drugs						
Amitriptyline	10–25 [13–93][a]	+	+++	+++	++	++
Dosulepin (dothiepin)	14–40	++	+	+	++	++
Clomipramine	16–20	+	+++	++	++	++ (<10%)
Imipramine	4–18 [12–61][b]	++	+++	++	++	++ (>10%)
Lofepramine	5 [12–61][b]	+++	+	+	+	0
Nortriptyline	13–93	+++	+	++	0	+
Venlafaxine	5 [11][c]	+++	+++	0	0	+
SSRIs						
Fluoxetine	2–3 days [7–15 days][d]	0	++	0	0	0
Fluvoxamine	15	0	++	0	0	0
Nefazodone	3–4	0	++	0	0	0
Paroxetine	20	0	++	+[g]	0	0
Sertraline	26 [36]	0	++	0	0	0

Pharmacological activity: 0 = none; + = slight; ++ = moderate; +++ = marked.

a. nortriptyline; b. desipramine; c. desmethylvenlafaxine; d. norfluoxetine 7–15 days.

Sedative effects are more common in physically ill patients, particularly if receiving other psychoactive drugs, including opioids. Apart from paroxetine, SSRIs do not have antimuscarinic properties and are less cardiotoxic in overdosage.[9,10] Although dose titration is generally easier, SSRIs have characteristic adverse effects of their own, notably nausea and vomiting; they are also more expensive. Prescribing more than one antidepressant at the same time is *not* recommended. Compound preparations of an antidepressant and an anxiolytic are also *not* recommended because the dose of the individual components cannot be adjusted separately. Further, whereas antidepressants are generally given continuously over several months, anxiolytics are prescribed on a short-term basis. Although anxiety is often present in depressive illness and may be the presenting symptom, the use of **antipsychotics** or **anxiolytics** may mask the true diagnosis. They should therefore be used with caution, although they are useful adjuncts in agitated depression. Maintenance treatment helps to prevent a recurrence of depression and is recommended for patients who have had ⩾3 depressive episodes in the preceding 5 years.[11]

There is little place for MAOIs in palliative care. A potentially fatal excitatory crisis may occur if tyramine-containing foods are eaten (Table 4.8) or another serotonergic drug is prescribed concurrently, notably **pethidine** (Box 4.D). This interaction is precipitated by an increased concentration of cerebral serotonin; *it does not occur with other opioids* (Box 4.E).[12–14]

CSM advice: Hyponatraemia (usually in the elderly and possibly due to inappropriate secretion of antidiuretic hormone) has been associated with all types of antidepressants and should be considered in all patients who develop drowsiness, confusion or convulsions while taking an antidepressant.

Box 4.D   Serotonin syndrome[15]

Highest risk	**Significant risk**	**Dubious association**
MAOI +	SSRI +	Carbamazepine
pethidine	dextromethorphan	Fentanyl
dextromethorphan	tramadol	Pentazocine
tricyclic	tryptophan	
SSRI	lithium	
tryptophan	Buspirone	
lithium	Bromocriptine	
levodopa	'Ecstasy'	
	(methylene di-oxymethamfetamine)	

Can also be caused by a single drug,[16] or in overdose.[17]

Clinical features
Restlessness, agitation, delirium, tachycardia, myoclonus, hyperreflexia, tremor, shivering and hyperthermia (>40.5°C). Hyperthermia is a bad prognostic sign.
Onset generally within a few hours of drug/dose changes and most resolve in 24h.
Recurrent mild symptoms may occur for weeks before a full-blown syndrome.
Hypertension (and headache), convulsions and death have been reported.

Treatment
Discontinue serotonergic medication
Symptomatic measures (based on animal studies and clinical reports):

* **paracetamol** as an antipyretic

* external cooling if hyperthermia

* **propranolol** 20mg q8h[18] *or* ⎫
                          ⎬ have antiserotonergic properties
* **cyproheptadine** 4–8mg PO q2h–q4h p.r.n. ⎭

* **midazolam** 5–10mg SC p.r.n. for myoclonus and convulsions.

Box 4.E A misleading report about morphine and MAOIs[12]

A patient who regularly took a MAOI and trifluoperazine 20mg daily was given pre-operative promethazine 50mg IM and morphine 1mg IV followed by two doses of morphine 2.5mg IV. About 3min later she became unresponsive and hypotensive (systolic pressure 40mm Hg); responding within 2min to IV naloxone. Although repeatedly referenced as such, this was *not* a MAOI-related serotonin syndrome, it was a hypotensive response to IV morphine in someone chronically taking trifluoperazine, an α-adrenergic antagonist.

Table 4.8 Tyramine-containing foods associated with MAOI-related serotonin syndrome

Alcohol	Meat or yeast extracts
red wine (white wine is safe)	Bovril
beer	Oxo
Broad bean pods	Marmite
Cheese	Pickled herring

Withdrawal

Abrupt cessation of antidepressant therapy (particularly a MAOI) after regular administration for ≥8 weeks may result in withdrawal phenomena.[19] Discontinuation reactions are distinct from recurrence of the primary psychiatric disorder. They generally start abruptly within a few days of stopping the antidepressant (or of reducing its dose) and may last up to 3 weeks. In contrast, a depressive relapse is uncommon in the first week after stopping an antidepressant, and symptoms tend to build up gradually and persist. Discontinuation symptoms are varied and differ depending on the class of antidepressant. Common symptoms include:

- gastro-intestinal disturbance (nausea, abdominal pain, diarrhoea)
- sleep disturbance (insomnia, vivid dreams, nightmares)
- general somatic distress (sweating, lethargy, headaches)
- affective symptoms (low mood, anxiety, irritability).

With SSRIs the commonest symptom appears to be dizziness/lightheadedness and sensory abnormalities (including numbness, paraesthesia, and electric shock-like sensations). Discontinuation reactions usually resolve within 24h of re-instating antidepressant therapy, whereas with a depressive relapse the response is slower.

To reduce the likelihood of discontinuation reactions the BNF recommends that antidepressants which have been continuously prescribed for ≥8 weeks should be gradually reduced over 4 weeks. Tapering is probably unnecessary when switching between SSRIs. If a discontinuation reaction is suspected, the antidepressant should be restarted and reduced more gradually. If mild, however, re-assurance alone may be adequate ± a benzodiazepine to overcome insomnia.

---

1 Max MB *et al.* (1992) Effects of desipramine, amitriptyline and fluoxetine on pain in diabetic neuropathy. *New England Journal of Medicine.* **326**: 1250–1256.

2 Watson CPN and Evans RJ (1985) A comparative trial of amitriptyline and zimelidine in postherpetic neuralgia. *Pain.* **23**: 387–394.

3 Lynch S *et al.* (1990) Efficacy of antidepressants in relieving diabetic neuropathy pain: amitriptyline vs. desipramine and fluoxetine vs. placebo. *Neurology.* **40** (suppl 1): 437.

4 Sindrup SH *et al.* (1990) The selective serotonin re-uptake inhibitor paroxetine is effective in the treatment of diabetic neuropathy symptoms. *Pain.* **42**: 135–144.

5 Goodnick PJ *et al.* (1997) Sertraline in diabetic neuropathy: preliminary results. *Annals of Clinical Psychiatry.* **9**: 255–257.

6 Onghena P and van Houdenhove B (1992) Antidepressant-induced analgesia in chronic non-malignant pain: a meta-analysis of 39 placebo-controlled studies. *Pain.* **49**: 205–219.

7 Zylicz Z *et al.* (1998) Paroxetine for pruritus in advanced cancer. *Journal of Pain and Symptom Management.* (in press).

8 Ashton CH (1998) Personal communication.

9 Schatzberg AF et al. (1997) Possible biological mechanisms of the serotonin reuptake inhibitor discontinuation syndrome. *Journal of Clinical Psychiatry*. **58** (suppl 7): 23–27.

10 Finley PR (1994) Selective serotonin reuptake inhibitors: pharmacologic profiles and potential therapeutic distinctions. *Annals of Pharmacotherapy*. **28**: 1359–1369.

11 Edwards JG (1998) Long term pharmacotherapy of depression. *British Medical Journal*. **316**: 1180–1181.

12 Barry BJ (1979) Adverse effects of MAO inhibitors with narcotics reversed with naloxone. *Anaesthesia and Intensive Care*. **7**: 194.

13 Browne B and Linter S (1987) Monoamine oxidase inhibitors and narcotic analgesics. A critical review of the implications for treatment. *British Journal of Psychiatry*. **151**: 210–212.

14 Stockley IH (1994) Monoamine oxidase inhibitors and morphine or methadone. In: Stockley IH (ed) *Drug Interactions*. (3rd edn) Blackwell Scientific Publications, Oxford. pp 642–644.

15 Sporer KA (1995) The serotonin syndrome. *Drug Safety*. **13**: 94–104.

16 Lejoyeux M et al. (1992) The serotonin syndrome. *American Journal of Psychiatry*. **149**: 1410–1411.

17 Kaminski CA et al. (1994) Sertraline intoxication in a child. *Annals of Emergency Medicine*. **23**: 1371–1374.

18 Guze BH and Baxter LR (1986) The serotonin syndrome: case responsive to propranolol. *Journal of Clinical Psychopharmacology*. **6**: 119–120.

19 Haddad P et al. (1998) Antidepressant discontinuation reactions. Are preventable and simple to treat. *British Medical Journal*. **316**: 1105–1106.

AMITRIPTYLINE   BNF 4.3.1

Class of drug: Tricyclic antidepressant.

Indications: Depression, panic disorder, nocturnal enuresis in children, [†]neuropathic pain, [†]urgency of micturition, [†]urge incontinence, [†]bladder spasms.

Contra-indications: Co-administration with a MAOI, recent myocardial infarction, arrhythmias (particularly heart block of any degree), mania, severe hepatic impairment.

Pharmacology

Amitriptyline exerts its antidepressant and analgesic effects by blocking the presynaptic re-uptake of serotonin and norepinephrine (noradrenaline). It may also act as a NMDA-receptor antagonist.[1] It has a sedative effect and this manifests immediately; improved sleep is the first benefit of therapy. The analgesic effect may manifest after 3–7 days, whereas the antidepressant effect may not be apparent for 2 weeks or more. A dose-response relationship has been shown for its analgesic effect.[2,3] There appears to be a 'therapeutic window' for amitriptyline in some patients.[4] Seven patients with postherpetic neuralgia or painful diabetic neuropathy had good relief with amitriptyline 20–100mg (median 50mg). With this dose the pain was reduced from severe to mild. When the dose was increased, the pain became severe again and, when decreased, the pain became mild again. Most patients, however, do not manifest this effect. Amitriptyline frequently causes increased appetite and weight gain – a bonus in palliative care but often an adverse effect for others. Up to 20% of patients fail to respond to amitriptyline (or related antidepressant drug); some of the failures relate to the dose being inadequate. However, because of the potential for adverse effects, low doses should be used initially in the frail elderly. *Plasma halflife* 10–25h; active metabolite nortriptyline 13–93h.

Cautions

Elderly, cardiac disease (particularly if history of arrhythmia), epilepsy, hepatic impairment, history of mania, psychoses (may aggravate), narrow-angle glaucoma, urinary hesitancy, history of urinary retention. Drowsiness may affect performance of skilled tasks, e.g. driving; effects of alcohol enhanced. Avoid abrupt withdrawal after prolonged use (see p.63). See also Appendix 3, p.213.

[†] unlicensed use.

Adverse effects

Antimuscarinic effects, sedation, delirium, postural hypotension, hyponatraemia; see also BNF 4.3. The use of amitriptyline in the elderly is associated with a doubling of the incidence of femoral fractures.[5]

Dose and use

Amitriptyline, like other tricyclic drugs, can be given as a single dose o.n. for all indications. If a patient experiences early morning drowsiness, or takes a long time settling at night, advise to take 2h before bedtime. A small number of patients are stimulated by amitriptyline and experience insomnia, unpleasant vivid dreams, myoclonus and physical restlessness. In these patients, change to a SSRI or administer amitriptyline o.m. Relatively small doses are often effective in relieving depression in debilitated cancer patients, e.g. amitriptyline 25–50mg o.n.; start with a small dose in the frail elderly (Table 4.9). Amitryptyline can also be given by IM or IV injection.

Table 4.9   Dose escalation timetables for amitriptyline

Dose (o.n.)	Elderly frail/ outpatient	Younger patient/ inpatient
10mg	Day 1	–
25mg	Day 3	Day 1
50mg	Week 2	Day 3
75mg	Week 3–4	Week 2
100mg	Week 5–6	Week 2
150mg	Week 7–8[a]	Week 3[a]

a. not often necessary in palliative care.

Supply

Tablets 10mg, 20 = 14p; 25mg, 20 = 9p; 50mg, 20 = 41p.
Solution 25mg/ml, 200ml = £14.40; 50mg/ml, 200ml = £15.75, available from Rosemont.
Injection 10mg/ml, 10ml vial = 54p.

1 Eisenach JC and Gebhart GF (1995) Intrathecal amitriptyline acts as an N-Methyl-D-Aspartate receptor antagonist in the presence of inflammatory hyperalgesia in rats. *Anesthesiology.* **83**: 1046–1054.
2 Max MB et al. (1987) Amitriptyline relieves diabetic neuropathy pain in patients with normal or depressed mood. *Neurology (NY).* **37**: 589–596.
3 McQuay HJ et al. (1993) Dose-response for analgesic effect of amitriptyline in chronic pain. *Anaesthesia.* **48**: 281–285.
4 Watson CPN (1984) Therapeutic window for amitriptyline analgesia. *Canadian Medical Association Journal.* **130**: 105–106.
5 Ray WA et al. (1987) Psychotropic drug use and the risk of hip fracture. *New England Journal of Medicine.* **316**: 363–369.

SERTRALINE   BNF 4.3.1

Class of drug: SSRI.

Indications: Depression, [†]neuropathic pain.

Contra-indications: Co-administration with a MAOI, mania.

[†] unlicensed use.   65

Pharmacology

SSRIs selectively block the presynaptic re-uptake of serotonin.[1,2] Compared with tricyclics, SSRIs are much less likely to cause weight gain, sedation, delirium, cardiac arrhythmias and heart block; they do not have antimuscarinic effects. SSRIs, however, may cause extrapyramidal effects. Sertraline, like other SSRIs, initially often causes nausea (but vomiting is uncommon) as a consequence of increased serotonergic activity in the gastro-intestinal tract and possibly via central $5HT_3$-receptors. $5HT_3$-receptor antagonists (see p.73) are effective anti-emetics in this situation,[3] as is cisapride, a $5HT_4$-receptor agonist.[4] Sertraline is as effective as amitriptyline in treating depression with anxiety; its antidepressant action may be enhanced by sodium valproate.[5] Sertraline has been shown to relieve diabetic neuropathic pain.[6]

Cautions

Epilepsy, hepatic impairment, renal impairment. Sertraline (or other SSRI) should not be started until 2 weeks after stopping a MAOI. Treatment should not be discontinued abruptly (Table 4.10). See also p.63 & Appendix 3, p.213.

Adverse effects

Anorexia, nausea (occasionally severe), diarrhoea, exacerbation of anxiety (initially), restlessness, headache.

Dose and use

Sertraline is easy to use because for most patients the starting dose does not need to be increased:
- the standard dose is 50mg o.m. preferably p.c.
- occasionally necessary to increase the dose to 100–200mg.

Supply

Tablets 50mg, 28 = £26.51; 100mg, 28 = £39.77.

Table 4.10   SSRI withdrawal syndrome[7]

Somatic symptoms	Psychological symptoms
Disequilibrium	*Core*
Dizziness	Anxiety/agitation
Vertigo	Crying spells
Ataxia	Irritability
Gastro-intestinal symptoms	*Other*
Nausea	Overactivity
Vomiting	Decreased concentration/slowed thinking
Flu-like symptoms	Memory problems
Fatigue	Depersonalization
Lethargy	Lowered mood
Myalgia	Delirium
Chills	
Sensory disturbance	
Paraesthesia	
Sensations of electric shock	
Sleep disturbances	
Insomnia	
Vivid dreams	

1 Finley PR (1994) Selective serotonin reuptake inhibitors: pharmacologic profiles and potential therapeutic distinctions. *Annals of Pharmacotherapy.* **28**: 1359–1369.

2 Leonard BE (1993) The comparative pharmacology of new antidepressants. *Journal of Clinical Psychiatry.* **54** [8 suppl]: 3–15.

3 Bailey JE *et al.* (1995) The $5-HT_3$ antagonist ondansetron reduces gastrointestinal side effects induced by a specific serotonin re-uptake inhibitor in man. *Journal of Psychopharmacology.* **9**: 137–141.

4 Bergeron R and Blier P (1994) Cisapride for the treatment of nausea produced by selective serotonin reuptake inhibitors. *American Journal of Psychiatry.* **151**: 1084–1086.

5 Dave M (1995) Antidepressant augmentation with valproate. *Depression.* **3**: 157–158.

6 Goodnick PJ et al. (1997) Sertraline in diabetic neuropathy: preliminary results. *Annals of Clinical Psychiatry.* **9**: 255–257.

7 Schatzberg AF et al. (1997) Serotonin reuptake inhibitor discontinuation syndrome: a hypothetical definition. *Journal of Clinical Psychiatry.* **58** (suppl 7): 5–10.

ANTI-EMETICS   BNF 4.6

Important factors to consider when prescribing anti-emetics include:
* mechanism of action of anti-emetic drugs (Figure 4.2; Tables 4.11 & 4.12)
* response to anti-emetics already given
* when more than one anti-emetic drug is needed, a combination of drugs with different actions should be used (e.g. cyclizine and haloperidol)
* combinations with antagonistic actions should not be used (e.g. cyclizine and metoclopramide)
* levomepromazine (methotrimeprazine) has multiple receptor effects and is sometimes more effective than drug combinations
* effects of anti-emetics on gastro-intestinal motility, i.e.
    prokinetic (metoclopramide, domperidone, cisapride)
    antikinetic (antimuscarinics, antihistaminic antimuscarinics)
* adjuvant use of antisecretory drugs (e.g. hyoscine butylbromide, octreotide)
* adjuvant use of corticosteroids (e.g. dexamethasone, prednisolone)
* adverse effects of drugs
* cost of drugs ($5HT_3$-receptor antagonists and octreotide are expensive)
* role of nondrug treatments.

Generally, the initial choice of an anti-emetic in palliative care lies between three drugs, namely **metoclopramide** (see p.71), **haloperidol** (see p.57) and **cyclizine** (see p.73). One of these should be prescribed both regularly and as needed (Box 4.F).

Table 4.11 Classification of drugs used to control nausea and vomiting

Putative site of action	Class	Example
Central nervous system		
Vomiting centre	Antimuscarinic	Hyoscine hydrobromide
	Antihistaminic antimuscarinic[a]	Cyclizine, dimenhydrinate, prochlorperazine
	$5HT_2$-receptor antagonist	Levomepromazine (methotrimeprozine)
Area postrema	D_2-receptor antagonist	Haloperidol, prochlorperazine, metoclopramide, domperidone
	$5HT_3$-receptor antagonist	Granisetron, ondansetron, tropisetron
Cerebral cortex	Benzodiazepine	Lorazepam
	Cannabinoid	Nabilone
	Corticosteroid	Dexamethasone
Gastro-intestinal tract		
Prokinetic	$5HT_4$-receptor agonist	Metoclopramide, cisapride
	D_2-receptor antagonist	Metoclopramide, domperidone
Antisecretory	Antimuscarinic	Hyoscine butylbromide, glycopyrrolate
	Somatostatin analogue	Octreotide, vapreotide
Vagal $5HT_3$-receptor blockade	$5HT_3$-receptor antagonist	Granisetron, ondansetron, tropisetron
Anti-inflammatory	Corticosteroid	Dexamethasone

a. the antihistamines and phenothiazines both have H_1-receptor antagonistic and antimuscarinic properties (see Table 4.12).

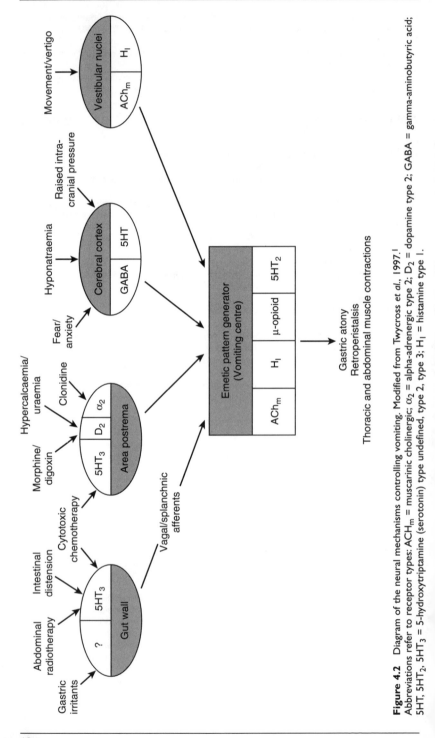

Figure 4.2 Diagram of the neural mechanisms controlling vomiting. Modified from Twycross et al., 1997.[1] Abbreviations refer to receptor types: ACH_m = muscarinic cholinergic; α_2 = alpha-adrenergic type 2; D_2 = dopamine type 2; GABA = gamma-aminobutyric acid; 5HT, $5HT_2$, $5HT_3$ = 5-hydroxytryptamine (serotonin) type undefined, type 2, type 3; H_1 = histamine type I.

Table 4.12 Receptor site affinities of selected anti-emetics[2–4]

	D_2-receptor antagonist	H_1-receptor antagonist	Muscarinic antagonist	$5HT_2$-receptor antagonist	$5HT_3$-receptor antagonist	$5HT_4$-receptor agonist
Metoclopramide	++	0	0	0	+	++
Domperidone	++[a]	0	0	0	0	0
Cisapride	0	0	0	0	0	+++
Ondansetron[b]	0	0	0	0	+++	0
Cyclizine	0	++	++	0	0	0
Hyoscine hydrobromide	0	0	+++	0	0	0
Haloperidol	+++	0	0	0	0	0
Prochlorperazine	++	+	0	0	0	0
Chlorpromazine	++	++	+	0	0	0
Levomepromazine (methotrimeprazine)	++	+++	++	+++	0	0

Pharmacological activity: 0 = none or insignificant; + = slight; ++ = moderate; +++ = marked.

a. domperidone does not cross the blood-brain barrier and therefore does not cause extrapyramidal effects

b. other $5HT_3$ -receptor antagonists, e.g. granisetron and tropisetron, have comparable receptor affinity.

Box 4.F First-line anti-emetics[5]

Prokinetic anti-emetic
For gastritis, gastric stasis, functional bowel obstruction:
metoclopramide 10mg q.d.s. PO/SC or 30–100mg/24h CSCI (see p.71).

Anti-emetic acting principally in area postrema
For most chemical causes of vomiting, e.g. morphine, hypercalcaemia, renal failure:
haloperidol 1.5mg o.n.–b.d. PO or 5mg/24h CSCI (see p.57).
Metoclopramide also has a central anti-dopaminergic action.

Anti-emetic acting principally in the vomiting centre
For mechanical bowel obstruction, raised intracranial pressure, motion sickness:
cyclizine 50mg PO t.d.s. or 150mg/24h CSCI (see p.73).
(In countries where cyclizine is not available, alternatives include **dimenhydrinate** and **diphenhydramine**.)

Do not prescribe a prokinetic drug and an antimuscarinic (anticholinergic) drug concurrently. The final common pathway for prokinetic drugs is cholinergic; antimuscarinic (anticholinergic) drugs (including cyclizine) block their prokinetic action.[6]

In inoperable bowel obstruction with large volume vomiting or associated intestinal colic, an antisecretory agent (which acts partly by reducing the volume of gastro-intestinal secretions) may be used either alone as a first-line manoeuvre, e.g. **hyoscine butylbromide** 60–120mg/24h CSCI, or in conjunction with **cyclizine**. If this proves inadequate, a trial of **octreotide** should be considered (see p.144).

Dexamethasone and **levomepromazine** (**methotrimeprazine**) are both useful options when first-line anti-emetics fail to relieve nausea and vomiting satisfactorily. Dexamethasone is normally *added* to an existing regimen (see p.138) whereas levomepromazine is normally *substituted* (see p.58). Sometimes it is necessary to use dexamethasone and levomepromazine concurrently. Other phenothiazines are still often used as anti-emetics, notably **prochlorperazine** and **chlorpromazine**. Prochlorperazine is generally effective against moderate chemical emetogenic stimuli in a dose of 5–10mg PO t.d.s.; suppositories and injections are also available. Chlorpromazine has an even broader spectrum of receptor affinity (Table 4.11) but does not share the potent $5HT_2$-receptor antagonism of levomepromazine – which should be used in preference to chlorpromazine when a broad-spectrum drug is indicated.

$5HT_3$-receptor antagonists, developed primarily to control chemotherapeutic vomiting, have a definite but limited role in palliative care (see p.73) **Cannabinoids** are used for otherwise intractable nausea and vomiting in AIDS patients, and in children and young adults receiving chemotherapy. Use in palliative care has also been reported.[7] A brain stem cannabinoid receptor and ligand have been identified, and there is evidence of a linkage to anti-inflammatory and opioid mechanisms.[8] Drug-induced nausea and vomiting can be problematic. It may be caused by several different mechanisms (Table 4.13), each of which calls for a distinct therapeutic response.

Table 4.13   Causes of drug-induced nausea and vomiting

Mechanism	Drugs
Gastric irritation	Antibiotics
	Iron supplements
	NSAIDs
	Tranexamic acid
Gastric stasis	Antimuscarinics (anticholinergics)
	Opioids
	Phenothiazines
	Tricyclics
Area postrema stimulation	Antibiotics
(chemoreceptor trigger zone)	Cytotoxics
	Digoxin
	Imidazoles
	Opioids
$5HT_3$-receptor stimulation	Antibiotics
	Cytotoxics
	SSRIs

1 Twycross RG et al. (1997) The use of low dose levomepromazine (methotrimeprazine) in the management of nausea and vomiting. *Progress in Palliative Care.* **5** (2): 49–53.

2 Dollery C (1991) *Therapeutic Drugs.* Churchill Livingstone, Edinburgh.

3 Dollery C (1992) *Therapeutic Drugs:* Supplement 1. Churchill Livingstone, Edinburgh.

4 Peroutka SJ and Snyder SH (1982) Antiemetics: neurotransmitter receptor bindings predicts therapeutic actions. *Lancet.* **i**: 658–659.

5 Twycross R and Back I (1998) The management of nausea and vomiting in advanced cancer. *European Journal of Palliative Care.* **5**: 39–45.

6 Schuurkes JAJ et al. (1986) Stimulation of gastroduodenal motor activity: dopaminergic and cholinergic modulation. *Drug Development Research.* **8**: 233–241.

7 Gonzalez-Rosales F and Walsh D (1997) Intractable nausea and vomiting due to gastro-intestinal mucosal metastases relieved by tetrahydrocannabinol (Dronabinol). *Journal of Pain and Symptom Management.* **14**: 311–314.

8 Mannix KA (1997) Palliation of nausea and vomiting. In: Doyle D, Hanks GWC, MacDonald N (eds) *Oxford Textbook of Palliative Medicine. (2nd edn)* Oxford University Press, Oxford. pp 489–499.

METOCLOPRAMIDE   BNF 4.6

Class of drug: Prokinetic anti-emetic.

Indications: Nausea and vomiting caused by gastric irritation (gastritis) or delayed gastric emptying, by stimulation of the area postrema (chemoreceptor trigger zone), by massive release of 5HT from enterochromaffin cells or platelets (see p.74).

Contra-indications: Concurrent administration with antimuscarinic drugs (block the cholinergic final common pathway of prokinetic drugs),[1] concurrent IV administration with 5HT$_3$-receptor antagonists (risk of cardiac arrhythmia).[2]

Pharmacology

Metoclopramide is a combined D$_2$-receptor antagonist and 5HT$_4$-receptor agonist. In daily doses above 100mg SC, it manifests 5HT$_3$-receptor antagonism. Metoclopramide is therefore a broad-spectrum anti-emetic but its clinical value mainly resides in its prokinetic properties (see p.6). As a centrally-acting D$_2$-receptor antagonist, it is second to haloperidol (see p.57) and, as a 5HT$_3$-receptor antagonist, it is second to the specific 5HT$_3$-receptor antagonists (see p.74).

Prokinetics act by triggering a cholinergic system in the gut wall. Opioids impede this action but antimuscarinic drugs, because they block the cholinergic receptors on the intestinal muscle fibres,[1] block the peripheral action of prokinetic drugs (see p.7). *Prokinetics and antimuscarinics should therefore not be given concurrently.* Domperidone and metoclopramide, however, would still exert an antagonistic effect at the dopamine receptors in the area postrema, but haloperidol would generally be a better choice in this situation (see p.57).

D$_2$-receptor antagonists block the dopamine brake on gastric emptying induced by stress, anxiety and nausea from any cause. In contrast, 5HT$_4$-receptor agonists have a direct excitatory effect which in theory gives them an advantage over the D$_2$-receptor antagonists particularly for patients with gastric stasis or functional bowel obstruction. When used for dysmotility dyspepsia, however, metoclopramide is no more potent than domperidone in standard doses.

Along with other drugs which block central dopamine receptors, there is a risk of developing acute dystonic reactions with facial and skeletal muscle spasms and oculogyric crises. These are more common in the young (particularly girls and young women), generally occur within a few days of starting treatment, and subside within 24h of stopping the drug. Because of this, metoclopramide is generally not used in children. An antimuscarinic drug will abort an attack, e.g. procyclidine 5–10 mg IV.

Bio-availability 50–80% PO.
Onset of action 10–15min IM; 15–60min PO.
Duration of action 1–2h (data for single dose and relating to gastric emptying).
Plasma halflife 2.5–5h.

Cautions

Serious drug interactions: a combination of IV metoclopramide and IV ondansetron occasionally causes cardiac arrhythmias.[2] 5HT$_3$-receptors influence various aspects of cardiac function, including inotropy, chronotropy and coronary arterial tone,[3] effects which are mediated by both parasympathetic and sympathetic nervous systems. Thus in any given patient, blockade of 5HT$_3$-receptors will produce effects dependent on the pre-existing serotonergic activity in both arms of the autonomic nervous system.

Metoclopramide is known to enhance the effects of catecholamines in patients with phaeo-chromocytomas and with essential hypertension.[4,5] Acute dystonia occurs in <5% of patients receiving metoclopramide in standard doses; the risk is greater if also receiving other drugs known to cause extrapyramidal effects, e.g. antipsychotics, 5HT$_3$-receptor antagonists, tricyclic antidepressants and SSRIs (see Appendix 5, p.227).

Adverse effects

Extrapyramidal effects, neuroleptic malignant syndrome. Occasionally drowsiness, restlessness, depression and diarrhoea.

Dose and use

Gastric irritation 10mg PO q.d.s. *or* 40–60mg/24h CSCI & 10mg PO/SC p.r.n.; also reduce or remove cause of gastritis and prescribe appropriate gastroprotective drugs.

Delayed gastric emptying as above, consider increasing to 100mg/24h CSCI or substitute **cisapride** 10–20mg b.d.

Stimulation of area postrema as above, but haloperidol generally preferable (*see* p.57).

For nausea and vomiting associated with 5HT release, a selective $5HT_3$-receptor antagonist should be used rather than high-dose metoclopramide (*see* BNF 4.6).

Supply
Tablets 10mg, 20 = 46p.
Solution 5mg/5ml, 100ml = £1.09.
Injection 5mg/ml, 2ml amp = 27p

---

1 Schuurkes JAJ et al. (1986) Stimulation of gastroduodenal motor activity: dopaminergic and cholinergic modulation. *Drug Development Research.* **8**: 233–241.

2 Baguley WA et al. (1997) Cardiac dysrhythmias associated with the intravenous administration of ondansetron and metoclopramide. *Anaesthesia and Analgesia.* **84**: 1380–1381.

3 Saxena PR and Villalon CM (1991) 5-Hydroxytryptamine: a chameleon in the heart. *Trends in Pharmacological Sciences.* **12**: 223–227.

4 Agabiti-Rosei E et al. (1995) Hypertensive crises in patients with phaeochromocytoma given metoclopramide. *Annals of Pharmacotherapy.* **29**: 381–383.

5 Kuchel O et al. (1985) Effect of metoclopramide on plasma catecholamine release in essential hypertension. *Clinical Pharmacology and Therapeutics.* **37**: 372–375.

DOMPERIDONE   BNF 4.6

Class of drug: Prokinetic anti-emetic.

Indications: Need for a prokinetic anti-emetic with D_2-receptor antagonism but without risk of extrapyramidal effects.

Pharmacology

Domperidone is a D_2-receptor antagonist which does not cross the blood-brain barrier. Its prokinetic effect is limited to the oesophago-gastric and gastroduodenal junctional areas; it also acts in the area postrema (chemoreceptor trigger zone). Domperidone can only correct the gastric dopamine brake; it has no positive prokinetic effect in its own right. It is therefore not as useful a prokinetic drug as metoclopramide and cisapride. Its use is further limited by the absence of a parenteral formulation; it is available, however, as a suppository. Its prokinetic effect is blocked by antimuscarinic drugs (see p.6).[1]

Bio-availability 13–17% PO; 12% PR.
Onset of action 30min.
Duration of action 8–16h.
Plasma halflife 14h.

Adverse effects

Actue dystonia (rare), rashes, reduced libido, gynaecomastia (raised prolactin concentration).

Dose and use

Given its long plasma halflife, domperidone can be taken b.d. even though the BNF recommends q4h–q8h:

- starting dose 20mg PO b.d.
- increase if necessary to 30mg PO q8h *or* 20mg PO q6h (these doses differ from BNF recommendations)
- 30mg PR = 10mg PO.

Supply
Tablets 10mg, 30 = £2.46.
Suspension sugar-free 5mg/5ml, 200ml = £1.80.
Suppositories 30mg, 30 = £7.95.

---

1 Schuurkes JAJ et al. (1986) Stimulation of gastroduodenal motor activity: dopaminergic and cholinergic modulation. Drug Development Research. **8**: 233–241.

CYCLIZINE   BNF 4.6

Class of drug: Antihistaminic antimuscarinic anti-emetic.

Indications: Nausea and vomiting associated with motion sickness, pharyngeal stimulation, [†]mechanical bowel obstruction and [†]raised intracranial pressure.

Pharmacology
Antihistaminics were originally introduced to control motion sickness following the observation that a patient with urticaria no longer became car sick during treatment with dimenhydrinate.[1] Studies were conducted in American servicemen crossing the Atlantic in the *General Ballou*, a modified freight ship without stabilizers which allowed the drugs to be classified according to relative efficacy. There is no correlation between efficacy in motion sickness and antihistamine potency. Antihistaminic anti-emetics exert their effect by acting upon the vomiting centre.
Bio-availability no data.
Onset of action <2h.
Duration of action 4–6h (and possibly longer in some patients).
Plasma halflife 5h early elimination phase with a prolonged late phase (data from 1 volunteer).[2]

Adverse effects
Drowsiness and antimuscarinic effects (*see* p.225).

Dose and use
Depending on circumstances, cyclizine can be given either PO or SC:
* 50–100mg PO b.d.–t.d.s. & p.r.n.
* 100–300mg/24h CSCI (typically 100–150mg) & 50mg SC p.r.n.
* usual maximum daily dose 200mg PO and CSCI.

Supply
Tablets 50mg, 20 = 99p.
Injection 50mg/ml, 1ml amp = 57p.

---

1 Gay LN and Carliner PE (1949) The prevention and treatment of motion sickness. Bulletin of Johns Hopkins Hospital. **49**: 470–491.
2 Griffin DS and Baselt RC (1984) Blood and urine concentrations of cyclizine by nitrogen-phosphorus gas-liquid chromatography. Journal of Analytical Toxicology. **8**: 97–99.

5HT$_3$-RECEPTOR ANTAGONISTS   BNF 4.6

Indications: Nausea and vomiting after surgery, chemotherapy and radiotherapy, [†]intractable vomiting due to chemical, abdominal and cerebral causes when usual approaches have failed, [†]pruritus associated with cholestasis and renal failure.

Contra-indications: Concurrent IV administration with IV metoclopramide (*see* p.71).

[†] unlicensed use.   73

Pharmacology

$5HT_3$-receptor antagonists were developed specifically to control emesis associated with highly emetogenic chemotherapy, e.g. cisplatin. They block the amplifying effect of excess 5HT on vagal nerve fibres and are therefore of specific value in situations where excessive amounts of 5HT are released from the body's stores (enterochromaffin cells and platelets) following chemotherapy or radiation-induced damage of the gut mucosa, bowel distension and renal failure (leaky platelets).

$5HT_3$-receptor antagonists also relieve nausea and vomiting after head injury and brain stem radiotherapy,[1,2] and in multiple sclerosis in patients with brain stem disease;[3] leakage of 5HT from the raphe nucleus probably accounts for the benefit seen in these circumstances. $5HT_3$-receptor antagonists are also effective in nausea and vomiting associated with acute gastro-enteritis.[4] In one patient who experienced persistent nausea after the insertion of an endo-oesophageal tube, a $5HT_3$-receptor antagonist brought about relief after failure with metoclopramide and cyclizine, and only temporary relief with domperidone.[5]

Ondansetron, the first $5HT_3$-receptor antagonist to be marketed, has been superseded by **granisetron** and **tropisetron**; these need only be given o.d., are as effective PO as by injection and are cheaper than recommended IV ondansetron regimens.[6,7] All $5HT_3$-receptor antagonists are expensive, however, and it is important not to price palliative care 'out of the market' by using them unnecessarily. Thus, if a $5HT_3$-receptor antagonist is not clearly effective within 3 days, it should be discontinued.[8,9] **Levomepromazine (methotrimeprazine)** is a much cheaper drug and can often substitute effectively for $5HT_3$-receptor antagonists (see p.58). For pharmacokinetic details see Table 4.14.

Table 4.14 Pharmacokinetic details of $5HT_3$-receptor antagonists

	Ondansetron	Granisetron	Tropisetron
Oral bio-availability	56–71%	60%	>95%
Onset of action PO	<30min	<30min	<30min
IV	<5min	<15min	<15min
Duration of action	12h	24h	24h
Plasma halflife	3h	10–11h	8h[a]

a. 32–45h poor metabolizers.

Adverse effects

Headache and constipation. Rarely, dystonic reactions (ondansetron), sensation of warmth or flushing, hiccup.

Dose and use

For chemotherapeutic vomiting, see BNF 4.6. In palliative care, granisetron 1–2 mg PO/SC o.d. or tropisetron 5mg PO/SC o.d. for 3 days initially; if of benefit, continue indefinitely unless cause self-limiting. For intractable vomiting, a $5HT_3$-receptor antagonist may need to be co-administered with **haloperidol**.[8,10] Doses for pruritus are comparable.[11]

Supply

Tablets granisetron 1mg, 10 = £91.40; 2mg, 10 = £182.86
Paediatric liquid sugar-free granisetron 1mg/5ml, 50ml = £91.43.
Sterile solution granisetron 1mg/ml, for dilution and use as injection or infusion, 1ml vial = £12; 3ml amp = £36.
Capsules tropisetron 5mg, 10 = £126.74.
Injection tropisetron 1mg/ml, 5ml amp = £14.31.

1 Kleinerman KB et al. (1993) Use of ondansetron for control of projectile vomiting in patients with neurosurgical trauma: two case reports. *Annals of Pharmacotherapy.* **27**: 566–568.

2 Bodis S et al. (1994) The prevention of radiosurgery-induced nausea and vomiting by ondansetron: evidence of a direct effect on the central nervous system chemoreceptor trigger zone. *Surgical Neurology.* **42**: 249–252.

3 Rice GPA and Ebers G (1995) Ondansetron for intractable vertigo complicating acute brain-stem disorders. *Lancet.* **345**: 1182–1183.

4 Cubeddu LX et al. (1997) Antiemetic activity of ondansetron in acute gastroenteritis. *Alimentary Pharmacology and Therapeutics.* **11**: 185–191.

5 Fair R (1990) Ondansetron in nausea. *Pharmaceutical Journal.* **245**: 514.

6 Gralla RJ et al. (1997) Can an oral antiemetic regimen be as effective as intravenous treatment against cisplatin: results of a 1054 patient randomized study of oral granisetron versus IV ondansetron. *Proceedings of ASCO.* **16**: 178.

7 Perez EA et al. (1997) Efficacy and safety of oral granisetron versus IV ondansetron in prevention of moderately emetogenic chemotherapy-induced nausea and vomiting. *Proceedings of ASCO.* **16**: 149.

8 Cole RM et al. (1994) Successful control of intractable nausea and vomiting requiring combined ondansetron and haloperidol in a patient with advanced cancer. *Journal of Pain and Symptom Management.* **9**: 48–50.

9 Currow DC et al. (1997) Use of ondansetron in palliative medicine. *Journal of Pain and Symptom Management.* **13**: 302–307.

10 Pereira J and Bruera E (1996) Successful management of intractable nausea with ondansetron: a case study. *Journal of Palliative Care.* **12** (2): 47–50.

11 Sanger G J and Twycross R (1996) Making sense of emesis, pruritus, 5HT- & 5HT$_3$-receptor antagonists. *Progress in Palliative Care.* **4**: 7–8.

HYOSCINE   BNF 4.6

Class of drug: Antimuscarinic antispasmodic and antisecretory.

Indications: [†]Inoperable bowel obstruction, [†]sialorrhoea (drooling), [†]death rattle.

Contra-indications: Narrow-angle glaucoma (unless moribund).

Pharmacology

Hyoscine (scopolamine) is a naturally occurring belladonna alkaloid with smooth muscle relaxant (antispasmodic) and antisecretory properties. It is available as **hydrobromide** and **butylbromide** (Buscopan) salts. Unlike the hydrobromide, hyoscine butylbromide does not cross the blood-brain barrier and so does not cause drowsiness, or have a central anti-emetic action. Because hyoscine butylbromide is poorly absorbed PO, tablets should be used only for mild–moderate bowel colic. Repeated administration of hyoscine hydrobromide leads to cumulation; occasionally this results paradoxically in an agitated delirium. Despite a plasma halflife of several hours, the duration of the antisecretory effect in volunteers after a single dose is only about 1h (butylbromide) and 2h (hydrobromide).[1] However, particularly after repeat injections and in moribund patients, a mean duration of effect of 10–15h has been observed.[2] Both hyoscine butylbromide and hydrobromide relieve death rattle in 50–60% of patients. However, provided time is taken to explain the cause of the rattle to the relatives and there is ongoing support, relatives' distress is relieved in >90% of cases.[2] Hyoscine hydrobromide by any route and hyoscine butylbromide SC can also be used in other situations where an antimuscarinic may be beneficial. Injections of hyoscine butylbromide are cheaper than hyoscine hydrobromide.

    For pharmacokinetic details see Table 4.15.

[†] unlicensed use.

Table 4.15   Pharmacokinetic details of hyoscine salts

	Hyoscine butylbromide	Hyoscine hydrobromide
Bio-availability	8–10% PO	(?) 60–80% SL
Onset of action PO	1–2h	–
SL	–	10–15min
IM	3–5min	3–5min
Duration of action IM (spasmolytic)	15min	15min
(antisecretory)	1–9h	1–9h
Plasma halflife	5–6h	5–6h

Cautions
As for all antimuscarinic drugs (see p.225). Blocks the final common (cholinergic) pathway through which prokinetic drugs act.[3]

Adverse effects
Antimuscarinic effects (see p.225). Central anticholinergic syndrome (excitement, ataxia, hallucinations, behavioural abnormalities and drowsiness).

Dose and use
For patients with obstructive symptoms without colic, **metoclopramide** *should be tried before hyoscine butylbromide because the obstruction may well be more functional than mechanical (see p.71).* Hyoscine butylbromide is generally given SC (Table 4.16). For mild–moderate colic not associated with intestinal obstruction there may be a place for PO tablets. For sialorrhoea, an alternative oral antimuscarinic may be better and more convenient, e.g. **amitriptyline** (see p.64), **orphenadrine** (see p.82), **propantheline** (see p.6), **thioridazine** (see p.59).

Table 4.16   Dose recommendations for SC hyoscine butylbromide

Indication	Stat dose	Initial infusion rate/24h	Common range
Inoperable bowel obstruction with colic[3,4]	20mg	60mg	60–120mg[a]
Death rattle	20mg	20–40mg	20–40mg

a. maximum dose = 300mg/24h.

With death rattle, an antisecretory drug is best started sooner rather than later because it does not affect existing pharyngeal secretions. There is less impact when the rattle is secondary to pneumonia[5] and little effect in pulmonary oedema. Some PCUs use hyoscine hydrobromide in preference to hyoscine butylbromide:
• hyoscine hydrobromide 400–600µg stat and 1.2–2.4mg/24h CSCI *or*
• transdermal hyoscine hydrobromide 500µg–1mg/72h.[6]
In resistant cases, more benefit may sometimes be obtained with **glycopyrollate** (see p.175).
   Hyoscine hydrobromide is available as an OTC preparation for SL use (to prevent motion sickness); it provides an alternative route of administration in palliative care. **Hyoscyamine** is an alternative SL preparation in some countries where hyoscine hydrobromide is not available. Hyoscyamine is the laevo-isomer of **atropine**; because the dextro-isomer is virtually inactive, hyoscyamine is approximately twice as potent as atropine.

Supply
Tablets hyoscine butylbromide 10mg, 56 = £2.59 (*not generally recommended*).
Tablets SL hyoscine hydrobromide 0.3mg (Kwells), 12 = £1.20.
Transdermal patch hyoscine hydrobromide 500µg/72h, 2 = £2.84.

Injection **hyoscine hydrobromide** 400µg, 1ml amp = £2.67; 600µg, 1ml amp = £2.69.
Injection **hyoscine butylbromide** 20mg/ml, 1ml amp = 20p.

1 Herxheimer A and Haefeli L (1966) Human pharmacology of hyoscine butylbromde. *Lancet.* **ii**: 418–421.
2 Hughes A *et al.* (1997) Management of 'death rattle'. *Journal of Pain and Symptom Management.* **12**: 271–272.
3 Schuurkes JAJ *et al.* (1986) Stimulation of gastroduodenal motor activity: dopaminergic and cholinergic modulation. *Drug Development Research.* **8**: 233–241.
4 Baines MJ (1997) ABC of palliative care: nausea and vomiting. *British Medical Journal.* **315**: 1148–1150.
5 Bennett MI (1996) Death rattle: an audit of hyoscine (scopolamine) use and review of management. *Journal of Pain and Symptom Management.* **12**: 229–233.
6 Dawson HR (1989) The use of transdermal scopolamine in the control of death rattle. *Journal of Palliative Care.* **5** (1): 31–33.

ANTICONVULSANTS   BNF 4.8

Indications: Epilepsy, [†]neuropathic pain, [†]terminal agitation (phenobarbital).

Pharmacology
Anticonvulsants act in three ways:
• inhibit the excessive firing of neurones
• inhibit the excitatory mechanisms (predominantly the glutamatergic system)
• potentiate inhibitory mechanisms (predominantly the GABAergic system).

Some anticonvulsants act by two or more mechanisms, and the different actions may be synergistic (Box 4.G). The mechanism of action of **ethosuximide** is nonsynaptic and possibly relates to the modulation of calcium channel function. It is effective in petit mal absences and myoclonic seizures; it is *ineffective* against grand mal (tonic–clonic) seizures and may unmask them if given alone to patients experiencing seizures of mixed type (see Data Sheet). The pharmacokinetic details of anticonvulsants are summarized in Table 4.17.

Table 4.17 Pharmacokinetic details of anticonvulsants

Drug	Oral bio-availability (%)	T_{max} (h)	Protein binding (%)	Plasma halflife (h)
Carbamazepine	80	4–8	75	8–24
Clobazam	100	0.5–2	85	10–30
Clonazepam	80–100	1–4	80–90	30–40
Diazepam	80–100	1–3	95–98	24–48
Gabapentin	60[a]	2–3	0	6
Lamotrigine	95–100	1–3	56	23–36
Phenobarbital	95–100	4–12	50	72–144
Phenytoin	90–95	4–8	90	9–40[a]
Valproate	100	1–2[b]	90	7–17
Vigabatrin	80–90	1	0	6

a. dose or plasma concentration-dependent
b. 3–8h for e/c tablets.

Box 4.G   Mechanisms of action of some anticonvulsants

Non-synaptic action
Sodium-channel blockers ('membrane stabilizers'):

- carbamazepine
- lamotrigine
- phenytoin

Presynaptic action

- carbamazepine
- gabapentin
- lamotrigine
- phenytoin
- sodium valproate

Increased release of GABA:

- sodium valproate

Postsynaptic action
Activation of inhibitory receptor-channel complex (Figure 4.3):

- benzodiazepines (via receptor)
- phenobarbital (activates chloride channel)
- sodium valproate (? GABA agonist)

Inhibition of excitatory receptor-channel complex (Figure 4.4):

- MK 801 (unsuitable for clinical use)
- ketamine (unsuitable for use as an anticonvulsant)

Perisynaptic action
Inhibition of GABA transaminase:

- vigabatrin

Interactions
Interactions between anticonvulsants are complex and may enhance toxicity without a corresponding increase in anti-epileptic effect. Interactions are generally caused by *hepatic enzyme induction or hepatic enzyme inhibition* (Box 4.H); displacement from protein binding sites is not generally a problem. These interactions are highly variable and unpredictable. Plasma monitoring is advisable with combination therapy.

Other important interactions include:

- effect of carbamazepine enhanced by dextropropoxyphene (in co-proxamol)
- some SSRIs increase plasma carbamazepine concentration; *paroxetine and sertraline do not*[1]
- some SSRIs increase valproic acid concentration; *paroxetine does not*[2] but no specific interaction studies have been done with sertraline and valproic acid
- carbamazepine accelerates the metabolism of tricyclic antidepressants
- sodium valproate inhibits the metabolism of tricyclic antidepressants[4]
- effect of tramadol decreased by carbamazepine.

See also Appendix 3, p.213.

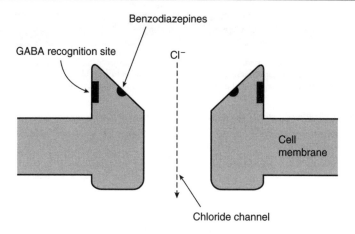

Figure 4.3 Simplified diagram of GABA (inhibitory) receptor-channel complex.[3]

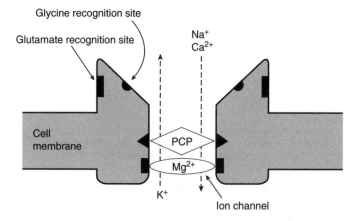

Figure 4.4 Simplified diagram of NMDA (excitatory) receptor-channel complex. The channel is blocked by Mg^{2+} when the membrane potential is at its resting level (voltage-dependent block) and by drugs which act at the phencyclidine (PCP) binding site in the glutamate-activated channel, e.g. MK 801 (use-dependent block).[3]

Cautions

Driving: patients suffering from epilepsy may drive a motor vehicle (but not a heavy goods or public service vehicle) provided that they have had a seizure-free period of 1 year or, if subject to seizures only while asleep, have sustained a 3-year period without seizures while awake. Patients affected by drowsiness should not drive or operate machinery.

Box 4.H   Drug interactions between anticonvulsants[a]

Carbamazepine often lowers plasma concentration of clonazepam, lamotrigine, phenytoin (but may also raise), topiramate and valproate. Sometimes lowers plasma concentration of ethosuximide and primidone (but tendency for corresponding increase in phenobarbital level).

Ethosuximide sometimes raises plasma concentration of phenytoin.

Lamotrigine sometimes raises plasma concentration of an active metabolite of carbamazepine.

Phenobarbital or **primidone** often lowers plasma concentration of carbamazepine, clonazepam, lamotrigine, phenytoin (but may also raise) and valproate. Sometimes lowers plasma concentration of ethosuximide.

Phenytoin often lowers plasma concentration of carbamazepine, clonazepam, lamotrigine, topiramate and valproate. Often raises plasma concentration of phenobarbital. Sometimes lowers plasma concentration of ethosuximide and primidone (by increasing conversion to phenobarbital).

Topiramate sometimes raises plasma concentration of phenytoin.

Valproate often raises plasma concentration of an active metabolite of carbamazepine and of lamotrigine, phenobarbital and phenytoin (but may also lower). Sometimes raises plasma concentration of ethosuximide and primidone (and tendency for significant increase in phenobarbital level).

Vigabatrin often lowers plasma concentration of phenytoin. Sometimes lowers plasma concentration of phenobarbital and primidone.

a. See Appendix 3, p.213.

Adverse effects

Carbamazepine: generally fewer adverse effects than phenytoin or phenobarbital: dose-related reversible diplopia, blurring of vision, nystagmus, dizziness, ataxia, drowsiness, headache.[5] Adverse effects may be reduced by giving a smaller dose more often (see below).
Phenobarbital: drowsiness, mental depression, ataxia, allergic skin reactions; paradoxical excitement, restlessness and delirium in the elderly.
Phenytoin: nausea and vomiting, nystagmus, delirium, dizziness, slurred speech, ataxia, coarse facies, acne, hirsutism, gingival hypertrophy and tenderness.
Sodium valproate: gastric irritation, nausea, tremor, ataxia, drowsiness, hepatic impairment leading rarely to fatal hepatic failure.

Dose and use

Combination therapy should generally be avoided in most patients because:
* no evidence of additive therapeutic effect
* drug interactions
* toxicity may be enhanced.

Epilepsy
Carbamazepine is a first-line drug for simple and complex partial seizures and for tonic–clonic seizures secondary to a focal discharge. It has a wider therapeutic index than phenytoin and the relationship between dose and plasma concentration is linear, but monitoring of plasma concentrations may be helpful in determining optimum dose. With regular administration, the plasma halflife reduces from about 36h to 16–24h as a result of auto-induction by hepatic enzymes. Plasma concentrations increase after each dose even when a steady-state has been attained – suffcient to cause or exacerbate adverse effects.[6] It is therefore better to give

carbamazepine in a lower dose more frequently than a higher dose less often, e.g. 50–100mg q.d.s. initially, rather than 100–200mg b.d.:

* starting dose 100–200mg o.d.–b.d.
* increments of 100–200mg every 2 weeks
* usual maximum daily dose = 800–1200mg in divided doses, occasionally 1.6–2g
* m/r preparations are best taken b.d.

Neuropathic pain

Sodium valproate 200–500mg o.n. initially, increasing if necessary by stages to 1g daily.[7,8] **Carbamazepine** is used in the same way as for epilepsy. **Gabapentin** is of benefit in some patients, e.g. 100–300mg t.d.s.[9] **Phenytoin** is rarely prescribed for pain relief despite its historic use in trigeminal neuralgia.

Terminal agitation

Phenobarbital is needed on rare occasions for terminal anguish not responding to CSCI midazolam 60mg and *either* haloperidol 30mg/24h *or* levomepromazine (methotrimeprazine) 200mg/24h:

* dilute 200mg/1ml (in propylene glycol) injection to 10ml with WFI
* give a stat dose of 100–200mg IV
* then 600–1200mg/24h CSCI.

Also used as an anticonvulsant in patients who cannot swallow but in whom sedation with midazolam is inappropriate:

* if a stat dose is indicated, give 100mg SC/IM
* then 200–400mg/24h CSCI.

Cautions

Withdrawal: abrupt cessation of long-term anti-epileptic therapy, particularly barbiturates and benzodiazepines, should be avoided because rebound seizures may be precipitated. If it is decided to discontinue anti-epileptic therapy, it should be done *slowly over six months or more* (Table 4.18). In adults the risk of relapse on stopping treatment is 40–50%.[10] Substituting one anti-epileptic drug regimen for another should also be done cautiously, withdrawing the first drug only when the new regimen has been introduced.

Table 4.18 Recommended monthly reductions of anti-epileptics[11]

Drug	Reduction
Carbamazepine	100mg
Clobazam	10mg
Clonazepam	0.5mg
Ethosuximide	250mg
Gabapentin	400mg
Lamotrigine	25mg
Phenobarbital	15mg
Phenytoin	50mg
Sodium valproate	200mg
Topiramate	25mg
Vigabatrin	500mg

Supply

Tablets carbamazepine 100mg, 20 = 58p; 200mg, 20 = £1.07; 400mg, 20 = £2.11.
Tablets m/r carbamazepine 200mg, 20 = £1.72; 400mg, 20 = £3.38.
Liquid sugar-free carbamazepine 100mg/5ml, 300ml = £5.72.
Suppositories carbamazepine 125mg (equivalent to 100mg PO), 5 = £7.50; 250mg (equivalent to 200mg PO), 5 = £10.00.
Capsules gabapentin 100mg, 20 = £4.57; 300mg, 20 = £10.60; 400mg, 20 = £12.27.
Injection phenobarbital 200mg/ml, 1ml amp = 99p.
Capsules phenytoin 25mg, 20 = 39p; 50mg, 20 = 40p; 100mg, 20 = 56p; 300mg, 20 = £1.69.
Tablets phenytoin 50mg, 20 = 26p; 100mg, 20 = 31p.

Suspension **phenytoin** 30mg/5ml, 100ml = 71p.
Injection **phenytoin** 50mg/ml, 5ml amp = £4.07.
Tablets e/c **sodium valproate** 200mg, 20 = £1.18; 500mg, 20 = £2.94.
Solution **sodium valproate** 200mg/5ml, 100ml = £1.96.

---

1 Invicta Pharmaceuticals study 226, data on file.
2 Andersen BB *et al.* (1991) No influence of the antidepressant paroxetine on carbamazepine, valproate and phenytoin. *Epilepsy Research.* **10** (2–3): 201–204.
3 Richens A (1991) The basis of treatment of epilepsy: neuropharmacology. In: Dam M (ed) *A practical approach to epilepsy.* Pergamon Press, Oxford. pp 75–85.
4 Fu C *et al.* (1994) Valproate/nortriptyline interaction. *Journal of Clinical Psychopharmacology.* **14** (3): 205–206.
5 Hoppener RJ *et al.* (1980) Correlation between daily fluctuations of carbamazepine serum levels and intermittent side effects. *Epilepsia.* **21**: 341–350.
6 Tomson T (1984) Interdosage fluctuations in plasma carbamazepine concentration determine intermittent side effects. *Archives of Neurology.* **41**: 830–834.
7 Budd K (1989) Sodium valproate in the treatment of pain. In: Chadwick D (ed) *Fourth international symposium on sodium valproate and epilepsy.* Royal Society of Medicine, London. pp 213–216.
8 Twycross R (1997) *Symptom Management in Advanced Cancer.* Radcliffe Medical Press, Oxford.
9 Rosner H *et al.* (1996) Gabapentin adjunctive therapy in neuropathic pain states. *The Clinical Journal of Pain.* **12**: 56–58.
10 Hopkins A and Shorvon S (1995) Definitions and epidemiology of epilepsy. In: Hopkins A, Shorvon S, Cascino G (eds) *Epilepsy.* (2nd edn) Chapman and Hall Medical, London. pp 1–24.
11 Chadwick DW (1995) The withdrawal of antiepileptic drugs. In: Hopkins A, Shorvon S, Cascino G (eds) *Epilepsy.* (2nd edn) Chapman and Hall Medical, London. pp 215–220.

ORPHENADRINE   BNF 4.9.2

Class of drug: Antimuscarinic antiparkinsonian.

Indications: Parkinson's disease, parkinsonism, [†]sialorrhoea (drooling), [†]extrapyramidal dystonia.

Contra-indications: Glaucoma, prostatic hypertrophy, *tardive dyskinesia* (see p.227).

Pharmacology

Orphenadrine and other antimuscarinic antiparkinsonian drugs are used primarily in Parkinson's disease. They are less effective than **levodopa** in established Parkinson's disease although they often usefully supplement its action. Patients with mild symptoms, particularly where tremor predominates, may be treated initially with antimuscarinic drugs, levodopa being added or substituted as symptoms progress. Antimuscarinic drugs exert their antiparkinsonian effect by correcting the relative central cholinergic excess which occurs in parkinsonism as a result of dopamine deficiency. In most patients their effects are only moderate, reducing tremor and rigidity to some extent but without significant action on bradykinesia. They exert a synergistic effect when used with levodopa and are also useful in reducing sialorrhoea.

Antimuscarinic drugs reduce the symptoms of drug-induced parkinsonism (seen mainly with antipsychotic drugs) but there is no justification for giving them prophylactically (see p.227). *Tardive dyskinesia is not improved by antimuscarinic drugs and may be made worse.* No major differences exist between antimuscarinic drugs but orphenadrine sometimes has a mood-elevating effect. Some people tolerate one antimuscarinic better than another. **Procyclidine** and **benzatropine** may be given parenterally and are effective emergency treatment for severe acute drug-induced dystonic reactions (see p.227).
Onset of action 30–60min.
Duration of action 12–24h.
Plasma halflife 18h.

[†] unlicensed use.

Cautions

Hepatic or renal impairment, cardiovascular disease. Avoid abrupt discontinuation.

Adverse effects

Antimuscarinic effects (see p.225). Nervousness, euphoria, insomnia occasionally. In a psychotic patient receiving a phenothiazine, the addition of orphenadrine to reverse a drug-induced movement disorder may precipitate a toxic confusional psychosis as a result of the summation of antimuscarinic effects.

Dose and use

- starting dose 50mg b.d.–t.d.s.
- increase by 50mg every 3 days if necessary
- maximum recommended daily dose = 400mg.

Supply

Tablets 50mg, 20 = 48p.
Solution 50mg/5ml, 200ml = £7.00.

ANALGESICS

Principles governing the use of analgesics

Paracetamol

Nonsteroidal anti-inflammatory drugs (NSAIDs)
Diclofenac
Diflunisal
Flurbiprofen
Ibuprofen
*Ketorolac
Naproxen

Weak opioids
Codeine phosphate
Dextropropoxyphene
Dihydrocodeine
Tramadol

Strong opioids
Morphine
Diamorphine
Buprenorphine
Fentanyl
*Hydromorphone
*Methadone
*Oxycodone
*Phenazocine

Naloxone

Principles governing the use of analgesics

Analgesics comprise three classes, namely **nonopioid** (paracetamol and NSAIDs), **opioid** (weak and strong) and **adjuvant** (e.g. corticosteroids, antidepressants, anticonvulsants, muscle relaxants). The principles governing their use are encapsulated in the WHO Method for Relief of Cancer Pain:[1]

'By the mouth' 'Individualized treatment'
'By the clock' 'Use adjuvant drugs'
'By the ladder' (Figure 5.1) 'Attention to detail'.

The concept behind the analgesic ladder is 'broad-spectrum analgesia', i.e. drugs from each of the three classes of analgesic are used appropriately either singly or in combination, to maximize their impact (Figure 5.2). Generally, however, the benefits of the WHO ladder should be exploited before introducing, or substituting, an adjuvant analgesic. The nonopioids and opioids are featured in this section; adjuvant analgesics are discussed elsewhere (see Index).

1 World Health Organization (1986) *Cancer Pain Relief*. World Health Organization, Geneva.

*specialist use only.

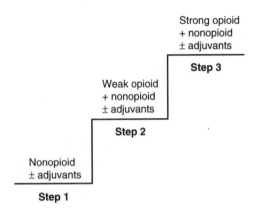

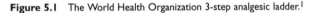

Figure 5.1 The World Health Organization 3-step analgesic ladder.[1]

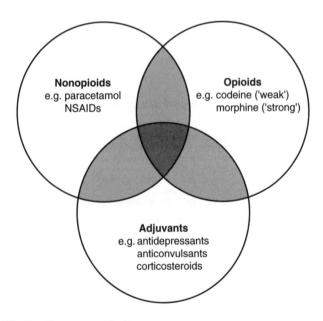

Figure 5.2 Broad-spectrum analgesia.

PARACETAMOL

Class: Nonopioid analgesic.

Indications: Mild–moderate pain, pyrexia.

Pharmacology

Paracetamol is a synthetic nonopioid analgesic which inhibits COX in the brain.[1] It also has a peripheral effect.[2] Like the NSAIDs, paracetamol is antipyretic; unlike the NSAIDs, it has no anti-inflammatory effect in joints. Features which distinguish paracetamol from NSAIDs include:

- adverse effects are uncommon
- does not injure the gastric mucosa
- is well tolerated by patients with peptic ulcers
- does not affect plasma uric acid concentration
- has no effect on platelet function.

In addition, paracetamol can be taken by 2/3 of patients who are hypersensitive to aspirin.[3] Because NSAIDs are mainly peripheral in action and paracetamol central, the two can be used in combination with an additive effect. The main drawback with paracetamol is the frequency of administration (q4h–q6h).

Paracetamol metabolism is age- and dose-dependent. Only 2–5% of a therapeutic dose of paracetamol is excreted unchanged in the urine; the remainder is metabolized mainly by the liver. At therapeutic doses, >80% of paracetamol is metabolized to glucuronide and sulphate conjugates. About 10% is converted by cytochrome P450-dependent hepatic mixed-function oxidase to a highly reactive metabolite. In turn, this metabolite is rapidly inactivated by conjugation with glutathione and excreted in the urine after further metabolism as cysteine and mercapturic acid conjugates. Large overdoses of paracetamol can exhaust stores of glutathione and leave the highly reactive metabolite to bind irreversibly with vital cell elements, which may result in acute hepatic necrosis.[4] Plasma paracetamol concentrations and halflife are within the normal range in chronic renal disease, although the sulphate and glucuronide conjugates accumulate because of reduced renal excretion.

The threshold dose for liver toxicity is about 250mg/kg (about 15g in a 60kg person). Patients with increased iso-enzyme activity or a decreased glutathione synthesis (seen with malnutrition or hepatic impairment) are at greatest risk. The smallest fatal overdose reported is 18g and many have survived with doses of up to 25g. Above this level, death is increasingly likely unless specific treatment is instituted. Antidotes such as **IV acetylcysteine** or **oral methionine** (both precursors of glutathione) protect the liver if given within 10–12h of paracetamol ingestion; acetylcysteine may be effective for 24h or even longer.[5]

Bio-availability 60–70% PO; 30–40% PR (with delayed peak plasma concentration) .
Onset of action 0.5h.
Duration of action 4–6h.
Plasma halflife 2–4h.

Cautions

Severe hepatic impairment (particularly if associated with alcohol dependence and malnutrition). In patients on anticoagulants, a regular intake of paracetamol ≥1300mg/day for a week may result in an increase in the INR to >6, and necessitate a reduction in the dose of concurrently administered coumarin anticoagulants.[6] A total weekly dose of paracetamol of ≤2g, however, does not affect the INR. The underlying mechanism is not clear, but may relate to interference with the hepatic synthesis of factors II, VII, IX and X.

Adverse effects

All rare: cholestatic jaundice,[7,8] thrombocytopenia, agranulocytosis, allergic reactions.[9,10]

Dose and use

Typical oral dose regimens range from 500–1000mg q6h–q4h: *the latter dose exceeds the 4g maximum daily dose recommended in the BNF but is often used with morphine q4h.* Paracetamol is available in several combination preparations with weak opioids (*see* p.102).

Supply
Tablets 500mg, 20 = 9p.
Tablets dispersible 500mg, 20 = 75p.
Suspension 250mg/5ml, 200ml = £1.48p.
Suppositories 500mg, 10 = £9.90; 1g, 10 = £12.00, manufactured by Burton-on-Trent Hospital for Aurum Pharmaceuticals.

1 Flower RJ and Vane JR (1972) Inhibition of prostaglandin synthetase in brain explains the antipyretic actions of paracetamol. *Nature.* **240**: 410–411.
2 Moore UJ et al. (1992) The efficacy of locally applied aspirin and acetaminophen in postoperative pain after third molar surgery. *Clinical Pharmacology and Therapeutics.* **52**: 292–296.
3 Settipane RA et al. (1995) Prevalence of cross-sensitivity with acetaminophen in aspirin-sensitive asthmatic subjects. *Journal of Allergy and Clinical Immunology.* **96**: 480–485.
4 Prescott LF (1986) Effects of non-narcotic analgesics on the liver. *Drugs.* **32** (suppl 4): 129–147.
5 British National Formulary (1998) Emergency treatment of poisoning. In: *British National Formulary, No. 35.* British Medical Association, London. pp 20–22.
6 Hylek EM et al. (1998) Acetaminophen and other risk factors for excessive warfarin anticoagulation. *Journal of the American Medical Association.* **279**: 657–662.
7 Waldum HL et al. (1992) Can NSAIDs cause acute biliary pain with cholestasis? *Journal of Clinical Gastroenterology.* **14**: 328–330.
8 Wong V et al. (1993) Paracetamol and acute biliary pain with cholestasis. *Lancet.* **342**: 869.
9 Stricker BH et al. (1985) Acute hypersensitivity reactions to paracetamol. *British Medical Journal.* **291**: 938–939.
10 Leung R et al. (1992) Paracetamol anaphylaxis. *Clinical and Experimental Allergy.* **22**: 831–833.

NONSTEROIDAL ANTI-INFLAMMATORY DRUGS (NSAIDs)   BNF 4.7.1 & 10.1.1

NSAIDs are of particular benefit for pains associated with inflammation, e.g. soft tissue infiltration and bone metastases. Because inflammation leads to central sensitization and increased pain, NSAIDs will sometimes play a crucial role in relieving cancer-related neuropathic pain.[1,2]

Ibuprofen, diclofenac and **naproxen** are the most widely used NSAIDs in palliative care. Availability, fashion, relative cost, patient convenience and adverse effects profile all dictate choice as much as efficacy. **Flurbiprofen** is the NSAID of choice at Sobell House, and **diclofenac** at Hayward House. Specific circumstances may indicate a specific choice, e.g. **diflunisal** (see p.96) and **ketorolac** (see p.98). NSAIDs act at several sites, both peripheral and central. The central analgesic effects of NSAIDs have not been fully elucidated and it is possible that clinically important differences may emerge when more data are available. Further, it is not known whether some cancer patients obtain more benefit from one particular NSAID as is anecdotally reported in rheumatoid arthritis.

NSAIDs inhibit cyclo-oxygenase (COX), an important enzyme in the arachidonic acid cascade, which results in the production of tissue and inflammatory PGs.[3] Inhibition of PG synthesis does not account for the total analgesic effect of NSAIDs, although it appears to explain most of the adverse effects. In postdental extraction pain, most weak COX inhibitors are significantly superior to aspirin and most strong inhibitors inferior (Table 5.1). COX exists in two forms; COX-1 is constitutive (i.e. present in all normal tissues), whereas COX-2 is normally undetectable in most tissues but massively induced by inflammation (Figure 5.3). By producing selective COX-2 inhibitors, it is hoped to reduce the gastric toxicity of NSAIDs. COX-1 inhibition alone, however, does not explain the differential impact of NSAIDs on the gastro-intestinal tract; uncoupling of oxidative phosphorylation is possibly more important.[4] COX-2 is normally present in the kidney,

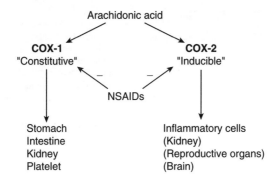

Figure 5.3 Important sites of COX-1 and COX-2 production; – indicates inhibition.

Table 5.1 Analgesic efficacy of orally administered NSAIDs in dental pain compared to aspirin 650mg[5]

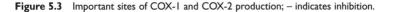

Significantly superior[a]	Not significantly different	Significantly inferior
Azapropazone (3)	Diclofenac (1)	Fenbufen (1)
Diflunisal (3)	Etodolac (1)	Nabumetone (1)
Flurbiprofen (1)	Sulindac (1)	
Ketoprofen (2)		
Ketorolac (3)		
Naproxen (3)		
Tolmetin (3)		

a. numbers in parentheses indicate capacity to inhibit PG synthesis: 1 = potent; 2 = moderate; 3 = weak.

female reproductive organs and brain. The possibility that selective COX-2 inhibitors (yet to be marketed) may cause renal dysfunction must not be ignored.

NSAIDs differ in their effect on platelet function. In patients undergoing chemotherapy or with thrombocytopenia from other causes, it is best to use a NSAID which has no effect on platelet function (Table 5.2).

Table 5.2   NSAIDs and platelet function

Drug	Effect on platelets	Comment
Aspirin	+	*Irreversible* platelet dysfunction (acetylation of platelet COX-1)
Nonacetylated salicylates	−	No effect at recommended doses (choline magnesium trisalicylate, diflunisal, salsalate)
Nonselective COX inhibitors	+	Reversible platelet dysfunction (includes all other long-established NSAIDs)
Preferential COX-2 inhibitors	−	Meloxicam,[6] nimesulide[7]
Selective COX-2 inhibitors	−	None presently marketed

Cautions

Recent peptic ulceration, hypovolaemia, cardiac failure, renal and hepatic impairment. Concurrent use with coumarin anticoagulants (Box 5.A). Drug interactions are summarized in Table 5.3 (see also Appendix 3, p.213). Of particular importance is the interaction with **methotrexate**, a weak organic acid which is 60–80% excreted unchanged by the kidney.[8] Concurrent administration with a second drug which interferes with its excretion increases the plasma concentration and toxicity of methotrexate; such drugs include NSAIDs, penicillins and co-trimoxazole. An interaction with NSAIDs is seen in only a few patients but two deaths have occurred with **aspirin** and life-threatening neutropenia with several other NSAIDS.[8] In most patients concurrent treatment is safe. Toxicity is dose-related; it is much less likely with chronic low-dose methotrexate in rheumatoid arthritis than with high-dose pulses of cancer chemotherapy.

Box 5.A   Anticoagulants and NSAIDs[9]

No interaction normally occurs with ibuprofen, diclofenac and naproxen but isolated cases have been described with **diclofenac**, **ketoprofen**, **tiaprofenic acid** and **tolmetin**.

Flurbiprofen potentiates oral anticoagulants sufficient to cause bleeding in a few patients.

All NSAIDs cause gastro-intestinal irritation and possible bleeding, and should be used with care in patients taking oral anticoagulants.

Adverse effects

The adverse effects have been categorized as type A ('augmented' effects) and type B ('bizarre' effects).[10] Type A effects are predictable and dose-dependent, whereas type B are unpredictable and dose-independent (Tables 5.4 & 5.5).

Table 5.3 Pharmacokinetic interactions with NSAIDs[11]

Drug affected	NSAIDs implicated	Effect	Clinical implications
NSAIDs affecting other drugs			
Oral anticoagulants	Azapropazone Oxyphenbutazone Phenylbutazone	Inhibition of metabolism of warfarin, increasing anticoagulant effect	Avoid this group of NSAIDs or monitor closely
Lithium	Probably all NSAIDs (? except sulindac, aspirin)	Inhibition of renal excretion of lithium, increasing lithium serum concentrations and increasing risk of toxicity	Use sulindac or aspirin if NSAID unavoidable; monitor lithium concentration and reduce dose accordingly
Oral hypoglycaemic	Azapropazone Oxyphenbutazone Phenylbutazone	Inhibition of metabolism of sulphonylurea drugs, prolonging halflife and increasing risk of hypoglycaemia	Avoid this group of NSAIDs
Phenytoin	Oxyphenbutazone Phenylbutazone	Inhibition of metabolism of phenytoin, increasing plasma concentration and risk of toxicity	Avoid this group of NSAIDs
	Other NSAIDs	Displacement of phenytoin from plasma protein	Careful interpretation of phenytoin concentration; measurement of unbound concentration may be helpful
Methotrexate	Salicylates Other NSAIDs (less so)	Reduced clearance of methotrexate, increasing plasma concentration and risk of severe toxicity	Avoid aspirin and other salicylates during chemotherapy; probably safe between pulses Use other NSAIDs with caution *Generally not a problem with low-dose chronic methotrexate therapy used in rheumatoid arthritis*
Sodium valproate	Aspirin ? other NSAIDS	Inhibition of valproate metabolism, increasing plasma concentration	Avoid aspirin; with other NSAIDs reduce dose of sodium valproate if toxicity suspected
Digoxin	All NSAIDs	Potential reduction in renal function (particularly in very young and very old) reducing digoxin clearance and increasing plasma concentration and risk of toxicity (no interaction if renal function normal)	Avoid NSAIDs if possible; if not, check digoxin plasma concentration and plasma creatinine

continued

Table 5.3 Continued

Drug affected	NSAIDs implicated	Effect	Clinical implications
Aminoglycosides	All NSAIDs	Reduction in renal function in susceptible individuals, reducing aminoglycoside clearance and increasing plasma concentration	Monitor plasma concentration and adjust dose
Other drugs affecting NSAIDs			
Antacids	Indometacin	Variable effects: • aluminium-containing antacids reduce rate and extent of absorption of indometacin • sodium bicarbonate increases rate and extent of absorption of indometacin	Other NSAIDs are not significantly affected by concurrent use of antacids,[9] and could be substituted for indometacin
Probenecid	Probably all NSAIDs	Reduction in metabolism and renal clearance of NSAIDs and glucuronide metabolites which are hydrolyzed back to parent drug	May be used therapeutically to increase the response
Barbiturates	Phenylbutazone ? other NSAIDs	Increased metabolic clearance of NSAIDs	May require higher dose of NSAID
Cholestyramine	Naproxen ? other NSAIDs	Anion exchange resin binds NSAIDs in gut reducing rate (? and extent) of absorption	Separate administration by 4h; may need higher dose of NSAID
Metoclopramide	Aspirin	Increased rate and extent of absorption of aspirin in patients with migraine	May be used therapeutically to speed onset of action of aspirin

Table 5.4 Type A reactions to NSAIDs[10]

Organ/system	Clinical reaction
Blood	Decreased platelet adhesiveness
Gastro-intestinal tract	Dyspepsia
	Haemorrhage
	Peptic ulceration
	Perforation
Kidney	Salt and water retention
	Interstitial nephritis
Lung	Bronchospasm

Table 5.5 Type B reactions to NSAIDs[10]

Organ/system	Clinical reaction	NSAIDs
Immunological	Anaphylaxis	Most NSAIDs
Skin	Morbilliform rash	Fenbufen
	Angioedema	Ibuprofen
		Azapropazone
		Piroxicam
Blood	Thrombocytopenia	Diclofenac
		Ibuprofen
		Piroxicam
	Haemolytic anaemia	Mefenamic acid
		Diclofenac
	Agranulocytosis	Phenylbutazone
	Aplastic anaemia	Phenylbutazone
Gastro-intestinal	Diarrhoea	Mefenamic acid
		Flufenamic acid
Liver	Reye's syndrome	Aspirin
	Hepatitis	Diclofenac
		Piroxicam
CNS	Aseptic meningitis	Ibuprofen

Gastro-intestinal toxicity is by far the most serious adverse effect of NSAIDs. It is a class effect but propensity varies between NSAIDs (Table 5.6). Various risk factors have been identified (Table 5.7). Being over 60 may not be a true risk factor; it may relate to the fact that many elderly people take aspirin as prophylaxis against thrombosis. This might also explain why heart disease was found to be a risk factor (odds ratio $\approx$ 2) in another study.[12]

Table 5.6 Risk of NSAID-related gastroduodenopathy

Lowest	Intermediate	Highest
Ibuprofen	Aspirin (dispersible and e/c)	Aspirin (coarse granules)
Meloxicam	Diclofenac	Azapropazone
Nimesulide	Diflunisal	Ketorolac
	Flurbiprofen	Piroxicam
	Indometacin	
	Ketoprofen	
	Naproxen	

Table 5.7   Risk factors for NSAID-related gastroduodenopathy[13]

Group		Odds ratio
Overall		3
Treatment	<1 month	8
	1–3 months	3
	>3 months	2
Age >60		6
Previous peptic ulceration		5
High dose		4–8
Concomitant corticosteroids		4–5
Concomitant anticoagulants		13

Aspirin-induced asthma is related to COX inhibition. Aspirin-sensitive subjects possibly differ from other people with asthma by depending more on the bronchodilating activity of PGE_2 than on the β-adrenergic system. Aspirin inhibits the production of PGE_2 with the result that more arachidonic acid is available as a substrate for leukotriene production. Leukotrienes C_4 and D_4 are known to be potent bronchoconstrictors and mucus secretagogues. Other unidentified bronchoconstrictors could also be involved.[14] Although a class effect, bronchospasm has not been observed with **choline salicylate**, **sodium salicylate**, **azapropazone** and **benzydamine**.

All NSAIDs cause salt and water retention which may result in ankle oedema; they therefore antagonize the action of diuretics. NSAIDs may also cause acute or acute-on-chronic renal failure particularly in patients with hypovolaemia from any cause, e.g. diuretics, fever, dehydration, vomiting, diarrhoea, haemorrhage, surgery.

The risk of NSAID-induced renal failure increases in situations where the plasma concentrations of vasoconstrictor substances such as angiotensin II, norepinephrine (noradrenaline) and vasopressin are increased, e.g. in heart failure, cirrhosis and nephrotic syndrome. The inhibition of renal PG production by NSAIDs prevents the protective vasodilatory mechanism for safeguarding renal blood flow from functioning effectively.[15] Early studies which suggested that **sulindac** has little or no effect on renal PG synthesis have not been substantiated by subsequent reports.[16] Whether **meloxicam** and **nimesulide** have less effect on renal function than other NSAIDs remains to be seen from postmarketing surveillance. Sporadic cases of interstitial nephritis (± nephrotic syndrome or ± papillary necrosis) have been reported with most NSAIDs.

Apart from biliary and renal colic,[17] NSAIDS should be given PO in patients who can swallow. There is no evidence of greater efficacy by other routes.[18] Topical NSAIDs are of value for the relief of pain associated with soft tissue trauma, e.g. strains and sprains.[19]

1 Dellemijn PL et al. (1994) Medical therapy of malignant nerve pain. A randomised double-blind explanatory trial with naproxen versus slow-release morphine. *European Journal of Cancer.* **30A** (9): 1244–1250.

2 Ripamonti C et al. (1996) Continuous subcutaneous infusion of ketorolac in cancer neuropathic pain unresponsive to opioid and adjuvant drugs. A case report. *Tumori.* **82**: 413–415.

3 Flower RJ and Vane JR (1972) Inhibition of prostaglandin synthetase in brain explains the antipyretic activity of paracetamol. *Nature.* **240**: 410–411.

4 Somasundaran S et al. (1995) The biochemical basis of nonsteroidal anti-inflammatory drug-induced damage to the gastrointestinal tract: a review and a hypothesis. *Scandinavian Journal of Gastroenterology.* **30**: 289–299.

5 McCormack K and Brune K (1991) Dissociation between the antinociceptive and anti-inflammatory effects of the nonsteroidal anti-inflammatory drugs: a survey of their analgesic efficacy. *Drugs.* **41**: 533–547.

6 Guth B et al. (1996) Therapeutic doses of meloxicam do not inhibit platelet aggregation in man. *Rheumatology in Europe.* **25** (Suppl 1): Abs. 443.

7 Cullen L et al. (1997) Selective suppression of cyclo-oxygenase-2 during chronic administration of nimesulide in man. *Presented at 4th International Congress on essential fatty acids and eicosanoids.* Edinburgh.

8 Stockley IH (1996) *Drug interactions. (4th edn)* Pharmaceutical Press, London. pp 505–506.

9 Stockley IH (1996) *Drug interactions. (4th edn)* The Pharmaceutical Press, London. p 278.

10 Rawlins MD (1997) Non-opioid analgesics. In: Doyle D, Hanks GWC, MacDonald N (eds) *Oxford Textbook of Palliative Medicine (2nd edn)*. Oxford University Press, Oxford. pp 355–361.

11 Tonkin AL and Wing LMH (1988) Interactions of nonsteroidal anti-inflammatory drugs. In: Brooks PM (ed) *Bailliere's Clinical Rheumatology. Anti-rheumatic drugs, Vol 2, No. 2*. Bailliere Tindall, London. pp 455–483.

12 Silverstein FE *et al.* (1995) Misoprostol reduces serious gastrointestinal complications in patients with rheumatoid arthritis receiving nonsteroidal anti-inflammatory drugs. *Annals of Internal Medicine.* **123**: 241–249.

13 Gabriel SE *et al.* (1991) Risk for serious gastrointestinal complications related to use of nonsteroidal anti-inflammatory drugs: a meta-analysis. *Annals of Internal Medicine.* **115**: 787–796.

14 Capron A *et al.* (1985) New functions for platelets and their pathological implications. *International Archives of Allergy and Applied Immunology.* **77**: 107–114.

15 MacDonald TM (1994) Selected side-effects: 14. Non-steroidal anti-inflammatory drugs and renal damage. *Prescribers' Journal.* **34**: 77–80.

16 Eriksson L-O *et al.* (1990) Effects of sulindac and naproxen on prostaglandin excretion in patients with impaired renal function and rheumatoid arthritis. *American Journal of Medicine.* **89**: 313–321.

17 Lundstam SOA *et al.* (1982) Prostaglandin-synthetase inhibition with diclofenac sodium in treatment of renal colic: comparison with use of a narcotic analgesic. *Lancet.* **i**: 1096–1097.

18 Tramer MR *et al.* (1998) Comparing analgesic efficacy of non-steroidal anti-inflammatory drugs given by different routes in acute and chronic pain: a qualitative systematic review. *Acta Anaesthesiologica Scandinavica.* **42**: 71–79.

19 Moore RA *et al.* (1998) Quantitative systematic review of topically applied non-steroidal anti-inflammatory drugs. *British Medical Journal.* **316**: 333–338.

DICLOFENAC   BNF 10.1.1

Class of drug: Nonopioid analgesic, NSAID.

Indications: Pain (particularly that associated with tissue inflammation), [†]neoplastic fever.

Contra-indications: Active peptic ulceration, hypersensitivity to aspirin or other NSAID (urticaria, rhinitis, asthma, angioedema).

Pharmacology

Diclofenac is an acetate NSAID.[1] It is rapidly and completely absorbed but the peak plasma concentration is delayed for several hours if taken p.c. About 10% of patients experience adverse effects (mainly gastric intolerance) which are generally mild and transient; diclofenac needs to be withdrawn in only 2%.[2] Age, renal impairment and hepatic impairment do not have any significant effect on plasma concentrations of diclofenac, although metabolite concentrations increase in severe renal impairment. The principal metabolite, hydroxydiclofenac, possesses little anti-inflammatory effect. Diclofenac does not normally interact with coumarin anticoagulants (see p.90) or oral hypoglycaemic agents. Although diclofenac is a potent reversible inhibitor of platelet aggregation *in vitro*, typical oral doses have no effect on platelet adhesiveness or bleeding time.[2] Further, although IV diclofenac has a measurable effect on bleeding time, most subjects remain within the normal range. Diclofenac is never, or hardly ever, associated with certain sporadic adverse effects seen with many other NSAIDs, e.g. acute pancreatitis, aseptic meningitis, cutaneous reactions and photosensitivity. Diclofenac is the NSAID of choice at Hayward House.

Oral bio-availability no data.
Onset of action 20–30min.
Duration of action 8h.
Plasma halflife 1–2h.

[†] unlicensed use.

Cautions and adverse effects: See p.90.

Dose and use
- 50mg b.d.–t.d.s.
- m/r 100mg o.d.
- m/r 75mg b.d. or 150mg o.d.

Although the manufacturer's UK licence is for ≤150mg/day, some patients obtain greater benefit with no increase in adverse effects from 200mg/day, e.g. m/r 100mg b.d. In some centres diclofenac is given by CSCI if a non-oral route is necessary; it must be given in a separate syringe driver because it is immiscible with other drugs.

Diclofenac is also given by injection:
- 75mg SC/IM stat and 150mg/24h CSCI in patients unable to take oral medication
- 75mg IM p.r.n. for biliary and renal colic.[3,4]

(**Tenoxicam** may be a more convenient option for some patients who need a parenteral NSAID; this has a plasma halflife of 72h and can be given 20mg o.d. as a bolus injection.)

Supply
Tablets e/c 50mg, 20 = £1.67.
Tablets dispersible 50mg, 20 = £4.90.
Tablets e/c **Arthrotec 50**, diclofenac 50mg + misoprostol 200µg, 20 = £4.99.
Tablets e/c **Arthrotec 75**, diclofenac 75mg + misoprostol 200µg, 20 = £5.86.
Capsules m/r 75mg, 20 = £4.65; 100mg, 20 = £6.69.
Suppositories 50mg, 20 = £4.20; 100mg, 20 = £7.52.
Injection 75mg/3ml, 3ml amp = 83p.

1 John VA (1979) The pharmacokinetics and metabolism of diclofenac sodium (Voltarol) in animals and man. *Rheumatology and Rehabilitation.* Suppl 2: 22–37.
2 Todd PA and Sorkin EM (1988) Diclofenac sodium: a reappraisal of its pharmacodynamic and pharmacokinetic properties, and therapeutic efficacy. *Drugs.* **35**: 244–285.
3 Lundstam SOA et al. (1982) Prostaglandin-synthetase inhibition with diclofenac sodium in treatment of renal colic: comparison with use of a narcotic analgesic. *Lancet.* **i**: 1096–1097.
4 Thompson JF et al. (1989) Rectal diclofenac compared with pethidine injection in acute renal colic. *British Medical Journal.* **299**: 1140–1141.

DIFLUNISAL

BNF 10.1.1

Class of drug: Nonopioid analgesic, NSAID.

Indications: Pain (particularly that associated with tissue inflammation), [†]neoplastic fever.

Contra-indications: Active peptic ulceration, hypersensitivity to aspirin or other NSAID (urticaria, rhinitis, asthma, angioedema).

Pharmacology
Diflunisal is a salicylic acid derivative which causes less gastrotoxicity than equivalent doses of aspirin. It is well absorbed with a peak plasma concentration after about 2h. Steady-state concentration is reached after 3–4 days with a dose of 125mg b.d., after 7–9 days with 500mg b.d. With each doubling of dose, the plasma concentration increases about 3 times.[1] Bio-availability is reduced by the regular use of aluminium-containing antacids, although this effect is less marked if taken with or after food. Diflunisal is metabolized by conjugation to glucuronide and excreted in the urine. Diflunisal decreases plasma uric acid concentration. It affects platelet function only in doses >500mg b.d.

Onset of action 20–30min.
Duration of action 8–12h.
Plasma halflife 8–12h; up to 115h in severe renal impairment.

† unlicensed use.

Cautions and adverse effects: See p.90.

Dose and use
- 250–500mg b.d.
- increase to 500mg t.d.s. if necessary.

Supply
Tablets 250mg, 20 = £1.80; 500 mg, 20 = £3.61.

---

1 Cooper SA (1983) New peripherally-acting oral analgesic agent. *Annual Review of Pharmacology and Toxicology.* **23**: 617–647.

FLURBIPROFEN   BNF 10.1.1

Class of drug: Nonopioid analgesic, NSAID.

Indications: Pain (particularly that associated with tissue inflammation), [†]neoplastic fever.

Contra-indications: Active peptic ulceration, hypersensitivity to aspirin or other NSAID (urticaria, rhinitis, asthma, angioedema).

Pharmacology
Flurbiprofen is a propionic acid derivative and a highly potent COX inhibitor. In animal studies, it is 8–20 times more potent than aspirin. Flurbiprofen is rapidly and well absorbed; peak plasma concentrations are attained 90min after a single dose. It is excreted in the urine both as unchanged drug and a number of hydroxylated metabolites. In addition to its analgesic use, flurbiprofen has been used to relieve frequency caused by instability of the detrusor muscle of the bladder.[1] Flurbiprofen is the NSAID of choice at Sobell House.
Onset of action 20–30min.
Duration of action 8–16h.[2]
Plasma halflife 3–12h.

Cautions and adverse effects: See p.90.

Dose and use
- 50–100mg b.d.–t.d.s.
- m/r 200mg o.d.
Suppositories can be used in patients who are unable to swallow tablets.

Supply
Tablets 50mg, 20 = £1.65; 100mg, 20 = £3.13.
Capsules m/r 200mg, 20 = £7.26.
Suppositories 100mg, 20 = £4.83.

---

1 Cardozo LD *et al.* (1980) Evaluation of flurbiprofen in detrusor instability. *British Medical Journal.* **280**: 281–282.
2 Kowanko JC *et al.* (1981) Circadian variations in the signs and symptoms of rheumatoid arthritis and in the therapeutic effectiveness of flurbiprofen at different times of day. *British Journal of Clinical Pharmacology.* **11**: 477–484.

[†] unlicensed use.

IBUPROFEN

BNF 10.1.1

Class of drug: Nonopioid analgesic, NSAID.

Indications: Pain (particularly that associated with tissue inflammation), [†]neoplastic fever.

Contra-indications: Active peptic ulceration, hypersensitivity to aspirin or other NSAID (urticaria, rhinitis, asthma, angioedema).

Pharmacology

Ibuprofen acts predominantly as an analgesic in doses up to 1200mg daily; its anti-inflammatory properties are more evident at higher doses. Ibuprofen is rapidly and well absorbed; doses of 2400mg daily are well tolerated by most patients. Ibuprofen is also safe in overdose; no deaths have been reported with ibuprofen alone, even with a single dose of 40g.[1] Ibuprofen is 3 times more potent than aspirin, i.e. 200mg is equivalent to 600mg of aspirin; higher doses of ibuprofen have a greater analgesic effect than standard doses of aspirin.

Onset of action 20–30min; peak plasma concentrations <2h.
Duration of action 4–6h.
Plasma halflife 2h.

Cautions and adverse effects: See p.90.

Dose and use
- 400mg t.d.s.–q.d.s.
- increase to 600mg q.d.s. if necessary.

Supply
Ibuprofen 200mg tablets are available OTC.
Tablets 400mg, 20 = 29p; 600mg, 20 = 44p.
Tablets m/r 800mg, 20 = £3.61.
Syrup 100mg/5ml, 500ml = £7.34.
Granules effervescent 600mg/sachet, 20 = £5.15; *contains Na+ 9 mmol/sachet.*

---

1 Busson M (1984) Update on ibuprofen: review article. *Journal of International Medical Research.* 14: 53–62.

*KETOROLAC

BNF 10.1.1

Class of drug: Nonopioid analgesic, NSAID.

Indications: *Oral,* short-term postoperative pain relief; *parenteral,* [†]severe pain associated with soft tissue and bone metastases poorly responsive to maximum doses of other NSAIDs combined with a strong opioid.

Contra-indications: Active peptic ulceration or history of peptic ulceration, gastro-intestinal bleeding, suspected or confirmed cerebrovascular bleeding, haemorrhagic diatheses, asthma, hypersensitivity to aspirin or other NSAID, syndrome of nasal polyps and angioedema and bronchospasm (partial or complete), creatinine >160μmol/L, hypovolaemia. Concurrent prescription with anticoagulants, other NSAID, oxypentifylline, probenecid and lithium.

Pharmacology

Ketorolac is a cyclic propionate structurally related to the acetate NSAIDs tolmetin and indometacin.[1,2] It is available as ketorolac trometamol which is more water-soluble. Over 99% of

---

* specialist use only. [†] unlicensed use.

the oral dose is absorbed and about 75% of a dose is excreted in the urine within 7h, and over 90% within 2 days, nearly 2/3 as unmodified ketorolac.[2] The rest is excreted in the faeces. Because of its propensity to cause gastric haemorrhage, the licence for ketorolac is restricted to short-term use for postoperative pain. In palliative care, however, ketorolac is sometimes used for extended periods.[3–6]

The analgesic and anti-inflammatory activity of ketorolac resides mainly in the laevorotatory isomer. The analgesic effect is far greater than the antipyretic and anti-inflammatory properties. In animal studies, ketorolac is about 350 times more potent than aspirin as an analgesic but only 20 times more potent as an antipyretic.[3] As an anti-inflammatory ketorolac is about 1/2 as potent as indometacin and twice as potent as naproxen. Like most NSAIDs, ketorolac inhibits platelet aggregation.

Oral bio-availability >80%; peak plasma concentrations 30min PO, 45min IM.
Onset of action 30min PO, 30min IM.
Duration of action 6h PO, 4–6h IM.
Plasma halflife 5h; 6–7h in the elderly.[7]

Cautions

Hepatic impairment. Interacts with furosemide (frusemide) (decreased diuretic response), ACE inhibitors (increased risk of renal impairment), methotrexate and lithium (decreased clearance), probenecid (increased ketorolac levels and halflife), oxypentifylline (increased bleeding tendency).

Adverse effects

See p.90. Bleeding and pain at injection site (less with CSCI).

Dose and use

Ketorolac is used by some PCUs when a parenteral NSAID is indicated. Ketorolac can be given by intermittent injections 20–30mg SC t.d.s. but these are uncomfortable, and it is better given by CSCI. It is generally given for a short period (<3 weeks) while arranging and awaiting benefit from more definitive therapy (e.g. radiotherapy). However, when all other options have been exhausted, ketorolac has been used for 6 months without adverse effects.[6]

- usual starting dose 60mg/24h CSCI (also recommended maximum dose in ≥65 year-olds and those ≤50kg)
- increase by 15mg/24h to 90mg/24h if necessary
- co-prescribe **misoprostol** 200µg t.d.s–q.d.s
- use **lansoprazole** 30mg o.d. or **omeprazole** 20mg o.d. for patients unable to tolerate misoprostol.

If normal saline is used, ketorolac 60–120mg/10ml is compatible with diamorphine.[4] *Ketorolac is incompatible with cyclizine, midazolam, haloperidol, morphine, pethidine, hydroxyzine and promethazine* (see Section 14, p.183).[2] (Alternative NSAIDs for parenteral use include **diclofenac** (see p.95) and **tenoxicam**; the latter has a plasma halflife of 72h and may be given 20mg o.d. as a bolus injection.)

Supply

Tablets 10mg, 20 = £6.52.
Injection 30mg/ml, 1ml amp = £1.28.

1 Buckley MM-T and Brogden RN (1990) Ketorolac: a review of its pharmacodynamic and pharmacokinetic properties, and therapeutic potential. *Drugs*. **39**: 86–109.
2 Litvak KM and McEvoy GK (1990) Ketorolac: an injectable nonnarcotic analgesic. *Clinical Pharmacy*. **9**: 921–935.
3 Blackwell N *et al*. (1993) Subcutaneous ketorolac: a new development in pain control. *Palliative Medicine*. **7**: 63–65.
4 Myers KG and Trotman IF (1994) Use of ketorolac by continuous subcutaneous infusion for the control of cancer related pain. *Postgraduate Medical Journal*. **70**: 359–362.
5 Middleton RK *et al*. (1996) Continuous infusion: a case report and review of the literature. *Journal of Pain and Symptom Management*. **12**: 190–194.

6 Hughes A et al. (1997) Ketorolac: continuous subcutaneous infusion for cancer pain. Journal of Pain and Symptom Management. 13: 315–316.
7 Greenwald RA (1992) Ketorolac: an innovative nonsteroidal analgesic. Drugs of Today. 28: 41–61.

NAPROXEN   BNF 10.1.1

Class of drug: Nonopioid analgesic, NSAID.

Indications: Pain (particularly that associated with tissue inflammation), [†]neoplastic fever.

Contra-indications: Active peptic ulceration, hypersensitivity to aspirin or other NSAID (urticaria, rhinitis, asthma, angioedema).

Pharmacology

Naproxen is a propionic acid derivative. It is completely absorbed PO and PR, although slower PR. Plasma concentrations do not increase with doses >500mg b.d. because of rapid urinary excretion.[1] Naproxen sodium 550mg is equivalent to 500mg naproxen. Naproxen sodium is more rapidly absorbed, resulting in higher plasma concentrations and an earlier onset of action.[2]
Bio-availability 99%.
Onset of action 20–30min.
Duration of action 6–8h with single dose; ≥12h with multiple doses.
Plasma halflife 12–15h.

Cautions and adverse effects: See p.90.

Dose and use

- typically 250–500mg b.d.
- can be taken as a single daily dose, either o.m. or o.n.
- increase to 500mg t.d.s. if necessary; this is higher than the usual maximum dose of 1g daily (recommended in the Data Sheet and the BNF) but is comparable to doses used for severe rheumatoid arthritis.

Suppositories can be used in patients who are unable to swallow or retain ingested tablets.

Supply

Tablets 250mg, 20 = £1.55; 500mg, 20 = £3.22.
Tablets m/r 500mg, 20 = £5.46.
Suspension 125mg/5ml, 240 ml = £3.82; *contains Na+ 1.7mmol/5ml.*
Suppositories 500mg, 20 = £4.78.

1 Simon LS and Mills JA (1980). Nonsteroidal anti-inflammatory drugs; Part 2. New England Journal of Medicine. 302: 1237–1243.
2 Sevelius H et al. (1980) Bioavailability of naproxen sodium and its relationship to clinical analgesic effects. British Journal of Clinical Pharmacology. 10: 259–263.

WEAK OPIOIDS   BNF 4.7.2

The division of opioids into 'weak' and 'strong' is to a certain extent arbitrary. By IM injection, all the weak opioids can provide analgesia equivalent, or nearly equivalent, to morphine 10mg. Generally, however, **codeine**, **dextropropoxyphene** and **dihydrocodeine** are not used parenterally.

[†] unlicensed use.

Weak opioids are said to have a 'ceiling' effect for analgesia. This is an oversimplification; whereas mixed agonist-antagonists such as **pentazocine** have a true ceiling effect, the maximum effective dose of weak opioid agonists is arbitrary. At higher doses there are progressively more adverse effects, notably nausea and vomiting, which outweigh any additional analgesic effect. For example, the amount of dextropropoxyphene in compound tablets was chosen so that only a small minority of patients would experience nausea and vomiting with two tablets. This adds a further constraint; in practice the upper dose limit is set by the number of tablets which a patient will accept, possibly only 2–3 of any preparation. There is little to choose between the weak opioids in terms of efficacy (Table 5.8). Codeine and dihydrocodeine are more constipating and, for this reason, co-proxamol is preferred at most palliative care units in the UK. **Meptazinol** and **tramadol** are not widely used in the UK. The following general rules should be observed:
• a weak opioid should be *added to*, not substituted for, a nonopioid
• if a weak opioid is inadequate when given regularly, change to a strong opioid (i.e. morphine)
• do not 'kangaroo' from weak opioid to weak opioid.

Table 5.8   Weak opioids

Drug	Bio-availability (%)	Time to maximum concentration (h)	Plasma halflife (h)	Duration of analgesia (h)[a]	Potency ratio with codeine
Codeine	40 (12–84)	1–2	2.5–3.5	4–5	1
Dextropropoxyphene	40	2–2.5	6–12[b]	6–8	7/8[c]
Dihydrocodeine	20	1.6–1.8	3.5–4.5	3–4	4/3
Meptazinol	<10	0.5–2	2[d]	3–4	2/5[e]
Pentazocine	20	1	3	2–3	1[e]
Tramadol	70	2	6	4–6	2[e]

a. when used in usual doses for mild–moderate pain
b. increased >50% in elderly
c. multiple doses; single dose = 1/2–2/3
d. multiple doses in elderly = 3.5–5h
e. estimated on basis of potency ratio with morphine.

CODEINE PHOSPHATE   BNF 3.9.1 & 4.7.2

Class: Weak opioid analgesic.

Indications: Pain unrelieved by nonopioids alone, diarrhoea, cough.

Pharmacology
Codeine (methylmorphine) is an opium alkaloid, about 1/10 as potent as morphine. An increasing analgesic response has been reported with IM doses up to 360mg.[1] In practice, however, codeine is used PO in doses of 20–60mg, generally in combination with a nonopioid. Its oral to parenteral potency ratio is 2:3, about double that of morphine. The main metabolite is codeine-6-glucuronide (which has comparable weak binding to the μ receptor), together with small amounts of nor-codeine, morphine, morphine-3-glucuronide and morphine-6-glucuronide. It has been suggested that codeine is mainly a prodrug of morphine because, in animals, codeine lacks significant anal-gesic activity if demethylation is blocked.[2] The amount of codeine biotransformed to morphine varies from 2–10%.[3] In humans, however, it has been shown that at least part of the analgesic effect of codeine is a direct one.[4]
Oral bio-availability 40% (12–84%).[5]
Onset of action 30–60min for analgesia; 1–2h for antitussive effect.
Duration of action 4–8h.
Plasma halflife 2.5–3.5h.[5]

Cautions and adverse effects
As for other opioids (see p.107).

Dose and use
Codeine is commonly given in a compound preparation with a nonopioid, typically 2 tablets q6h–q4h. The codeine content of these preparations is either low (8mg) or high (30mg); patients with inadequate relief will therefore benefit by changing to a higher strength preparation. When given alone, the dose is generally 30–60mg q6h–q4h. Higher doses can be given but equivalent doses of morphine are more reliable and less constipating. Codeine tablets are an effective antitussive; codeine linctus provides an alternative mode of administration in a dose of 15mg/5ml. The dose is tailored to need, e.g. 15–30mg p.r.n.–q4h. To control diarrhoea, a dose of 30–60mg is used, also p.r.n.–q4h according to circumstances (see also **loperamide**, p.14). It does not make sense to prescribe codeine to patients already taking morphine; if a greater antitussive or antidiarrhoeal effect is needed, the dose of morphine should be increased.

Supply
Tablets 15mg, 20 = 35p; 30mg, 20 = 39p; 60mg, 20 = 97p.
Compound tablets see Table 5.9.
Syrup 25mg/5ml, 100ml = 87p.
Linctus 15mg/5ml, 100ml = 38p.
Diabetic linctus 15mg/5ml, 100ml = 68p.
Injections of codeine are available but are not recommended.

Table 5.9 Compound preparations containing codeine phosphate

Generic name	Codeine content	Nonopioid content	Net price
Co-codaprin 8/400 *tablets*	8mg	aspirin 400mg	20 = 26p
Co-codaprin 8/400 *dispersible tablets*	8mg	aspirin 400mg	20 = 54p
Co-codamol 8/500 *tablets*	8mg	paracetamol 500mg	20 = 23p
Co-codamol 8/500 *dispersible tablets*	8mg	paracetamol 500mg	20 = 65p
Co-codamol 30/500 *tablets*	30mg	paracetamol 500mg	20 = £1.50
Co-codamol 30/500 *effervescent tablets*[a]	30mg	paracetamol 500mg	20 = £1.89

a. contain 13.6mmol Na$^+$/tablet; avoid in renal impairment or cardiac failure.

1 Beaver WT (1966) Mild analgesics: a review of their clinical pharmacology (part II). *American Journal of Medical Science.* **251**: 576–599.
2 Cleary J et al. (1994) The influence of pharmacogenetics on opioid analgesia: studies with codeine and oxycodone in the Sprague-Dawley/Dark Agouti rat model. *Journal of Pharmacology and Experimental Therapeutics.* **271**: 1528–1534.
3 Hanks G and Cherry N (1997) Opioid analgesic therapy. In: Doyle D, Hanks GWC, MacDonald N (eds) *Oxford Textbook of Palliative Medicine. (2nd edn)* Oxford University Press, Oxford. pp 331–355.
4 Quiding H et al. (1993) Analgesic effect and plasma concentrations of codeine and morphine after two dose levels of codeine following oral surgery. *European Journal of Clinical Pharmacology.* **44**: 319–323.
5 Persson K et al. (1992) The postoperative pharmacokinetics of codeine. *European Journal of Clinical Pharmacology.* **42**: 663–666.

DEXTROPROPOXYPHENE   BNF 4.7.2

Class: Weak opioid analgesic.

Indications: Pain unrelieved by nonopioids alone.

Pharmacology

Propoxyphene is a synthetic derivative of methadone and its analgesic properties reside in the dextro-isomer, dextropropoxyphene. It is a μ agonist with receptor affinity similar to that of codeine. It is also a weak NMDA-receptor antagonist.[1] Dextropropoxyphene undergoes extensive first-pass hepatic metabolism; this is dose-dependent and systemic availability increases with increasing doses.[2] The principal metabolite, norpropoxyphene, is also analgesic but crosses the blood-brain barrier to a much lesser extent. Both dextropropoxyphene and norpropoxyphene achieve steady-state plasma concentrations 5–7 times greater than those after the first dose. Randomized controlled trials in patients with postsurgical pain, arthritis and musculoskeletal pain collectively show no added benefit when dextropropoxyphene is combined with paracetamol compared with paracetamol alone.[3] Such reports have led to doubts about the general efficacy of dextropropoxyphene. However, dextropropoxyphene 65mg has been shown to have a definite analgesic effect in several placebo-controlled trials, and a dose-response curve has been established (Figure 5.4; placebos do not have a dose-response curve), thereby confirming its efficacy.[4] Dextropropoxyphene causes less nausea and vomiting, drowsiness and dry mouth than low-dose morphine, particularly during initial treatment.[5]

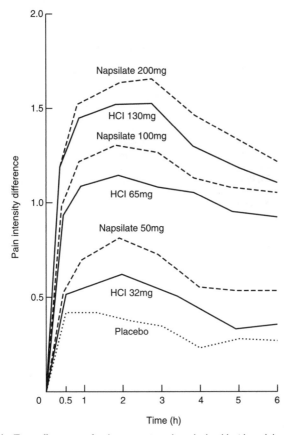

Figure 5.4 Time-effect curves for dextropropoxyphene hydrochloride and dextropropoxyphene napsilate.[4]

The relative potency of a single dose of dextropropoxyphene is 1/2–2/3 that of codeine.[2] When given regularly, dextropropoxyphene can be regarded as equipotent with codeine and dihydrocodeine. It is marketed as either the hydrochloride salt or as napsilate; dextropropoxyphene **napsilate** 100mg is equivalent to dextropropoxyphene **hydrochloride** 65mg, the difference relating to the different molecular weights of the two salts.
Onset of action 20–30min.
Duration of action 4–6h.
Plasma halflife 6–12h, increasing to >50h in elderly patients;[6] norpropoxyphene = 23h.

Cautions and adverse effects
As for other opioids (see p.107). Dextropropoxyphene may enhance the effect of oral anticoagulants, carbamazepine and other CNS depressants (including alcohol).

Dose and use
In the UK, used almost exclusively in compound tablets with paracetamol as **co-proxamol** 2 tablets t.d.s.–q4h, & p.r.n.

Supply
Tablets co-proxamol 32.5/325 (dextropropoxyphene hydrochloride 32.5mg, paracetamol 325mg), 20 = 25p.
Capsules dextropropoxyphene hydrochloride 65mg (as napsilate 100mg), 20 = £1.64 (DHS).

---

1 Ebert B et al. (1995) In: Current concepts in acute, chronic and cancer pain management. New York.
2 Perrier D and Gibaldi M (1972) Influence of first-pass effect on the systemic availability of propoxyphene. Journal of Clinical Pharmacology. 12: 449–452.
3 Li Wan Po A and Zhang WY (1997) Systematic overview of co-proxamol to assess analgesic effects of addition of dextropropoxyphene to paracetamol. British Medical Journal. 315: 1565–1571.
4 Beaver WT (1984) Analgesic efficacy of dextropropoxyphene and dextropropoxyphene-containing combinations: a review. Human Toxicology. 3: 191s–220s.
5 Mercadante S et al. (1998) Dextropropoxyphene versus morphine in opioid-naïve cancer patients with pain. Journal of Pain and Symptom Management. 15: 76–81.
6 Crome P et al. (1984) Pharmacokinetics of dextropropoxyphene and nordextropropoxyphene in elderly hospital patients after single and multiple doses of Distalgesic. Preliminary analysis of results. Human Toxicology. 3: 43s–48s.

DIHYDROCODEINE   BNF 4.7.2

Class: Weak opioid analgesic.

Indications: Pain unrelieved by nonopioids alone.

Pharmacology
Dihydrocodeine is a semisynthetic analogue of codeine. Like codeine it is an analgesic, antitussive and antidiarrhoeal. Its potency relative to SC morphine 10mg varies from 30–70mg.[1] By injection 60mg provides significantly more analgesia than 30mg but 90mg provides little more than 60mg. Dihydrocodeine is approximately twice as potent as codeine parenterally but, because its oral bio-availability is low, the two drugs are essentially equipotent by mouth.[2]
Bio-availability 20%.
Onset of action 30min.
Duration of action 3–6h.
Plasma halflife 3.5–4.5h.

Cautions and adverse effects

As for other opioids (see p.107). Like morphine and codeine, dihydrocodeine is more toxic in renal failure, probably because of cumulation of an active glucuronide.[3]

Dose and use

The usual starting dose is 30mg q6h–q4h, increasing to 60mg q6h–q4h. The higher dose is associated with a significant increase in adverse effects.[4]

Supply

Tablets 30mg, 20 = 56p.
Tablets m/r 60mg, 20 = £2.35; 90mg, 20 = £3.70; 120mg, 20 = £4.94.
Solution 10mg/5ml, 150ml = £2.40.
Injection CD 50mg/ml, 1ml amp = £1.49.

---

1 Palmer RN *et al.* (1966) Incidence of unwanted effects of dihydrocodeine bitartrate in healthy volunteers. *Lancet.* **ii**: 620–621.

2 Anonymous (1991) Dihydrocodeine (tartrate). In: Dollery C (ed) *Therapeutic Drugs.* Churchill Livingstone, Edinburgh. pp D133–136.

3 Barnes JN *et al.* (1985) Dihydrocodeine in renal failure: further evidence for an important role of the kidney in the handling of opioid drugs. *British Medical Journal.* **290**: 740–742.

4 McQuay HJ *et al.* (1993) A multiple dose comparison of ibuprofen and dihydrocodeine after third molar surgery. *British Journal of Oral and Maxillofacial Surgery.* **31**: 95–100.

TRAMADOL   BNF 4.7.2

Class: Weak opioid analgesic.

Indications: Pain unrelieved by nonopioids.

Pharmacology

Tramadol is a synthetic centrally acting analgesic. It has both opioid and nonopioid properties.[1,2] The latter are related to stimulation of neuronal serotonin release and inhibition of presynaptic re-uptake of norepinephrine (noradrenaline) and serotonin. Naloxone only partially reverses the analgesic effect of tramadol.[1] Tramadol is converted in the liver to O-desmethyltramadol which is itself an active substance, 2–4 times more potent than tramadol. Further biotransformation results in inactive metabolites which are excreted by the kidneys. A comparison of receptor site affinities and mono-amine re-uptake inhibition illustrates the unique combination of properties which underlie the action of tramadol (Table 5.10 & 5.11); it is necessary to invoke synergism to explain its analgesic effect. Tramadol causes much less constipation and respiratory depression than equi-analgesic doses of morphine.[3] Its dependence liability is also considerably less,[4] and it is not a CD.[5] By injection, tramadol is 1/10 as potent as morphine. By mouth, because of much better bio-availability, it is 1/5 as potent; it can be regarded as double strength codeine.

Oral bio-availability 75%; >90% with multiple doses.[6]
Onset of action 30min.
Duration of action 4–6h.
Plasma halflife 6.3h; active metabolite 7.4h.

Table 5.10   Opioid receptor affinities: K_i (μM) values[1] [a]

	Mu	Delta	Kappa
Morphine	0.0003	0.09	0.6
Dextropropoxyphene	0.03	0.38	1.2
Codeine	0.2	5	6
Tramadol	2	58	43

a. the lower the K_i value, the greater the receptor affinity.

Table 5.11 Inhibition of mono-amine uptake: K_i (μM) values[1] [a]

	Norepinephrine (noradrenaline)	Serotonin
Imipramine	0.0066	0.021
Tramadol	0.78	0.99
Dextropropoxyphene Codeine Morphine	IA[b]	IA[b]

a. the lower the K_i value, the greater the receptor affinity
b. IA = inactive at 10uM.

Cautions
Epilepsy, raised intracranial pressure, severe renal or hepatic impairment. Use with caution in patients taking medication which lowers seizure threshold, notably tricyclic antidepressants and SSRIs. Carbamazepine decreases the effect of tramadol.

Adverse effects
Similar to other opioids but generally less at recommended dose, i.e. ≤400mg/24h. Convulsions have been reported in patients receiving tramadol after rapid IV injection.

Dose and use
• usual oral doses are 50–100mg q4h–q6h
• maximum recommended dose = 400mg/day; higher doses have been given, e.g. 600mg/day, and sometimes more.

Supply
Capsules 50mg, 20 = £3.04.
Tablets soluble 50mg, 20 = £3.19.
Tablets m/r 100mg, 20 = £6.37; 150mg, 20 = £9.56; 200mg, 20 = £12.75.
Injection 50mg/ml, 2ml amp = £1.30.

1 Raffa RB et al. (1992) Opioid and nonopioid components independently contribute to the mechanism of action of tramadol, an 'atypical' opioid analgesic. *Journal of Pharmacology and Experimental Therapeutics.* **260**: 275–285.
2 Lee CR et al. (1993) Tramadol: a preliminary review of its pharmacodynamic and pharmacokinetic properties, and therapeutic potential in acute and chronic pain states. *Drugs.* **46**: 313–340.
3 Wilder-Smith CH and Bettiga A (1997) The analgesic tramadol has minimal effect on gastrointestinal motor function. *British Journal of Clinical Pharmacology.* **43**: 71–75.
4 Preston KL et al. (1991) Abuse potential and pharmacological comparison of tramadol and morphine. *Drug and Alcohol Dependence.* **27**: 7–18.
5 Radbruch L et al. (1996) A risk-benefit assessment of tramadol in the management of pain. *Drug Safety.* **15**: 8–29.
6 Gibson TP (1996) Pharmacokinetics, efficacy and safety of analgesia with a focus on tramadol HCl. *American Journal of Medicine.* **101** (suppl 1A): 47S–53S.

STRONG OPIOIDS   BNF 4.7.2

Globally, morphine remains the strong opioid of choice;[1] other strong opioids are used mainly when morphine is not readily available or when the patient has intolerable adverse effects with morphine (see p.110). Differences between opioids relate in part to differences in receptor affinity (Table 5.12).

Table 5.12 Receptor affinity of opioid analgesics and naloxone[2,3]

Drug	Receptor type		
	Mu	Kappa	Delta
Morphine ⎫			
Fentanyl ⎬	A	–	–
Hydromorphone ⎭			
Oxycodone	A(?)	A(?)	–
Methadone	A	–	A
Buprenorphine	pA	Ant	A
Pentazocine	pA	A	ant
Pethidine	a	–	–
Naloxone	Ant	Ant	Ant

A = strong agonist; a = weak agonist; Ant = strong antagonist; ant = weak antagonist; pA = partial agonist; – = negligible or no activity.

Strong opioids tend to cause the same range of adverse effects (Table 5.13), although to a varying degree. *Because pain is a physiological antagonist to the central depressant effects of morphine,* strong opioids do not cause clinically important respiratory depression in cancer patients in pain when used correctly.[4] Further, in contrast to postoperative patients, cancer patients with pain:
• generally have already been receiving a weak opioid (i.e. are not opioid naive)
• take medication by mouth (slower absorption, lower peak concentration)
• titrate the dose upwards step by step (less likelihood of an excessive dose being given).
It is therefore extremely rare to need to use **naloxone** (a specific opioid antagonist) in palliative care (see p.123). Because of the possibility of an additive sedative effect, care needs to be taken when strong opioids and psychotropic drugs are used concurrently.

Table 5.13 Adverse effects of opioid analgesics

Common initial	*Occasional*
Nausea and vomiting	Dry mouth
Drowsiness	Sweating
Unsteadiness	Pruritus
Delirium (confusion)	Hallucinations
	Myoclonus
Common ongoing	*Rare*
Constipation	Respiratory depression
Nausea and vomiting	Psychological dependence

Tolerance to strong opioids is not a practical problem. The fear of patients developing psychological dependence (addiction) is unfounded and should not limit the use of strong opioids for cancer pain. Caution in this respect should be reserved for patients with a present or past history of substance abuse; even then strong opioids should be used when there is clinical need. Physical dependence does not prevent a reduction in the dose of a strong opioid if the patient's pain ameliorates, e.g. as a result of radiotherapy or a nerve block.[5]

Pethidine and **dextromoramide** have short durations of action and are not recommended for round-the-clock prophylactic analgesia. Because of its rapid onset of action, some centres use dextromoramide for breakthrough pain in patients taking regular morphine, or as prophylactic additonal analgesia before a painful dressing or other procedure. However, at other centres, such procedures are timed to coincide with the peak plasma concentration after a regular or p.r.n. dose of morphine. **Pentazocine** should not be used; it is a weak opioid by mouth and often causes psychotomimetic effects (dysphoria, depersonalization, frightening dreams, hallucinations). When converting from an alternative strong opioid to oral morphine, the initial dose depends on the relative potency of the two drugs (Table 5.14).

Opioid substitution

In patients who have intolerable adverse effects with morphine (see p.110), it may be necessary to substitute an alternative strong opioid. For adverse effects such as cognitive failure, hallucinations or myoclonus, *hydromorphone** and *oxycodone (where available) have been used. However, for patients experiencing opioid-induced hyperexcitability,[6-8] **methadone** is preferable (see p.120). Methadone is also the opioid of choice for patients with morphine poorly-responsive neuropathic pain.[9]

Table 5.14 Approximate oral analgesic equivalence to morphine[a]

Analgesic	Potency ratio with morphine	Duration of action (h)[b]
Codeine	1/10	3–6
Dihydrocodeine		
Pethidine	1/8	2–4
Tramadol	1/5[c]	4–6
Dipipanone (in Diconal UK)	1/2	4–6
Papaveretum	2/3[d]	3–5
Oxycodone	1.5–2[c]	3–4
Dextromoramide	[2][e]	2–3
Levorphanol	5	4–6
Phenazocine	5	6–8
Methadone	5–10[f]	8–12
Hydromorphone	7.5	4–5
Buprenorphine (sublingual)	60	6–8
Fentanyl (transdermal)	150	72

a. multiply dose of opioid by its potency ratio to determine the equivalent dose of morphine sulphate

b. dependent in part on severity of pain and on dose; often longer-lasting in very elderly and those with renal dysfunction

c. tramadol and oxycodone are both relatively more potent by mouth because of high bio-availability; parenteral potency ratios with morphine are 1/10 and 3/4 respectively

d. papaveretum (strong opium) is standardized to contain 50% morphine base; potency expressed in relation to morphine sulphate

e. dextromoramide: a single 5mg dose is equivalent to morphine 15mg in terms of peak effect but is shorter-acting; overall potency ratio adjusted accordingly

f. methadone: a single 5mg dose is equivalent to morphine 7.5mg. Has a variable long plasma halflife and broad-spectrum receptor affinity resulting in a much higher than expected potency ratio when given repeatedly.[10]

1 World Health Organization (1986) *Cancer Pain Relief.* World Health Organization, Geneva.

2 Hill RG (1992) Multiple opioid receptors and their ligands. *Frontiers of Pain.* **4**: 1–4.

3 Corbett AD *et al.* (1993) Selectivity of ligands for opioid receptors. In: Herz A (ed) *Opioids I.* Springer Verlag, London. pp 657–672.

4 Borgbjerg FM *et al.* (1996) Experimental pain stimulates respiration and attenuates morphine-induced respiratory depression: a controlled study in human volunteers. *Pain.* **64**: 123–128.

5 Twycross RG (1994) *Pain relief in advanced cancer. (2nd edn)* Churchill Livingstone, Edinburgh. pp 339–342.

6 Sjogren P *et al.* (1993) Hyperalgesia and myoclonus in terminal cancer patients treated with continuous intravenous morphine. *Pain.* **55**: 93–97.

7 Sjogren P *et al.* (1994) Disappearance of morphine-induced hyperalgesia after discontinuing or substituting morphine with other opioid antagonists. *Pain.* **59**: 313–316.

* specialist use only.

8 Hagen N and Wanson R (1997) Strychnine-like multifocal myoclonus and seizures in extremely high-dose opioid administration: treatment strategies. *Journal of Pain and Symptom Management*. **14**: 51–58.
9 Morley JS and Makin MK (1998) The use of methadone in cancer pain poorly responsive to other opioids. *Pain Reviews*. **5**: 51–58.
10 Bruera E *et al.* (1996) Opioid rotation in patients with cancer pain. *Cancer*. **78**: 852–857.

MORPHINE   BNF 4.7.2

Class of drug: Strong opioid analgesic.

Indications: Pain poorly-responsive to the combined use of a weak opioid and a nonopioid, [†]diarrhoea, [†]cough, [†]dyspnoea.

Contra-indications: None, if titrated carefully against a patient's pain.

Pharmacology

Morphine is the main pharmacologically active constituent of opium. Its effects are mediated by specific opioid receptors, mainly within the CNS (see p.107); peripherally its main action is on smooth muscle. It is readily absorbed by all routes of administration. When given regularly, the oral to SC potency ratio is normally between 1:2 and 1:3; the same ratio holds true for IM and IV injections.[1,2] The liver is the principal site of morphine metabolism.[3] Metabolism also occurs in other organs,[4] notably the CNS.[5] Glucuronidation is rarely impaired in hepatic failure,[2] and morphine is well tolerated in most patients with hepatic impairment;[6] although with impairment severe enough to prolong the prothrombin time, the plasma halflife of morphine may be increased[4] and the dose of morphine may need to be reduced or given less often, i.e. q6h–q8h. The major metabolites of morphine are morphine-3-glucuronide (M3G) and morphine-6-glucuronide (M6G);[7] M6G binds to opioid receptors whereas M3G does not. M6G contributes substantially to the analgesic effect of morphine in humans, can cause nausea and vomiting,[8] and respiratory depression.[9]

Oral bio-availability 35% (ranging from 16-68%).
Onset of action 20–30min.
Duration of action 3–6h.
Plasma halflife 1.5–4.5h PO; 1.5h IV.

Adverse effects: Table 5.13 (see p.107) & Table 5.15.

Dose and use

Morphine should generally be given together with a nonopioid. Morphine is administered as tablets ('normal release' 10mg, 20mg, 50mg) or aqueous solutions (10mg/5ml, 100mg/5ml). An increasing range of m/r preparations is available – tablets, capsules and suspensions. There are no generic m/r morphine tablets. Because of differing pharmacokinetic profiles, it is best to keep individual patients on the same brand. Most are administered b.d., some o.d. Patients can be started on either an ordinary (normal release) or a m/r preparation (Box 5.B).

When adjusting the dose of morphine, generally increase by 33–50%. 2/3 of patients never need more than 30mg q4h (or m/r morphine 100mg q12h); the rest need up to 200mg q4h (or m/r morphine 600mg q12h), and occasionally more. Instructions must be clear: extra p.r.n. morphine does not mean that the next dose of regular morphine is omitted. The p.r.n. dose is the same as the q4h dose of morphine and *is increased when the regular dose is increased.* An antiemetic should be supplied, e.g. **haloperidol** 1.5mg stat & o.n (see p.57) and a laxative, e.g. **codanthrusate** or **senna + docusate** (see p.15).

Suppositories and enemas continue to be necessary in about 1/3 of patients. *Constipation may be more difficult to manage than the pain.* Warn patients about the possibility of initial drowsiness. If swallowing is difficult or vomiting persists, give 1/3 of the oral dose as CSCI **diamorphine** (or 1/2 the oral dose of morphine as CSCI morphine). Alternatively, morphine may be given PR (same dose as PO).

[†] unlicensed use.

Table 5.15 Potential intolerable effects of morphine[10]

For general adverse effects of opioid analgesics see Table 5.13, p.107.

Type	Effects	Initial action	Comment
Gastric stasis	Epigastric fullness, flatulence, anorexia, hiccup persistent nausea	Metoclopramide 10–20mg q4h; cisapride 10–20mg b.d.	If the problem persists, change to an alternative opioid
Sedation	Intolerable persistent sedation	Reduce dose of morphine; consider methylphenidate 10mg o.d.–b.d.	Sedation may be caused by other factors; stimulant rarely appropriate
Cognitive failure	Agitated delirium with hallucinations	Reduce dose of morphine and/or prescribe haloperidol 3–5mg stat & o.n.; if necessary switch to an alternative opioid	Some patients develop intractable delirium with one opioid but not with an alternative opioid
Myoclonus	Multifocal twitching ± jerking of limbs	Reduce dose of morphine but revert to former dose if pain recurs; consider a benzodiazepine	Unusual with typical oral doses; more common with high dose IV and spinal morphine
Hyperexcitability	Abdominal muscle spasms and symmetrical jerking of legs; whole-body allodynia and hyperalgesia manifesting as excruciating pain	Reduce dose of morphine; consider changing to an alternative opioid	A rare syndrome in patients receiving IT or high-dose IV morphine; occasionally seen with typical PO and SC doses
Vestibular stimulation	Incapacitating movement-induced nausea and vomiting	Cyclizine or dimenhydrinate or promethazine 25–50mg q8h–q6h	Rare; try an alternative opioid or levomepromazine (methotrimeprazine)
Histamine release cutaneous	Pruritus	Oral antihistamine (e.g. chlorphenamine (chlorpheniramine) 4mg b.d.–t.d.s.)	If the pruritus does not settle in a few days, prescribe an alternative opioid
bronchial	Bronchoconstriction → dyspnoea	IV/IM antihistamine (e.g. chlorphenamine (chlorpheniramine) 5–10mg) and a bronchodilator	Rare; change to a chemically distinct opioid immediately e.g. methadone or phenazocine

---

Box 5.B   Starting a patient on morphine PO

Oral morphine is indicated in patients with pain which does not respond to the optimized combined use of a nonopioid and a weak opioid.

The starting dose of morphine is calculated to give a greater analgesic effect than the medication already in use:

- if the patient was previously receiving a weak opioid, give 10mg q4h or m/r 30mg q12h
- if changing from an alternative strong opioid (e.g. fentanyl, methadone) a much higher dose of morphine may be needed (see p.108).

With frail elderly patients, however, consider starting on a lower dose (e.g. 5mg q4h) in order to reduce initial drowsiness, confusion and unsteadiness.

Upward titration of the dose of morphine stops when either the pain is relieved or intolerable adverse effects supervene. In the latter case, it is generally necessary to consider alternative measures. The aim is to have the patient free of pain and mentally alert.

M/r morphine may not be satisfactory in patients troubled by frequent vomiting or those with diarrhoea or an ileostomy.

Scheme 1: ordinary (normal release) morphine tablets or solution

- morphine given q4h 'by the clock' with p.r.n. doses of equal amount
- after 1–2 days, recalculate q4h dose based on total used in previous 24h (i.e. regular + p.r.n. use)
- continue q4h and p.r.n. doses
- increase the regular dose until treatment gives adequate relief from pain, maintaining availability of p.r.n. doses
- *a double dose at bedtime obviates the need to wake the patient for treatment during the night.*

Scheme 2: ordinary (normal release) morphine and m/r morphine

- begin as for Scheme 1
- when the q4h dose is stable, it is replaced with m/r morphine q12h, or o.d. if a 24h preparation is prescribed
- the q12h dose will be *three times* the previous q4h dose; an o.d. dose will be *six times* the previous q4h dose, rounded to a convenient number of tablets
- continue to provide ordinary morphine tablets or solution for p.r.n. use.

Scheme 3: m/r morphine when ordinary (normal release) morphine is unavailable

(In some countries, q12h m/r morphine is available but ordinary morphine preparations are not.)

- starting dose generally m/r morphine 20–30mg b.d.
- use a weak opioid or an alternative strong opioid for p.r.n. medication
- dose of m/r morphine adjusted until adequate relief throughout each 12h period
- if of benefit, maintain the availability of p.r.n. doses of a weak opioid or an alternative strong opioid.

Supply

Unless indicated otherwise, all morphine preparations are **CD**.
Oramorph oral solution 10mg/5ml **(POM)**, 100ml = £2.31; 250ml = £5.36; 500ml = £9.70.
Oramorph oral concentrate 100mg/5ml, 30ml = £6.47; 120ml = £24.15.
Oramorph unit dose vials 10mg/5ml **(POM)**, 25 = £3.31; 30mg/5ml, 25 = £9.30; 100mg/5ml, 25 = £31.00.
Sevredol tablets 10mg, 56 = £6.31; 20mg, 56 = £12.62; 50mg, 56 = £31.55.
M/r preparations (see Table 5.16).
Injection 10, 15, 20 and 30mg/ml, 1 and 2 ml amps (all) = 64–96p.
Suppositories (hydrochloride or sulphate) 10mg, 12 = £6.12; 15mg, 12 = £5.53; 20mg, 12 = £7.45; 30mg, 12 = £8.50.

Table 5.16   Prices of morphine m/r preparations for 30 days (£)

	Morcap	MST tablets	MST suspension	Oramorph SR	Zomorph capsules[a]	MXL capsules
5mg b.d.		4.50				
10mg b.d.		7.51		5.75	4.51	
15mg b.d.		13.16				
30mg o.d.						13.16
20mg b.d.	11.42		57.20			
30mg b.d.		18.03	59.44	13.80	10.82	
60mg o.d.						18.03
50mg b.d.	27.68					
60mg b.d.		35.16	118.88	26.89	21.10	
90mg o.d.						26.59
120mg o.d.						35.16
150mg o.d.						43.95
100mg b.d.	55.36	55.67	198.14	42.59	33.40	
200mg o.d.						55.67
200mg b.d.		111.35	396.28		66.80	

a. the contents of Zomorph capsules can be administered as a suspension or if preferred they can be added to hot liquids (e.g. soup). After 15min in water at 50°C, only 9% of the morphine is released (but 42% by 30min).[11]

1 Hanks GW et al. (1996) Morphine in cancer pain: modes of administration. *British Medical Journal.* **312**: 823–826.
2 Max MB and Payne R (Co-chairs) (1992) *Principles of analgesic use in the treatment of acute pain and cancer management.* American Pain Society. p 12.
3 Hasselstrom J et al. (1986) Morphine metabolism in patients with liver cirrhosis. *Acta Pharmacologica et Toxicologica.* (suppl V): abstract 101.
4 Mazoit J-X et al. (1987) Pharmacokinetics of unchanged morphine in normal and cirrhotic subjects. *Anesthesia and Analgesia.* **66**: 293–298.
5 Sandouk P et al. (1991) Presence of morphine metabolites in human cerebrospinal fluid after intracerebroventricular administration of morphine. *European Journal of Drug Metabolism and Pharmacology.* **16** (suppl 3): 166–171.
6 Regnard CFB and Twycross RG (1984) Metabolism of narcotics. *British Medical Journal.* **288**: 860.
7 McQuay HJ et al. (1990) Oral morphine in cancer pain: influences on morphine and metabolite concentration. *Clinical Pharmacology and Therapeutics.* **48**: 236–244.
8 Thompson PI et al. (1992) Morphine 6-glucuronide: a metabolite of morphine with greater emetic potency than morphine in the ferret. *British Journal of Pharmacology.* **106**: 3–8.
9 Osborne RJ et al. (1986) Morphine intoxication in renal failure: the role of morphine-6-glucuronide. *British Medical Journal.* **292**: 1548–1549.

10 Twycross R (1997) Update on analgesics. In: Kaye P (ed) *Tutorials in Palliative Medicine*. EPL Publications, Northampton. pp 94–131.

11 Data on file (1997) Link Pharmaceuticals.

DIAMORPHINE   BNF 4.7.2

Class of drug: Strong opioid analgesic.

Indications: As for morphine; used in the UK instead of parenteral morphine.

Contra-indications: As for morphine.

Pharmacology

Diamorphine (di-acetylmorphine, heroin) is a prodrug without intrinsic activity.[1] *In vivo* or in solution, it is rapidly de-acetylated to mono-acetylmorphine and then more slowly to morphine itself.[2] It is well absorbed by all routes of administration. Because of greater lipid-solubility, diamorphine and mono-acetylmorphine cross the blood-brain barrier more readily than morphine. This accounts for the observed potency difference between parenteral diamorphine and morphine. IM diamorphine is more than twice as potent as morphine; PO, however, the two opioids are almost equipotent. In terms of analgesic efficacy and effect on mood, diamorphine has no clinical advantage over morphine by oral or IM routes.[3–5] Diamorphine is much more soluble than morphine sulphate/hydrochloride and is the strong opioid of choice for parenteral use in the UK because large amounts can be given in very small volumes (Table 5.17).

Oral bio-availability probably zero; unknown percentage available as mono-acetylmorphine.
Onset of action 10–30min to peak analgesia IM.
Duration of action 3–4h.
Plasma halflife 3min; metabolized to active metabolites.

Table 5.17 Solubility of selected opioids[6]

Preparation	Amount of water needed to dissolve 1g at 25°C (ml)
Morphine	5000
Morphine hydrochloride	24
Morphine sulphate	21
Diamorphine hydrochloride	1.6[a]
Hydromorphone	3

a. 1g of diamorphine hydrochloride dissolved in 1.6ml has a volume of 2.4ml.

Morphine : diamorphine potency ratio

Diamorphine IM is 2–2.5 times more potent than morphine IM.[4,5,7] If diamorphine is only a prodrug, this is perhaps surprising. The following points provide an explanation:

- diamorphine is a prodrug for mono-acetylmorphine as well as morphine
- mono-acetylmorphine may well be more potent than morphine[8]
- by injection, hepatic first-pass metabolism is circumvented and more mono-acetylmorphine will be available
- diamorphine is highly lipophilic and crosses the blood-brain barrier more readily than morphine.

Adverse effects: See p.107.

Dose and use

The following conversion ratios are approximate but serve as a general guide:

- PO morphine to SC diamorphine, give 1/3 of the PO dose
- PO diamorphine to SC diamorphine, give 1/2 the PO dose.

Supply

Diamorphine hydrochloride is available for medicinal use only in the UK.

Tablets 10mg, 100 = £11.20.

Injection (powder for reconstitution) 5mg amp = £1.16; 10mg amp = £1.34; 30mg amp = £1.60; 100mg amp = £4.42; 500mg amp = £20.68.

1 Inturrisi CE et al. (1984) The pharmacokinetics of heroin in patients with chronic pain. New England Journal of Medicine. **310**: 1213–1217.
2 Barrett DA et al. (1992) The effect of temperature and pH on the deacetylation of diamorphine in aqueous solution and in human plasma. Journal of Pharmacy and Pharmacology. **44**: 606–608.
3 Twycross RG (1977) Choice of strong analgesic in terminal cancer: diamorphine or morphine? Pain. **3**: 93–104.
4 Beaver WT (1981) Comparison of the analgesic effect of intramuscular heroin and morphine in patients with cancer pain. Clinical Pharmacology and Therapeutics. **29**: 232.
5 Kaiko RF et al. (1981) Analgesic and mood effects of heroin and morphine in cancer patients with postoperative pain. New England Journal of Medicine. **304**: 1501–1505.
6 Hanks GW and Hoskin PJ (1987) Opioid analgesics in the management of pain in patients with cancer: a review. Palliative Medicine. **1**: 1–25.
7 Reichle CW et al. (1962) Comparative analgesic potency of heroin and morphine in postoperative patients. Journal of Pharmacology. **136**: 43–46.
8 Wright CI and Barbour FA (1935) The respiratory effects of morphine, codeine and related substances. Journal of Pharmacology and Experimental Therapeutics. **54**: 25–33.

BUPRENORPHINE   BNF 4.7.2

Class of drug: Strong opioid analgesic.

Indications: An alternative strong opioid particularly in patients with dysphagia.

Contra-indications: As for morphine.

Pharmacology

Buprenorphine is a potent partial μ agonist, κ antagonist and δ agonist. It is an alternative to oral morphine in the low to middle part of morphine's dose range. Subjective and physiological effects are generally similar to morphine. Buprenorphine is available as a *sublingual* tablet; ingestion markedly reduces bio-availability. Vomiting is more common after SL administration than after IM injection. Unlike most opioids, buprenorphine does not increase pressure within the biliary and pancreatic ducts.[1] Buprenorphine does slow intestinal transit,[2] but probably less so than morphine. In low doses, buprenorphine and morphine are additive in their effects; at very high doses, antagonism by buprenorphine may occur. There is no need, however, to prescribe both; use one or the other. Naloxone does not reverse the effect of buprenorphine when used in standard doses (see p.123). Serious respiratory depression, however, is unlikely to occur in clinical practice. The manufacturers recommend doxapram, a nonspecific respiratory stimulant, in the event of difficulties following massive self-poisoning. It is generally considered that there is an analgesic ceiling at a daily dose of 3–5mg; equivalent to 180–300mg of oral morphine/24h. In some countries, 1.6mg is regarded as the ceiling daily dose. Whether this represents genetic differences or local custom is not clear.

Bio-availability 90% SL (400µg SL is equivalent to 300µg IM).

Onset of action 30min; peak effect 3h.

Duration of action 6–9h.

Plasma halflife 3h.

Adverse effects: *See p.107.*

Dose and use
If previously receiving a weak opioid, a patient should start on 200µg q8h with the advice that, 'If it is not more effective than your previous tablets, take a further 200µg after 1h, and 400µg q8h after that.' With daily doses of over 3mg, patients may prefer to take fewer tablets q6h. Buprenorphine SL is about 60 times more potent than morphine PO. Thus when changing from an *unsatisfactory* buprenorphine regimen to morphine PO, the total daily dose of buprenorphine should be multiplied by 100 to give the appropriate *total daily dose* of morphine. Adverse effects, e.g. nausea, vomiting, constipation, drowsiness, need to be monitored as with morphine.

Supply
Tablets SL 200µg, 50 = £6; 400µg, 50 = £12.
Injection 300µg/ml, 1ml amp = 55p.

---

1 Staritz M et al. (1985) Pentazocine hampers bile flow. Lancet. i: 573–574.
2 Anonymous (1979) Buprenorphine injection (Temgesic). Drug and Therapeutics Bulletin. 17: 17–19.

FENTANYL   BNF 4.7.2

Class of drug: Strong opioid analgesic.

Indications: An alternative strong opioid in cases of intolerable adverse effects with morphine, severe morphine-induced constipation, and in patients who find it difficult to take oral medication.

Contra-indications: The need for rapid titration of strong opioid medication for severe pain.

Pharmacology
Fentanyl, like morphine, is mainly a strong µ agonist. It is widely used IV as a peri-operative analgesic. Transdermal patches are available for cancer pain management. Steady-state plasma concentrations of fentanyl are achieved after 36–48h.[1] Time to reach a minimal effective plasma concentration ranges from 3–23h.[1] After removal of a patch, the elimination plasma halflife is almost 24h.[2] Rescue medication will be necessary during the first 24h. If effective analgesia does not last for 3 days, the correct response is to increase the patch strength. Even so, some patients do best if the patch is changed every 2 days.[3] The manufacturer recommends a conversion ratio for morphine and fentanyl of 150:1 but some centres use a ratio conversion of 100:1 when deciding the initial patch strength. [4]

Transdermal fentanyl is less constipating than morphine.[3,5,6] Thus, when converting from morphine to fentanyl, the dose of laxative should be halved and subsequently adjusted according to need. Some patients experience withdrawal symptoms when changed from oral morphine to transdermal fentanyl despite satisfactory pain relief, i.e. colic, diarrhoea and nausea together with sweating and restlessness. These symptoms are easily treatable by using rescue doses of morphine until they resolve after a few days.

Transdermal fentanyl can be continued until the death of the patient, and the dose varied as necessary. Rescue medication will continue to be ordinary morphine tablets or solution (or an alternative 'normal release' strong opioid preparation). If a patient is unable to swallow, it is important to give adequate rescue doses of an alternative strong opioid (Box 5.C).

Cautions
The rate of absorption of fentanyl from the patch may be increased in febrile patients, or if the skin under the patch becomes vasodilated because of an external heat source such as an electric blanket or heat pad.

Box 5.C   Parenteral rescue medication for patients receiving transdermal fentanyl

Divide the delivery rate ('patch size') of transdermal fentanyl (μg/h):

- by 3 and give as SC morphine (mg)
- by 5 and give as SC diamorphine (mg)
- by 15 and give as SC hydromorphone (mg).

Adverse effects
Typical opioid adverse effects (see p.107); constipation less, and may be less emetogenic.

Dose and use
The use of fentanyl patches is summarized in Box 5.D. Some centres adjust the patch strength on a *daily* basis during the initial period of dose titration.[7] With inpatients, a fentanyl patch chart to record observations is helpful (Box 5.E).

Supply
Patches **(for 3 days)** 25μg/h, 5 = £28.97; 50μg/h, 5 = £54.11; 75μg/h, 5 = £75.43; 100μg/h, 5 = £92.97.

Box 5.D   Guidelines for the use of transdermal fentanyl patches

1   Transdermal fentanyl is an alternative strong opioid which can be used in place of both PO morphine and SC morphine/diamorphine in the management of cancer pain.

2   Indications for using transdermal fentanyl include:

- intractable morphine-induced constipation
- intolerable adverse effects with morphine e.g. nausea and vomiting (despite the appropriate use of anti-emetics) and/or hallucinations (despite the use of haloperidol)
- 'tablet phobia' or difficulty swallowing oral preparations
- poor compliance with oral medication.

3   Transdermal fentanyl is *contra-indicated* in patients who need rapid titration of their medication for severe uncontrolled pain.

4   *Warning*: pain not relieved by morphine will *not* be relieved by fentanyl. If in doubt, seek specialist advice before prescribing transdermal fentanyl.

5   Transdermal fentanyl patches are available in four strengths: 25, 50, 75 and 100μg/h *for 3 days*:

- patients with inadequate relief from **codeine, dextropropoxyphene** or **dihydro-codeine ≥240 mg/day** should start on 25μg/h
- patients on **oral morphine**: *divide 24h dose in mg by 3* and choose nearest patch strength in μg/h
- patients on **SC diamorphine**: choose nearest patch strength in μg/h.

Note: these doses are slightly higher than the manufacturer's recommendations.

6   Apply the transdermal fentanyl patch to *dry, non-inflamed, non-irradiated, unshaven, hairless skin* on the upper arm or trunk; body hair may be clipped but not shaved. Some patients need micropore around the edges to ensure adherence.

continued

Box 5.D Continued

7 Systemic analgesic concentrations are generally reached within 12h; so:
- if converting from **4-hourly oral morphine**, continue to give regular doses for 12h
- if converting from **12-hourly morphine** preparations, apply the fentanyl patch at the same time as giving the final 12-hourly dose
- if converting from a *syringe driver*, maintain the syringe driver for about 12h after applying the first patch.

8 Steady-state plasma concentrations of fentanyl are achieved only after 36–48h; the patient should use rescue doses liberally during the first 3 days, particularly during the first 24h. Rescue doses should be approximately half the fentanyl patch strength given as normal-release morphine in mg. [Example: with fentanyl 50μg/h, give morphine 20–30mg p.r.n.]

9 After the first 48h, if a patient continues to need 2 or more rescue doses of morphine, the patch strength should be increased by 25μg/h. When using the manufacturer's recommended starting doses, about 50% of patients need to increase the patch strength after the first 3 days.

10 If the patient continues to experience breakthrough pain on the third day after patch application, increase the patch strength and review.

11 About 10% of patients experience opioid withdrawal symptoms when changed from morphine to transdermal fentanyl. Patients should be warned that they may experience symptoms 'like gastric flu' for a few days after the change, and to use rescue doses of morphine for these symptoms.

12 Fentanyl is less constipating than morphine; halve the dose of laxatives when starting fentanyl and titrate according to need. Some patients develop diarrhoea; if troublesome, use rescue doses of morphine to control it, and completely stop laxatives.

13 Fentanyl probably causes less nausea and vomiting than morphine but, if necessary, prescribe haloperidol 1.5mg stat & nocte.

14 In febrile patients, the rate of absorption of fentanyl increases, and occasionally causes toxicity, principally drowsiness. Absorption may also be enhanced by an external heat source over the patch, e.g. electric blanket or hot-water bottle; patients should be warned about this. Patients may shower with a patch but should not soak in a hot bath.

15 Remove patches after 72h; change the position of the new patches so as to rest the underlying skin for 3–6 days.

16 A reservoir of fentanyl accumulates in the skin under the patch, and significant blood levels persist for 24h, sometimes more, after removing the patch. This only matters, of course, if transdermal fentanyl is discontinued.

17 In moribund patients, it is best to continue transdermal fentanyl and give rescue doses of SC diamorphine based on the 'rule of 5', i.e. divide the patch strength by 5 and give as **mg of diamorphine**. [Example: with fentanyl 100μg/h, use diamorphine 20mg as needed.]

18 In moribund patients, should it be decided to replace the patch by **continuous SC diamorphine**:
- give *half the patch strength as mg/24h* rounded up to a convenient ampoule size
- after 24h, give *the whole of the previous patch strength as mg/24h* rounded up to a convenient ampoule size.

19 Transdermal fentanyl patches are unsatisfactory in some patients, generally because of failure to remain adherent or allergy to the silicone medical adhesive.

20 Used patches still contain fentanyl. After removal, fold the patch with the adhesive side inwards and discard in a sharps container (hospital) or dustbin (home); wash hands. Ultimately, any unused patches should be returned to a pharmacy.

Box 5.E Fentanyl patch chart: nursing record

Nottingham City Hospital NHS Trust
HAYWARD HOUSE
Fentanyl Patch Chart

Patient name:

Date of birth:

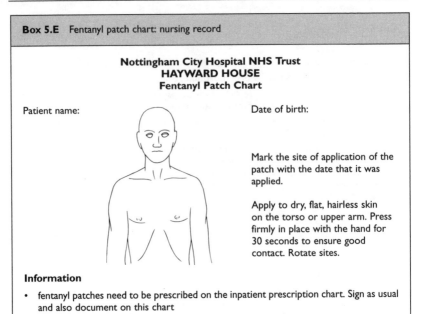

Mark the site of application of the patch with the date that it was applied.

Apply to dry, flat, hairless skin on the torso or upper arm. Press firmly in place with the hand for 30 seconds to ensure good contact. Rotate sites.

Information

- fentanyl patches need to be prescribed on the inpatient prescription chart. Sign as usual and also document on this chart

- a nurse should check that each patch is still in place at 1000h and 2200h and sign. Comments should be made if a problem is found, stating action taken (e.g. patch lifted so needed to be secured with Tegaderm)

- fentanyl patches should be replaced every 72 hours. After removal, fold patches in half with the adhesive side inwards and discard in a sharps bin, witnessed by a second nurse and signed for.

Date and time patch applied	Strength and number of patches Site	Signature	B.d. observations				Removal and destruction Date/Time/Sign Comments
			1000h	Sign	2200h	Sign	
Example					23/2 ✓	AS	26/2/98
23/2/98	25mcg/h × 1	S Thorp	24/2 ✓	ST	24/2 ✓	MB	1000h
1000h	Left arm		25/2 ✓	ST	25/2 ✓	MB	S Thorp
			26/2 ✓	AS			A Smith

1 Gourlay GK et al. (1989) The transdermal administration of fentanyl in the treatment of post-operative pain: pharmacokinetics and pharmacodynamic effects. Pain. 37: 193–202.

2 Portenoy RK et al. (1993) Transdermal fentanyl for cancer pain. Anesthesiology. 78: 36–43.

3 Donner B et al. (1998) Long-term treatment of cancer pain with transdermal fentanyl. Journal of Pain and Symptom Management. 15: 168–175.

4 Donner B et al. (1996) Direct conversion from oral morphine to transdermal fentanyl: a multicenter study in patients with cancer pain. Pain. 64: 527–534.

5 Ahmedzai S and Brooks D (1997) Transdermal fentanyl versus sustained-release oral morphine in cancer pain: preference, efficacy, and quality of life. Journal of Pain and Symptom Management. 13: 254–261.

6 Grond S et al. (1997) Transdermal fentanyl in the long-term treatment of cancer pain: a prospective study of 50 patients with advanced cancer of the gastrointestinal tract or the head and neck region. Pain. 69: 191–198.

7 Korte W et al. (1996) Day-to-day titration to initiate transdermal fentanyl in patients with cancer pain: short- and long-term experiences in a postoperative study of 39 patients. Journal of Pain and Symptom Management. 11: 139–146.

*HYDROMORPHONE   BNF 4.7.2

Class of drug: Strong opioid analgesic.

Indications: An alternative strong opioid in cases of intolerable adverse effects with morphine.

Contra-indications: As for morphine.

Pharmacology

Hydromorphone is an analogue of morphine with similar pharmacokinetic and pharmacodynamic properties. By mouth and by injection it is about 7.5 times more potent than morphine.[1] Hydromorphone provides useful analgesia for about 4h. As with morphine, there is wide interpatient variation in bio-availability. The main metabolite is hydromorphone-3-glucuronide; hydromorphone-6-glucuronide is not formed.[2] Two minor metabolites, dihydro-isomorphine and dihydromorphine, are pharmacologically active and are metabolised to 6-glucuronides. By the spinal route in opioid naive subjects, hydromorphone causes much less pruritus than morphine, 11% v 44%.[3]

Oral bio-availability 37–62%.[2]
Onset of action 20–30min.
Duration of action 4–5h.
Plasma halflife 2.5h early elimination phase with a prolonged late phase.

Adverse effects: See p.107.

Dose and use

Hydromorphone is available in many countries in a range of preparations for oral and parenteral administration. In the UK, hydromorphone is available as ordinary capsules (1.3 and 2.6mg = morphine 10 and 20mg) and m/r capsules (2, 4, 8, 16, 24mg = m/r morphine 15, 30, 60, 120, 180mg). In some countries (but not the UK), hydromorphone is available in high potency ampoules containing 10mg/ml and 20mg/ml to facilitate use in continuous SC infusions.

Supply

Capsules 1.3mg, 56 = £8.67; 2.6mg, 56 = £17.34.
Capsules m/r 2mg, 56 = £18.42; 4mg, 56 = £25.24; 8mg, 56 = £49.22; 16mg, 56 = £93.52; 24mg, 56 = £140.30.

1 McDonald CJ and Miller AJ (1997) A comparative potency study of a controlled release tablet formulation of hydromorphone with controlled release morphine in patients with cancer pain. *European Journal of Palliative Care. Abstracts of the Fifth Congress.*

2 Babul N and Darke AC (1992) Putative role of hydromorphone metabolites in myoclonus. *Pain.* **51**: 260–261.

3 Chaplan SR *et al.* (1992) Morphine and hydromorphone epidural analgesia. *Anesthesiology.* **77**: 1090–1094.

*METHADONE   BNF 4.7.2

Class of drug: Strong opioid analgesic.

Indications: Intolerable adverse effects with morphine, [†]morphine hyperexcitability, [†]morphine poorly-responsive pain, [†]pain relief in severe renal failure.[1,2]

Contra-indications: As for morphine.

Pharmacology

Methadone is a mixed μ and δ agonist and a NMDA-receptor antagonist.[3] Its effects are generally similar to those of morphine despite substantial structural differences. Its central effects are mediated via CNS opioid receptors; peripherally it acts directly on smooth muscle. Methadone is a racemic mixture; L-methadone is responsible for almost all the analgesic effect, whereas D-methadone is a useful antitussive. Methadone is a basic and lipophilic drug which is well absorbed from all routes of administration. There is a high volume of distribution with only about 1% of the drug in the blood. Methadone accumulates in tissues when given repeatedly, creating an extensive reservoir.[4] Protein binding (principally to a glycoprotein) is 60–90%;[5] this is double that of morphine. Both volume of distribution and protein binding contribute to the long plasma halflife, and cumulation is a potential problem. Methadone is metabolized chiefly in the liver to several metabolites.[6] About half of the drug and its metabolites are excreted by the intestines and half by the kidneys; most of the latter unchanged.[7] Renal and hepatic impairment do not affect methadone clearance.[8,9]

In single doses, methadone PO is about 1/2 as potent as IM,[10] and IM a single dose of methadone is marginally more potent than morphine. With repeated doses, methadone is several times more potent. It is also longer acting; with chronic administration, analgesia lasts 6–12h and sometimes more. Some patients who obtain only poor relief with morphine but severe adverse effects (drowsiness, delirium, nausea and vomiting) obtain good relief with relatively low-dose methadone with few or no adverse effects. Methadone may be particularly beneficial for neuropathic pain because of its NMDA antagonism. Methadone is also used in selected patients with chronic renal failure who have developed excessive drowsiness and/or delirium with morphine because of cumulation of morphine-6-glucuronide.

Oral bio-availability 80% (range 40–100%).

Onset of action 30min.

Duration of action 4–24h.

Plasma halflife 8–75h;[11] longer in older patients; acidifying the urine results in a shorter halflife (20h) and raising the pH with sodium bicarbonate a longer halflife (>40h).[12]

Cautions

The lipid-solubility and long halflife of methadone means that cumulation to a significant extent is bound to occur, particulary in elderly patients; p.r.n. dose titration is generally necessary to avoid this potential hazard (see below).[13] MAOIs may prolong and enhance the respiratory depressant effects of methadone. Carbamazepine, phenobarbital, phenytoin and rifampicin increase the metabolism of methadone; amitriptyline and cimetidine decrease its metabolism. Methadone increases plasma zidovudine.

Adverse effects
See p.107. Local erythema and induration when given by CSCI.[14]

Dose and use
Dose titration is different from morphine. For 2–3 days patients are advised to take a dose q3h p.r.n.;[11,12] after which patients can be converted to either a b.d. or t.d.s regimen (Box 5.F).

Box 5.F Calculating the starting dose of methadone[2]

Stop morphine (or other strong opioid).

Give a fixed dose of methadone that is 1/10 of the 24h PO morphine dose when the 24h dose is <300mg.

When the 24h morphine dose is >300mg, the fixed methadone dose should be 30mg.

The fixed dose is taken PO p.r.n. *but not more frequently than q3h.*

On day 6, the amount of methadone taken over the previous 2 days is averaged and converted into a regular q12h dose (and q3h p.r.n.).

If p.r.n. medication continues to be needed, increase the dose of methadone by 1/2–1/3 every 4–6 days (e.g. 10mg b.d. → 15mg b.d.; 30mg b.d. → 40mg b.d.).

Supply
Tablets 5mg, 50 = £3.11.
Linctus 2mg/5ml, 500ml = £5.06.
Solution 1mg/ml, 10mg/ml, 20mg/ml, from Rosemont.
Injection 10mg/ml, 1ml amp = 86p; 2ml amp = £1.55; 3.5ml amp = £1.78; 5ml amp = £1.92.

---

1 Gannon C (1997) The use of methadone in the care of the dying. *European Journal of Palliative Care.* **4**: 152–158.
2 Morley JS and Makin MK (1998) The use of methadone in cancer pain poorly responsive to other opioids. *Pain Reviews.* **5**: 51–58.
3 Gorman AL et al. (1997) The d- and l-isomers of methadone bind to the non-competitive site on the N-methyl-D-aspartate (NMDA) receptor in rat forebrain and spinal cord. *Neuroscience Letters.* **223**: 5–8.
4 Robinson AE and Williams FM (1971) The distribution of methadone in man. *Journal of Pharmacy and Pharmacology.* **23**: 353–358.
5 Eap CB et al. (1990) Binding of D-methadone, L-methadone and DL-methadone to proteins in plasma of healthy volunteers: role of variants of XI-acid glycoprotein. *Clinical Pharmacology and Therapeutics.* **47**: 338–346.
6 Fainsinger R et al. (1993) Methadone in the management of cancer pain: a review. *Pain.* **52**: 137–147.
7 Inturrisi CE and Verebely K (1972) The levels of methadone in the plasma in methadone maintenance. *Clinical Pharmacology and Therapeutics.* **13**: 633–637.
8 Kreek MJ et al. (1980) Methadone use in patients with chronic renal disease. *Drug Alcohol Dependence.* **5**: 197–205.
9 Novick DM et al. (1981) Methadone disposition in patients with chronic liver disease. *Clinical Pharmacology and Therapeutics.* **30**: 353–362.
10 Beaver WT et al. (1967) A clinical comparison of the analgesic effects of methadone and morphine administered intramuscularly and of orally and parenterally administered methadone. *Clinical Pharmacology and Therapeutics.* **8**: 415–426.
11 Sawe J (1986) High-dose morphine and methadone in cancer patients: clinical pharmacokinetic consideration of oral treatment. *Clinical Pharmacology.* **11**: 87–106.

12 Nilsson MI et al. (1982) Pharmacokinetics of methadone during maintenance treatment adaptive changes during the induction phase. European Journal of Clinical Pharmacology. 22: 343–349.

13 Hendra TJ et al. (1996) Fatal methadone overdose. British Medical Journal. 313: 481–482.

14 Bruera E et al. (1991) Local toxicity with subcutaneous methadone: experience of two centers. Pain. 45: 141–143.

*OXYCODONE   BNF 4.7.2

Class of drug: Strong opioid analgesic.

Indications: Used abroad as an alternative strong opioid; in the UK used occasionally as suppository in patients with dysphagia (oxycodone pectinate).

Contra-indications: As for morphine.

Pharmacology

Oxycodone is a μ, κ agonist with similar properties to morphine.[1,2] Although oxycodone has no clinically important active metabolites, the maximum plasma concentration increases by 50% in renal failure causing more sedation.[3] Parenterally it is about 3/4 as potent as morphine. However, oral bio-availability is 2/3 or more, compared with about 1/3 for morphine. This means that oxycodone by mouth is about 1.5–2 times more potent than oral morphine.[4,5] Oxycodone is generally given q4h but could be given q6h in some patients. A range of oral m/r preparations is expected to be marketed shortly in the UK.
Bio-availability 70%.
Onset of action 20–30min.
Duration of action 4–6h.
Plasma halflife 3.5h; 4.5h in renal failure.

Adverse effects

Essentially the same as morphine (see p.107), but in one study constipation was more common and vomiting less common with oxycodone.[6]

Dose and use

Oxycodone pectinate is a primitive m/r formulation which converts a q4h drug into a q8h suppository; effectively superseded by SC morphine. If used, however, begin with a convenient dose PR, approximately 2/3 that of previous PO morphine.

Supply

Suppositories m/r 30mg from BCM Specials as a special order.

1 Glare PA and Walsh TD (1993) Dose-ranging study of oxycodone for chronic pain in advanced cancer. Journal of Clinical Oncology. 11: 973–978.

2 Poyhia R et al. (1993) Oxycodone: an alternative to morphine for cancer pain. A review. Journal of Pain and Symptom Management. 8: 63–67.

3 Kaiko R et al. (1996) Clinical pharmacokinetics of controlled-release oxycodone in renal impairment. Clinical Pharmacology and Therapeutics. 59: 130.

4 Heiskanen T et al. (1996) Double-blind, randomised, repeated dose, crossover comparison of controlled-release oxycodone and controlled-release morphine in cancer pain 1: pharmacodynamic profile. Abstracts of 8th World Congress on Pain. IASP Press, Seattle. pp 17–18.

5 Kaiko R et al. (1996) Analgesic onset and potency of oral controlled-release (CR) oxycodone and controlled-release morphine. Clinical Pharmacology and Therapeutics. 59: 130.

6 Heiskanen T and Kalso E (1997) Controlled-release oxycodone and morphine in cancer related pain. Pain. 73: 37–45.

*PHENAZOCINE   BNF 4.7.2

Class of drug: Strong opioid analgesic.

Indications: An alternative strong opioid in cases of morphine intolerance.

Contra-indications: As for morphine.

Pharmacology

Phenazocine is a μ agonist, with pharmacodynamic properties similar to those of morphine. It has a longer plasma halflife than morphine and need be given only q6h, sometimes only q8h. It is less emetogenic than morphine.

Bio-availability no data.
Onset of action 20min.
Duration of action 5–6h.
Plasma halflife no data.

Adverse effects: *See p.107.*

Dose and use

Phenazocine is available in the UK as a 5mg tablet for PO or SL use; this is equivalent to about morphine 25mg PO, i.e. too much for many patients if they have not previously been taking another strong opioid. For such patients, 2.5mg q.d.s. would be an appropriate starting dose. Individual doses of up to 20mg q4h have been used.

Supply

Tablets 5mg, 100 = £28.51.

NALOXONE   BNF 15.1

Class of drug: Opioid antagonist.

Indications: Reversal of life-threatening opioid-induced respiratory depression.

Pharmacology

Naloxone is a pure and potent opioid antagonist. It has a high affinity for morphine receptor sites and reverses the effect of opioid analgesics by displacement. The degree of displacement is dose-related. Partial antagonism may be obtained by using small doses. Activity after oral administration is low; it is only 1/15 as potent by mouth as by injection. Naloxone is rapidly metabolized by the liver, primarily to naloxone glucuronide which is excreted by the kidneys. The most important clinical property of naloxone is reversal of opioid-induced respiratory depression (and other opioid effects) caused by either an overdose of an opioid (including codeine and dextropropoxyphene) or an exaggerated response to conventional doses. Naloxone also reverses the opioid effects of pentazocine and other mixed agonist–antagonists; antagonism of buprenorphine is less complete because of the latter's high receptor affinity. *Naloxone is not effective against respiratory depression caused by nonopioids such as barbiturates.* Naloxone has also been shown to be of benefit in patients with chronic idiopathic constipation,[1] in septic shock,[2] morphine-induced peripheral vasodilatation,[3] ischaemic central neurological deficits [4,5] and poststroke central pain.[6]

Oral bio-availability 6%.
Onset of action 2–3min IV.
Duration of action 15–90min IV.
Plasma halflife 20min.

Cautions

Naloxone should *not* be used for drowsiness and/or delirium which is not life-threatening because of the danger of totally reversing the opioid analgesia and precipitating severe/agonizing pain and a major physical withdrawal syndrome.

Adverse effects

Nausea and vomiting. Occasionally severe hypertension, pulmonary oedema, tachycardia, cardiac arrest;[7] doses as small as 100–400µg of naloxone have been implicated.[8] The mechanism of these sporadic events may be related to the centrally-mediated catecholamine responses to opioid reversal.[9]

Dose and use

Naloxone is best given IV but, if not practical, may be given IM or SC. After IV injection, antagonism lasts for between 15 and 90min. The BNF contains two entries for naloxone. One relates to overdosage by addicts and recommends *0.8-2mg* IV every 2–3min up to a total of 10mg if necessary, with the possibility of an ongoing IV infusion.

The other relates to reversal of respiratory depression caused by the medicinal use of opioids. In this circumstance, *100–200µg* IV should be given, with increments of *100µg* every 2min until respiratory function is satisfactory. Further IM doses should be given after 1–2h if there is concern that further absorption of the opioid will result in delayed respiratory depression. Even lower doses have been recommended (Box 5.G). *It is important to titrate dose against respiratory function and not the level of consciousness because total antagonism will cause a return of severe pain with hyperalgesia and, if physically dependent, severe physical withdrawal symptoms and marked agitation.*

Box 5.G   Naloxone for iatrogenic opioid overdose (based on the recommendations of the American Pain Society)[10]

If respiratory rate ≥8/min and the patient easily rousable and not cyanosed, adopt a policy of 'wait and see'; consider reducing or omitting the next regular dose of morphine.

If respiratory rate <8/min, patient barely rousable/unconscious and/or cyanosed:

- dilute a standard ampoule containing naloxone 400µg to 10ml with saline for injection
- administer 0.5ml (20µg) IV every 2min until the patient's respiratory status is satisfactory
- further boluses may be necessary because naloxone is shorter-acting than morphine (and other opioids).

Supply

Injection 400µg/ml, 1ml amp = 73p.

---

1 Kreek M-J et al. (1983) Naloxone, a specific opioid antagonist, reverses chronic idiopathic constipation. Lancet. i: 262–263.

2 Peters WP et al. (1981) Pressor effect of naloxone in septic shock. Lancet. i: 529–532.

3 Cohen RA and Coffman JD (1980) Naloxone reversal of morphine-induced peripheral vasodilatation. Clinical Pharmacology and Therapeutics. 28: 541–544.

4 Baskin DS and Hosobuchi Y (1981) Naloxone reversal of ischaemic neurological deficits in man. Lancet. ii: 272–275.

5 Bousigue J-Y et al. (1982) Naloxone reversal of neurological deficit. Lancet. ii: 618–619.

6 Ray DAA and Tai YMA (1988) Infusions of naloxone in thalamic pain. British Medical Journal. 296: 969–970.

7 Partridge BL and Ward CF (1986) Pulmonary oedema following low-dose naloxone administration. Anesthesiology. 65: 709–710.

8 Pallasch TJ and Gill CJ (1981) Naloxone associated morbidity and mortality. Oral Surgery. 52: 602–603.

9 Smith G and Pinnock C (1985) Editorial: naloxone – paradox or panacea? British Journal of Anesthesia. 57: 547–549.

10 Max MB and Payne R (1992) Principles of analgesic use in the treatment of acute pain and cancer pain. American Pain Society. p.41.

6: Drugs used in
INFECTIONS

The BNF Section 5 contains a comprehensive account of antibiotic use and many hospitals have antibiotic policies which govern local practice. Information presented here is limited to common situations in palliative care, some of which demand decisive immediate action. When in doubt, obtain advice from a microbiologist.

Metronidazole

Urinary tract infections

***Clostridium difficile* enteritis**

Cellulitis in a lymphoedematous limb

Ascending cholangitis

Candidal infection

METRONIDAZOLE   BNF 5.1.11 & 13.10.1

Class of drug: Amoebicidal antibiotic.

Indications: Anaerobic infection, malodour caused by anaerobic infection, pseudo-membranous colitis (see p.128).

Pharmacology

Metronidazole is highly active against anaerobic bacteria and protozoa. Although it has no activity against aerobic organisms *in vitro*, in mixed infections *in vivo* both aerobes and anaerobes disappear. Unlike most other antibiotics, resistance to metronidazole among anaerobes is uncommon. Metronidazole can be applied topically to malodourous fungating cancers and decubitus ulcers but is more expensive by this route.[1,2] The malodour is due to volatile fatty acids produced by anaerobic bacteria. **Tinidazole** is similar to metronidazole with a longer duration of action; it causes less gastro-intestinal disturbance but costs more.[3]
Bio-availability 100% PO; 60–80% PR; 20% PV.
Onset of action 20–60min PO; 5–12h PR.
Duration of action 8–12h.
Plasma halflife 6–11h.

Cautions

Metronidazole precipitates a disulfiram-like reaction with alcohol in 2–24% of patients.[4,5] Metabolites of metronidazole, like disulfiram, inhibit alcohol dehydrogenase, xanthine oxidase and aldehyde dehydrogenase. Inhibition of alcohol dehydrogenase leads to activation of microsomal enzyme oxidative pathways which generate ketones and lactate which may cause acidosis.[6] Xanthine oxidase inhibition can lead to norepinephrine (noradrenaline) excess.[6] Accumulation of acetaldehyde is probably responsible for most of the symptoms, e.g. flushing of the face and neck, headaches, epigastric discomfort, nausea and vomiting, and a fall in blood pressure. Patients should be warned that if they drink alcohol when taking metronidazole they may have an unpleasant reaction. Generally, however, this is little more than a moderate food aversion; the occasional patient may vomit profusely. The risk of a reaction with metronidazole PV is small because absorption is low.[7]

Adverse effects

Nausea and vomiting, unpleasant taste, furred tongue, gastro-intestinal disturbance, darkening of urine, anaphylaxis (rare).

Dose and use

Anaerobic infections

Metronidazole 400mg PO t.d.s. for 2 weeks; 400mg PO b.d. in elderly debilitated patients. Tablets should be taken with or after food but suspensions are taken on an empty stomach, i.e. 1h before meals. If malodour or other symptoms and signs of infection recur, retreat and after 2 weeks continue indefinitely with 200mg b.d.

Fungating tumours

Metronidazole applied topically as a gel, using either a crushed 200mg tablet in KJ jelly or liberal amounts of a commercially-produced gel.[1,2,8,9]

Ascending cholangitis (associated with a stent in the bile duct)

Metronidazole 400mg PO q8h and **cefuroxime** 1500mg IV q8h (see p.129).

Clostridium difficile enteritis (see p.128).

Supply

Tablets 200mg, 20 = 43p; 400mg, 20 = 97p.

Suspension 200mg/5ml, 100ml = £4.14.

Gel 0.75%, 15g = £4.70; 30g = £8.31.

Gel 0.8%, 15g = £4.95; 30g = £8.75; use tube once only.

Crushed tablets cost about 2p per topical application compared with about £5–£8 for a proprietary gel.

---

1 Newman V et al. (1989) The use of metronidazole gel to control the smell of malodorous lesions. *Palliative Medicine.* **3**: 303–305.

2 Editorial (1990) Management of smelly tumours. *Lancet.* **335**: 141–142.

3 Carmine AA et al. (1982) Tinidazole in anaerobic infections. A review of its antibacterial activity, pharmacological properties and therapeutic efficacy. *Drugs.* **24**: 85–117.

4 Penick SB et al. (1969) Metronidazole in the treatment of alcoholism. *American Journal of Psychiatry.* **125**: 1063–1066.

5 de Mattos H (1968) Relationship between alcoholism and the digestive system. *Hospital Rio-J.* **74**: 1669–1676.

6 Harries DP et al. (1990) Metronidazole and alcohol: potential problems. *Scottish Medical Journal* **35**: 179–180.

7 Plosker GL (1987) Possible interaction between ethanol and vaginally administered metronidazole. *Clinical Pharmacology.* **6**: 189–193.

8 Ashford R et al. (1984) Double-blind trial of metronidazole in malodorous ulcerating tumours. *Lancet.* **1**: 1232–1233.

9 Thomas S and Hay NP (1991) The antimicrobial properties of two metronidazole medicated dressings used to treat malodorous wounds. *Pharmaceutical Journal.* **246**: 264–266.

URINARY TRACT INFECTIONS   BNF 5.1.13

Urinary tract infections (UTIs) are more common in women than in men. *Escherichia coli* is the most common cause of UTI. Less common causes include *Proteus* and *Klebsiella spp. Pseudomonas aeruginosa* infections are generally associated with functional or anatomical abnormalities of the renal tract. *Staphylococcus epidermidis* and *Enterococcus faecalis* infection may complicate catheterization or instrumentation. Whenever possible a specimen of urine should be collected for culture and sensitivity testing before starting antibiotic therapy.

Treatment strategy

Initially use **Multistix 8SG** to decide whether a patient has a UTI. Each stick costs <20p (compare £20 for a MSU) and the result is available immediately (Box 6.A). If a UTI is suspected clinically and supported by the Multistix 8SG results:[1]

- send a MSU for culture and sensitivity
- start empirical treatment with **trimethoprim** 200mg PO b.d. *or* **IV cefuroxime** and/or **IV gentamicin** if systemically unwell (see BNF for dose regimens).

Recommendations vary in relation to duration of antibiotic treatment from 3 days for an uncomplicated UTI in a woman to 10 days for children, men, and women with fever and/or loin

---

Box 6.A   Using Multistix 8SG to diagnose urinary tract infections

Multistix 8SG measure urinary pH and specific gravity, and the presence and amount of:

- glucose
- ketone
- blood
- protein
- nitrate, a bacterial metabolite
- leucocytes, produced by inflammation/infection.

How to do the test

- take a mid-stream specimen of urine (MSU)
- dip the strip into the urine and remove immediately
- after 60 seconds read nitrate result   } the colours on the strips should
- after 2min read the leucocyte result   } be compared to the bottle colours.

Late readings are of no value.

Significance of the results

Leucocyte and nitrate positive	infection is probable; send MSU
Nitrate only positive	infection possible; MSU advisable
Leucocyte only positive	infection possible; MSU advisable
Leucocyte and nitrate negative	infection is unlikely; no need to send MSU unless definite urinary tract symptoms.

---

pain. In *catheterized patients* bacterial colonization is normal and is not necessarily harmful; it should not be investigated unless symptomatic. For patients who are about to be decatheterized, antibiotics for 48h before removal significantly reduces the risk of post-catheter bacteriuria.[2] In debilitated patients, and in those who find it difficult to take tablets, a single dose of **trimethoprim 300mg** is a useful compromise option;[3] the cure rate is 74% at 1 week and 71% at 6 weeks.[4]

Alternative approaches

Cranberry juice 33%: 180ml b.d. acidifies urine and inhibits bacterial adherence to the bladder mucosa.[5] The addition of ascorbic acid is not necessary, although sometimes recommended.
Methenamine hippurate: 1g b.d. acidifies urine and in catheterized patients it reduces sediment and catheter blockage, and the frequency of symptomatic UTIs.[6]

Supply

Tablets **trimethoprim** 100mg, 20 = 40p; 200mg, 20 = 69p.
Suspension sugar-free **trimethoprim** 50mg/5ml, 100ml = £1.77.
Tablets **methenamine hippurate** 1g, 20 = £2.47.

---

1 Schofield S *et al.* (1996) Is it a urinary tract infection? *Oxford Radcliffe Trust Medicines Information Leaflet.* No. 4: February.
2 Hustinx WNM *et al.* (1991) Impact of concurrent antimicrobial therapy on catheter-associated urinary tract infection. *Journal of Hospital Infection.* **18**: 45–56.
3 Bailey RS and Abbott GD (1978) Treatment of urinary tract infection with a single dose of trimethoprim-sulfamethoxazole. *CMA Journal.* **118**: 551–552.
4 Brumfitt W *et al.* (1982) Comparative trial of trimethoprim and co-trimoxazole in recurrent urinary infections. *Infection.* **10**: 280–284.

5 Avorn J et al. (1994) Reduction of bacteriuria and pyuria after ingestion of cranberry juice. *Journal of the American Medical Association.* **271**: 751–754.
6 Cronberg S et al. (1987) Prevention of recurrent acute cystitis by methenamine hippurate: double blind controlled crossover long term study. *British Medical Journal.* **294**: 1507–1508.

CLOSTRIDIUM DIFFICILE ENTERITIS

Pseudomembranous colitis is an uncommon complication of antibiotic therapy (Table 6.1). Symptoms generally begin within 1 week of starting antibiotic therapy or shortly after stopping, but may occur up to 1 month later. It is caused by colonization of the bowel by *Clostridium difficile* and the production of toxins A and B which cause mucosal damage.

Table 6.1   Pseudomembranous colitis

	Causal antibiotics	
Clinical features	Most prevalent	Highest incidence
Explosive foul-smelling watery diarrhoea + mucus ± blood	Ampicillin	Clindamycin
Abdominal pain	Amoxicillin	Lincomycin
Tenderness	Cephalosporins	
Fever	Ciprofloxacin	

Environmental control measures
Spread of *Clostridium difficile* is by the ingestion of spores which can be isolated from the environment around symptomatic patients. Environmental controls ('universal precautions') will prevent the spread of outbreaks:
• patients should be isolated while they have diarrhoea
• carers should use gloves and aprons, and thoroughly wash their hands after patient contact using either soap or alcohol-based products.

Treatment strategy
Clostridium difficile is strongly anaerobic and difficult to culture. Faecal tests to detect *Clostridium difficile* toxins can be used to confirm the diagnosis. If in doubt, endoscopy and rectal biopsy are of value, although a trial of therapy is more practical. **Metronidazole** is the treatment of choice. It is as effective as **vancomycin**[1,2] which is much more expensive and should be given only after seeking specialist advice. Vancomycin is generally reserved for patients with an ileus or those who are severely ill. About 20% of patients relapse, most within 3 weeks. This may be caused by germination of residual spores within the colon, re-infection with *Clostridium difficile* or further antibiotic treatment. Mild relapses often resolve spontaneously; repeat treatment with metronidazole is still recommended.[3,4] Repeated relapses require prolonged treatment with a slowly decreasing dose of vancomycin.[5] *Relapse due to resistance of Clostridium difficile to antibiotic treatment is extremely rare.*

Dose and use
• **metronidazole** 400mg t.d.s. for 10 days
• **vancomycin** 125mg q.d.s. for 10 days.

Supply
Capsules **vancomycin** 125mg, 10-day course = £126.16.
Injection (powder for reconstitution) **vancomycin** 500mg, 1 vial = £6.50.
The injection can be used to prepare an oral solution as a cheaper alternative to the capsules; add 10ml WFI to a vial and give 2.5ml q.d.s. with added flavouring (10-day course = £65.00).
For metronidazole preparations, see p.126.

1 Cherry RD et al. (1982) Metronidazole: an alternate therapy for antibiotic-associated colitis. *Gastroenterology.* **82**: 849–851.

2 Teasley DG et al. (1983) Prospective randomised trial of metronidazole versus vancomycin for Clostridium difficile-associated diarrhoea and colitis. *Lancet.* **2**: 1043–1046.

3 Joint Working Group Report (1994) The prevention and management of Clostridium difficile infection. Department of Health. Public Health Laboratory Service, London.

4 Tabaqchali S and Jumaa P (1995) Diagnosis and management of Clostridium difficile infections. *British Medical Journal.* **310**: 1375–1380.

5 Anonymous (1995) Antibotic-induced diarrhoea. *Drug and Therapeutics Bulletin.* **33** (3): 23–24.

CELLULITIS IN A LYMPHOEDEMATOUS LIMB

Acute inflammatory episodes are a feature of chronic lymphoedema. Static protein-rich lymph causes low-grade inflammation and this may be complicated by secondary infection.

Management strategy

A hot red tender area and a rapid increase in swelling suggest infection. Most patients feel unwell and are febrile. Treat promptly with rest, elevation and antibiotics. Because streptococcal infections are the most common, **phenoxymethylpenicillin** is the initial antibiotic of choice. **Erythromycin** is used for patients who are allergic to penicillin (Figure 6.1). For penicillin-resistant infections, flucloxacillin or cefradine is used (Figure 6.1). Some centres use **co-amoxiclav** instead but, although this is active against both streptococci and staphylococci and means taking fewer tablets (t.d.s. v q.d.s.), it causes more diarrhoea and rashes, and is more expensive.

Supply

Tablets **phenoxymethylpenicillin** 250mg, 20 = 33p.
Tablets e/c **erythromycin** 250mg, 20 = 82p; 500mg, 20 = £1.80.
Capsules **flucloxacillin** 250mg, 20 = £1.56; 500mg, 20 = £2.94.
Tablets **co-amoxiclav** 250/125 (amoxicillin 250mg/clavulanic acid 125mg), 21 = £9.79; co-amoxiclav 500/125, 21 = £14.30.
Tablets dispersible **co-amoxiclav** 250/125, 21 = £9.99.

1 Twycross R (1997) *Symptom Management in Advanced Cancer.* Radcliffe Medical Press, Oxford.

ASCENDING CHOLANGITIS

Ascending cholangitis may occur in patients with a partially obstructed or stented common bile duct. It often causes severe systemic disturbance and should be treated promptly with antibiotics.

Management strategy

Ascending cholangitis should be treated with a combination of an appropriate cephalosporin and metronidazole:
- **IV cefuroxime** 1500mg q8h for 48h
- **PO metronidazole** 400mg q8h (tablets with or after food; suspension on an empty stomach, i.e. 1h a.c.).

If oral administration unreliable because of nausea and vomiting, **metronidazole** should be given PR (1g q8h) or IV (500mg q8h). Prolonged rectal use causes proctitis; limit use by this route to 2–3 days.

Cefuroxime can be given IM if IV administration difficult, but 1500mg means an injection of 6 ml.

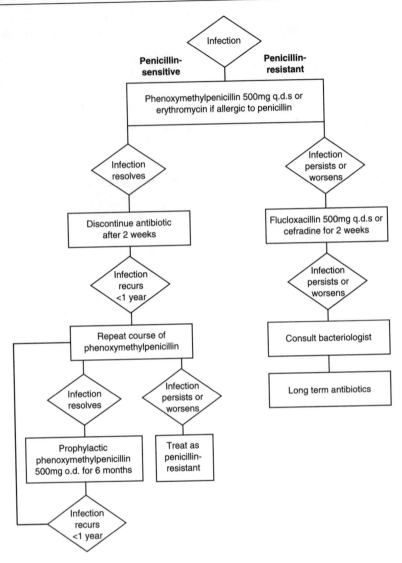

Figure 6.1 Antibiotic treatment for limb infection in obstructive lymphoedema.[1]

Supply
Injection (powder for reconstitution) **cefuroxime** 750mg, 1 vial = £2.64.
Tablets **metronidazole** 200mg, 20 = 43p; 400mg, 20 = 97p.
Suspension **metronidazole** 200mg/5ml, 100ml = £4.14.
Suppositories **metronidazole** 1g, 10 = £6.80.
IV infusion **metronidazole** 5mg/ml, 100ml = £3.41–£4.50.

CANDIDAL INFECTION   BNF 5.2

Oropharyngeal candidiasis is a relatively common fungal infection in debilitated patients, particularly in diabetics and those receiving corticosteroids and/or antibiotics. A systemically administered imidazole antifungal antibiotic, e.g. **ketoconazole** or **fluconazole**, is the treatment of choice. Some centres recommend topical oral **nystatin** as first-line treatment because of the emergence of resistance to the imidazole antifungals. However, treatment q.d.s. with concurrent *denture removal and cleaning q.d.s.* is difficult and, in hospital, more costly of nursing time.

Cautions

Serious drug interactions: when prescribing an imidazole antifungal (**fluconazole**, **itraconazole**, **ketoconazole** or **miconazole**), avoid concomitant administration with **astemizole**, **terfenadine** and **cisapride** (see p.9 & Appendix 3, p.213).

Dose and use
Typical regimens comprise:
• **nystatin** 100 000 units/ml q.d.s. for 1 week (BNF 5.2) or until 2 days after clinical cure (Data Sheet)
• **ketoconazole** 200mg o.d. for 5 days; if recurs, give a repeat course for 10 days[1]
• **fluconazole** 150mg stat (as effective as ketoconazole 200mg o.d. for 5 days)[1]
• **fluconazole** 50–100mg o.d. for 7–14 days if resistant to ketoconazole.
In immunocompromised people, higher doses and longer courses of **fluconazole** may be needed (see BNF 5.2). Systemic antifungals are also effective in treating vaginal candidiasis.

Supply
Suspension **nystatin** 100 000 units/ml, 7 days = £2.77.
Tablets **ketoconazole** 200mg, 5 = £2.62.
Suspension **ketoconazole** 100mg/5ml, 50ml = £3.58.
Capsules **fluconazole** 50mg, 7 = £16.61; 150mg, 1 = £7.12.
Suspension **fluconazole** 50mg/5ml, 35ml = £16.61; 200mg/5ml, 35ml = £66.42.

---

1 Regnard CFB (1994) Single dose fluconazole versus five-day ketoconazole in oral candidosis. *Palliative Medicine.* **8**: 72–73.

7: Drugs used in
ENDOCRINE DISORDERS

Bisphosphonates

Corticosteroids

Demeclocycline

Desmopressin

Drugs for diabetes mellitus

*Octreotide

Progestogens

Stanozolol

BISPHOSPHONATES   BNF 6.6.2

Indications: Hypercalcaemia, bone pain. Also used prophylactically to reduce the incidence of pain and pathological fracture *in breast cancer and myeloma*.

Pharmacology

Bisphosphonates inhibit osteoclast activity and thereby inhibit bone resorption, but have no impact on the effect of parathyroid-related protein (PTHrP) on renal tubular re-absorption of calcium. Bisphosphonates are generally given IV, at least initially, because of poor alimentary absorption. Bisphosphonates are adsorbed onto the bone surface where they remain bound to hydroxyapatite for weeks or months. A single infusion therefore has a prolonged duration of action on osteoclasts. The two most widely used bisphosphonates are **clodronate** and **pamidronate**. Bisphosphonates are expensive and some recommended regimens are very costly.

For onset of action, duration of action *see* Table 7.1.

Cautions

Serious drug interactions: symptomatic hypocalcaemia may occur if an aminoglycoside antibiotic is given concurrently with long-term oral clodronate therapy.[1]

Reduce dose and speed of infusion in patients with renal impairment.

Adverse effects

Transient pyrexia, influenza-like symptoms. Oral preparations may cause dyspepsia, abdominal pain, diarrhoea or constipation. Hypocalcaemia may occur but is generally asymptomatic.

Table 7.1   Bisphosphonates and the treatment of hypercalcaemia[2]

	Bisphosphonate	
	Sodium clodronate	Disodium pamidronate
Initial IV dose	(a) 1500mg (b) 300–600mg daily for 5 days	30–90mg
Onset of effect	<2 days	<3 days
Maximum effect	3–5 days	5–7 days
Duration of effect	(a) 10 days ± (b) 15 days ±	3 weeks ±
Restores normocalcaemia	40–80%	70–90%

Mechanism of action
  inhibits osteoclasts
  stimulates osteoblasts
	
	+
	–
		
		+
		+

Initial PO treatment	Effective	Effective but gastro-intestinal intolerance common
Maintenance	PO tablets generally prevent relapse	IV infusion every 3–4 weeks

Dose and use

Hypercalcaemia: the dose of **disodium pamidronate** depends on the initial corrected plasma calcium concentration (Box 7.A & Table 7.2):
- maximum recommended dose is 90mg IV/treatment
- infusion rate should not exceed *1mg/min*
- concentration should not exceed *60mg/250ml*
- repeat after 1 week if initial response inadequate
- repeat every 3–4 weeks according to plasma calcium concentration.

Box 7.A   Correcting plasma calcium concentrations (Oxford Radcliffe Hospital Trust)

Corrected calcium (mmol/L) = measured calcium + (0.022 × (42 – albumin g/L))
  e.g. measured calcium   = 2.45; albumin = 32
    corrected calcium   = 2.45 + (0.022 × 10) = 2.67 mmol/L

Table 7.2   IV pamidronate for hypercalcaemia[a]

Corrected plasma calcium concentration (mmol/L)	Dose (mg)
<3	15–30
3–3.5	30–60
3.5–4	60–90
>4	90

a. manufacturer's recommendations.

Metastatic bone pain: several regimens have been recommended for when more conventional methods have been exhausted:
- **disodium pamidronate** 90mg IV (50% of patients respond); if helpful repeat 60–90 mg every 3–4 weeks for as long as benefit is maintained.[3]
- **disodium pamidronate** 120mg IV, repeated p.r.n. every 2–4 months[4]
- **sodium clodronate** 1.5g IV initially, plus maintenance therapy 1600mg PO o.d.[5,6]

One prophylactic regimen recommends **disodium pamidronate** 90mg IV every 4 weeks in patients with one or more osteolytic bone metastasis ≥1 cm in diameter; *very costly.*[7]

Supply
Injection (powder for reconstitution) **disodium pamidronate** 15mg, vial = £27.27; 30mg, vial = £54.53; 90mg, vial = £155.80.
Injection **sodium clodronate** 30mg/ml, 10ml amp = £14.43.

1 Johnson MJ and Fallon MT (1998) Symptomatic hypocalcaemia with oral clodronate. *Journal of Pain and Symptom Management.* **15**: 140–142.
2 Ralston SH (1994) Pathogenesis and management of cancer associated hypercalcaemia. In: GW Hanks (ed) *Cancer Surveys, vol 21: Palliative Medicine: Problem areas in pain and symptom management.* Cold Spring Harbor Laboratory Press. pp 179–196.
3 Crosby V et al. (in press) *Journal of Pain and Symptom Management.*
4 Vinholes J et al. (1996) Metabolic effects of pamidronate in patients with metastatic bone disease. *European Journal of Cancer.* **5**: 159–175.
5 Vorreuther R (1993) Biphosphonates as an adjunct to palliative therapy of bone metastases from prostatic carcinoma. A pilot study on clodronate. *British Journal of Urology.* **72**: 792–795.
6 O'Rourke N et al. (1995) Double-blind, placebo-controlled, dose response trial of oral clodronate in patients with bone metastases. *Journal of Clinical Oncology.* **13**: 929–934.
7 Hortobagyi GN et al. (1996) Efficacy of pamidronate in reducing skeletal complications in patients with breast cancer and lytic bone metastases. *New England Journal of Medicine.* **335**: 1785–1791.

CORTICOSTEROIDS   BNF 6.3

Indications: See Table 7.3; inclusion does *not* mean that a corticosteroid is necessarily the treatment of choice.

Table 7.3 Indications for corticosteroids in advanced cancer

Specific	*Pain relief*
Anti-emetic	Raised intracranial pressure
Spinal cord compression	Nerve compression
Nerve compression	Spinal cord compression
Dyspnoea	Bone pain
pneumonitis (after radiotherapy)	
lymphangitis carcinomatosa	*Hormone therapy*
tracheal compression/stridor	Replacement
Superior vena caval obstruction	Anticancer
Obstruction of hollow viscus	
bronchus	*General*
ureter	To improve appetite
bowel (?)	To enhance sense of wellbeing
Radiation-induced inflammation	
Rectal discharge (give PR)	

Table 7.4 Selected pharmacokinetic details of commonly used corticosteroids[1,2]

Drug	Anti-inflammatory potency	Approximate equivalent dose (mg)	Sodium-retaining potency	Oral bio-availability %	Duration of action (h)	Plasma halflife (h)	Relative affinity for lung tissue	Daily dose (mg) above which adrenal suppression possible Males	Females
Hydrocortisone	1	20	1	96	8–12	1.5	1	20–30	15–25
Prednisolone	4	5	0.25	75–85	12–36	3.5	1.6	7.5–10	7.5
Dexamethasone	25–50[a]	0.5–1	<0.01	78	36–54	4.5	1	1–1.5	1
Betamethasone				98–100	24–48	6.5			

a. thymic involution assay.

Pharmacology

The adrenal cortex secretes hydrocortisone (cortisol) which has glucocorticoid activity and weak mineralocorticoid activity. It also secretes aldosterone which has mineralocorticoid activity. Thus, in deficiency states, physiological replacement is best achieved with a combination of **hydrocortisone** and **fludrocortisone**, a mineralocorticoid. When comparing the relative anti-inflammatory (glucocorticoid) potencies of corticosteroids, their water-retaining properties (mineralocorticoid effect) should also be borne in mind (Table 7.4). Hydrocortisone is not used for long-term disease suppression because large doses would be required and these would cause troublesome fluid retention. On the other hand, the moderate anti-inflammatory effect of hydrocortisone makes it the first choice corticosteroid for topical use in inflammatory skin conditions; adverse effects are minimal, both topical and systemic. **Prednisolone** is the most frequently used corticosteroid for disease suppression but **dexamethasone**, with high glucocorticoid activity but insignificant mineralocorticoid effect, is particularly suitable for high-dose therapy. It is 6–12 times more potent than prednisolone (e.g. 2mg of dexamethasone is approximately equivalent to 15–25mg of prednisolone) and has a long duration of action (Table 7.4). Some esters of **betamethasone** and of **beclometasone** exert a marked topical effect; use is made of this property with skin applications and bronchial inhalations.

For pharmacokinetic details, see Table 7.4.

Cautions

Diabetes mellitus, psychotic illness. Fourfold increased risk of peptic ulcer if co-administered with a NSAID (but no increased risk if used alone).[3] Corticosteroids antagonize oral hypoglycaemics and insulin (glucocorticoid effect), antihypertensives and diuretics (mineralocorticoid effect). Increased risk of hypokalaemia if high doses of corticosteroids are prescribed with β_2-sympathomimetics (e.g. salbutamol, terbutaline) or carbenoxolone. The metabolism of corticosteroids is accelerated by aminoglutethimide (dexamethasone only), anticonvulsants (carbamazepine, phenobarbital, phenytoin, primidone) and rifampicin. This effect is more pronounced with long-acting gluco-corticoids; phenytoin may reduce the bio-availability of dexamethasone to 25–50%, and larger doses (double or more) will be needed when prescribed concurrently.[4] Dexamethasone itself can affect plasma phenytoin concentrations (may either rise or fall); the effect of concurrent use should be monitored.

Adverse effects: See Table 7.5, Boxes 7.B & 7.C and Appendix 3, p.213.

Table 7.5 Adverse effects of corticosteroids

Glucocorticoid effects	Mineralocorticoid effects
Diabetes mellitus	Sodium and water retention
Osteoporosis	→ oedema
Avascular bone necrosis	Potassium loss
Mental disturbances	Hypertension
insomnia	
agitation	Cushing's syndrome
paranoid psychosis	Moonface
euphoria	Striae
depression	Acne
Muscle wasting and weakness (see Box 7.B)	
Peptic ulceration (if given with a NSAID)[3]	Steroid cataract
Infection (increased susceptibility)	If prednisolone 15mg or equivalent
candidiasis	taken daily for several years = 75% risk
septicaemia (may delay recognition)	
tuberculosis (may delay recognition)	
chickenpox and measles (increased severity)[a]	
Suppression of growth (in child)	

a. if exposed to infection, should be given immunoglobulin either varicella-zoster or normal.

Box 7.B   Corticosteroid myopathy[5,6]

Onset generally in the third month of treatment with dexamethasone ≥4mg daily or prednisolone ≥40mg daily. Can occur earlier and with lower doses.

If the chronological sequence fits with corticosteroid myopathy, a presumptive diagnosis should be made and the following steps taken:

- explanation to patient and family

- discuss need to compromise between maximizing therapeutic benefit and minimizing adverse effects

- halve corticosteroid dose (generally possible as a single step)

- consider changing from dexamethasone to prednisolone (nonfluorinated corticosteroids cause less myopathy)

- attempt further reductions in dose of corticosteroid at intervals of 1–2 weeks

- arrange for physiotherapy (disuse exacerbates myopathy)

- indicate that weakness should improve after 3–4 weeks (provided cancer-induced weakness does not supervene).

Box 7.C   Steroid pseudorheumatism

Patients receiving corticosteroids for rheumatoid arthritis occasionally develop diffuse pains, malaise and pyrexia, so-called steroid pseudorheumatism.[7]

It is sometimes also seen in cancer patients receiving large doses of corticosteroids or when a very high dose is reduced rapidly to a lower dose. Most likely to be affected are those:

- receiving 100mg of prednisolone daily for several days in association with chemotherapy

- with spinal cord compression given dexamethasone 100mg daily for several days.[8 a]

- on high doses of dexamethasone to reduce raised intracranial pressure associated with brain metastases

- reducing to an ordinary maintenance dose after a prolonged course.

a. such a high dose is in fact unnecessary; 10mg is as effective as 100mg.[9]

Dose and use
Apart from hydrocortisone, corticosteroids can be given in a single daily dose o.m.; this eases compliance and reduces the likelihood of corticosteroid-induced insomnia. Even so, temazepam or diazepam o.n. is sometimes needed to counter insomnia or agitation. The initial daily dose varies according to indication and fashion, e.g.:

Replacement therapy: **hydrocortisone** 20mg o.m., 10mg each evening with **fludrocortisone** 0.1–0.3mg o.m.

Anorexia: **dexamethasone** 2–4mg o.m. or **prednisolone** 15–30mg o.m.

Anti-emetic: e.g. **dexamethasone** 8–20mg o.m.

Raised intracranial pressure: **dexamethasone** 8–16mg o.m.

Spinal cord compression: **dexamethasone** 16mg o.m.–b.d. (second dose before 1300h).

It is important for patients to appreciate that corticosteroids given for more than 2 weeks should not be stopped abruptly (Box 7.D).

Box 7.D Patient information about corticosteroids

Following concern about severe chickenpox associated with systemic corticosteroids, the CSM has issued a notice that *every* patient prescribed a systemic corticosteroid should receive the **Patient Information Leaflet** supplied by the relevant manufacturer.

Steroid cards should also be issued where appropriate: they can be obtained from the local Health Authority in England and Wales. In Scotland steroid cards are available from Health Boards. In Northern Ireland they may be obtained from Central Services Agency, 27 Adelaide St, Belfast BT2 8FH.

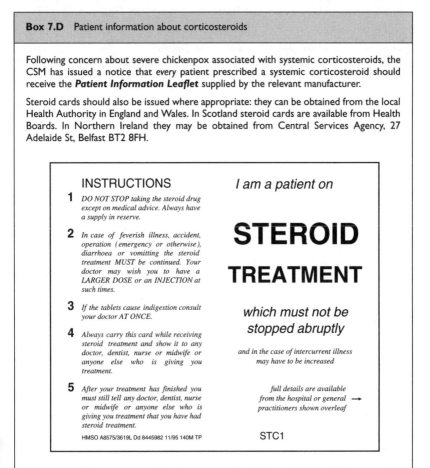

INSTRUCTIONS

1 *DO NOT STOP taking the steroid drug except on medical advice. Always have a supply in reserve.*

2 *In case of feverish illness, accident, operation (emergency or otherwise), diarrhoea or vomitting the steroid treatment MUST be continued. Your doctor may wish you to have a LARGER DOSE or an INJECTION at such times.*

3 *If the tablets cause indigestion consult your doctor AT ONCE.*

4 *Always carry this card while receiving steroid treatment and show it to any doctor, dentist, nurse or midwife or anyone else who is giving you treatment.*

5 *After your treatment has finished you must still tell any doctor, dentist, nurse or midwife or anyone else who is giving you treatment that you have had steroid treatment.*

HMSO A8575/3619L Dd 8445982 11/95 140M TP

I am a patient on

STEROID TREATMENT

which must not be stopped abruptly

and in the case of intercurrent illness may have to be increased

full details are available from the hospital or general → practitioners shown overleaf

STC1

Community pharmacists may also obtain steroid cards from the Royal Pharmaceutical Society of Great Britain.

Stopping corticosteroids

If after 7–10 days the corticosteroid fails to achieve the desired effect it should be stopped. It is often possible to stop corticosteroids abruptly, particularly if the duration of therapy is less than 3 weeks. Due to considerable variability between individuals, these recommendations should only be used as a guide. If there is uncertainty about the resolution of the underlying disease or symptom, withdrawal of corticosteroids should be guided by monitoring disease activity or the patient's symptoms. After whole-brain irradiation for primary or metastatic brain cancer, dexamethasone 4mg should be maintained for at least 1 week and the dose then reduced at the rate of 1mg/week.[9] In dying patients who are no longer able to swallow medication because they are moribund, it is generally acceptable to discontinue corticosteroids abruptly.

Occasionally a patient with intracranial disease who is not moribund requests the cessation of corticosteroids because of an unacceptable quality of life. Having ascertained that this is really what the patient wants, it is best to reduce the dexamethasone step by step on a daily basis because this gives the patient time to reconsider.[10] Additional p.r.n. analgesia should be prescribed for breakthrough headache. The situation should be monitored closely, with analgesia and anticonvulsant medication maintained by CSCI when the patient becomes unable to take oral medication.

If strong opioids depress ventilation, the increased $PaCO_2$ will result in intracranial vaso-dilatation and a rise in intracranial pressure; this may precipitate or exacerbate headache. If headache is suspected because of grimacing or general restlessness, p.r.n. medication should be given and the dose of the regular opioid increased until the patient appears comfortable. *It is important first to exclude the more common reasons for agitation in moribund patients, e.g. full bladder or rectum, pain and stiffness related to immobility.*

Supply
Tablets **prednisolone** 1mg, 20 = 19p; 5mg, 20 = 31p; 25mg, 20 = £1.52.
Tablets e/c **prednisolone** 2.5mg, 20 = 17p; 5mg, 20 = 28p.
Tablets soluble **prednisolone** 5mg, 20 = £1.15.
Tablets **dexamethasone** 500µg, 20 = 64p; 2mg, 20 = £1.73.
Injection **dexamethasone** 4mg/ml, 1ml amp = 83p; 2ml amp = £1.27.
Suspension **dexamethasone** from Rosemont (see Appendix 8, p.239).

1 Swartz SL and Dluhy RG (1978) Corticosteroids: clinical pharmacology and therapeutic use. *Current Therapeutics.* Sept: 145–170.
2 Demoly P and Chung KF (1998) Pharmacology of corticosteroids. *Respiratory Medicine.* **92**: 385–394.
3 Piper JM et al. (1991) Corticosteroid use and peptic ulcer disease: role of nonsteroidal anti-inflammatory drugs. *Annals of Internal Medicine.* **114**: 737–740.
4 Chalk JB (1984) Phenytoin impairs the bio-availability of dexamethasone in neurological and neurosurgical patients. *Journal of Neurology, Neurosurgery and Psychiatry.* **47**: 1087.
5 Dropcho EJ and Soong S-J (1991) Steroid induced weakness in patients with primary brain tumors. *Neurology.* **41**: 1235–1239.
6 Eidelberg G (1991) Steroid myopathy. In: Rottenberg DA (ed) *Neurological complications of cancer treatment.* Butterworth-Heinemann, Boston. pp 185–191.
7 Rotstein J and Good RA (1957) Steroid pseudorheumatism. *AMA Archives of Internal Medicine.* **99**: 545–555.
8 Greenberg HS et al. (1979) Epidural spinal cord compression from metastatic tumours: results with a new treatment protocol. *Annals of Neurology.* **8**: 361–366.
9 Committee on Safety of Medicines and Medicines Control Agency (1998) Withdrawal of systemic corticosteroids. *Current Problems in Pharmacovigilance.* **24**: 5–7.
10 Vecht CJ et al. (1994) Dose-effect relationship of dexamethasone on Karnofsky performance in metastatic brain tumors: *Neurology.* **24**: 5–7.

DEMECLOCYCLINE   BNF 5.1 & 6.5.2

Class of drug: Tetracycline antibiotic.

Indications: Symptomatic hyponatraemia caused by the syndrome of inappropriate ADH secretion (SIADH).

Management strategy
The diagnosis of SIADH is based on the following criteria.[1]
* hyponatraemia (<130mmol/L)
* low plasma osmolality (<270mosmol/L)
* raised urine osmolality (>100mosmol/L)
* urine sodium concentration:
    always >20mmol/L
    often >50mmol/L
* normal plasma volume.
In practice, a plasma sodium concentration of ≤120 mmol/L is sufficient to make a clinical diagnosis of SIADH in the absence of:
* severe vomiting
* diuretic therapy
* hypo-adrenalism

- diuretic therapy
- hypo-adrenalism
- hypothyroidism
- severe renal failure.

Treat the patient and not the biochemical results. If symptomatic, several options exist:
- treat the underlying cause if possible (e.g. chemotherapy in small cell lung cancer)
- restrict fluid intake to 700–1000ml/day to limit daily urine output to <500ml (can be difficult in practice)
- **demeclocycline** 300mg b.d.–q.d.s. (induces a nephrogenic diabetes insipidus).

Dose and use
Demeclocycline 300mg b.d.–q.d.s. on an empty stomach (e.g. 1h a.c.), avoiding milk, antacids and iron preparations. Warn the patient not to expose skin to direct sunlight or sunlamps because of the risk of photosensitivity.

Supply
Capsules 150mg, 20 = £4.13.

---

1 Saito T (1996) SIADH and other hyponatraemic disorders: diagnosis and therapeutic problems. *Japanese Journal of Nephrology.* **38**: 429–434.

DESMOPRESSIN   BNF 6.5.2

Class of drug: Vasopressin analogue.

Indications: Refractory nocturia not associated with infection.

Contra-indications: Renal impairment, cardiovascular disease, hypertension.

Pharmacology
Desmopressin is an analogue of the pituitary antidiuretic hormone, vasopressin. It increases water resorption by the renal tubules, thereby reducing urine volume. Desmopressin has a longer duration of action than **vasopressin** and **lypressin**, an alternative analogue.
Bio-availability 3.3–4.1% intranasal; 0.1–5% PO (PO compared to intranasal = 5%).
Onset of action 1h intranasal; 2h PO.
Duration of action 5–24h intranasal; 6–8h PO.
Plasma halflife 0.4–4h intranasal; 1.5–2.5h PO.

Cautions

Serious drug interactions: the concomitant use of drugs which increase the endogenous secretion of vasopressin increases the risk of symptomatic hyponatraemia, e.g. tricyclic antidepressants (see p.62).

Adverse effects
Water retention and hyponatraemia; in the most serious cases this may result in hyponatraemic convulsions. Patients should be warned to restrict fluids in the evenings; also to stop taking desmopressin if they develop persistent vomiting or diarrhoea. The effect of desmopressin is potentiated by indometacin (and possibly other NSAIDs).

Dose and use
Keep to the recommended starting doses to minimize the risk of hyponatraemic convulsions:
- starting doses 200–400µg PO o.n.; 10–20µg intranasally o.n.
- increase to higher dose only if lower one ineffective.

Supply
Tablets 100μg, 90 = £45.95; 200μg, 90 = £91.90.
Intranasal solution 100μg/ml, 2.5ml dropper bottle and catheter = £9.50.
Nasal spray 10μg/metered spray, 6ml = £28.00.

DRUGS FOR DIABETES MELLITUS   BNF 6.1

Indications: Diabetes mellitus not controlled by diet only.

Contra-indications: Chlorpropamide and **glibenclamide** should not be used in the frail elderly and those with renal or hepatic impairment. **Metformin** should not be used in patients with renal failure because of the risk of lactic acidosis; best avoided in all elderly debilitated patients, particularly those with associated hepatic or cardiac dysfunction.

Pharmacology
Glucose intolerance is one of the first metabolic consequences of cancer and is found in nearly 40% of nondiabetic cancer patients given an oral or IV glucose tolerance test.[1] Corticosteroids are the most common precipitant of diabetes in advanced cancer.[2] Thiazide diuretics and furosemide (frusemide) may also produce hyperglycaemia. In the noncancer population, patients newly presenting with diabetes are symptomatic (e.g. thirst) with a fasting blood glucose of ⩾12mmol/L. The renal threshold increases considerably with age, however, and it is common for older patients to be asymptomatic with a fasting blood glucose of 15–18mmol/L, occasionally more. In newly diagnosed symptomatic patients, a short-acting sulphonylurea such as **tolbutamide** or **gliclazide** should be prescribed with a realistic safe target (e.g. fasting blood glucose <12mmol/L). The dose should be reduced if the fasting blood glucose is consistently <8mmol/L. For pharmacokinetic details, *see* Table 7.6.

Table 7.6   Pharmacokinetic details of oral hypoglycaemics

	Tolbutamide	Gliclazide
Bio-availability	>95%	78%
Onset of action	1–3h	3–4h
Duration of action	⩽12h	12–24h
Plasma halflife	4.5–6.5h	10–12h

Insulin is not often needed in newly diagnosed diabetics with advanced cancer. Patients with pre-existing non-insulin dependent diabetes and on maximal doses of tolbutamide or gliclazide, sometimes require insulin in addition if prescribed a corticosteroid, e.g. **ultratard insulin** 10 units o.d. at 1800h. Less may be needed in an emaciated patient and more if obese. The dose is monitored to achieve a fasting blood glucose of 8–12mmol/L. With the appropriate dose of ultratard insulin, an inability to eat does not matter as it provides only a basal insulin supply. Note:

• it is unnecessary to maintain theoretically ideal blood glucose levels to avoid long-term complications
• rigid dietary control is not indicated when life expectancy is short
• when stable, monitoring is generally adequate with a *fasting blood glucose* fingerprick test twice a week.

Urine tests for glucose may well be adequate. For most patients, glycosuria 1+ and 2+ reflect satisfactory (asymptomatic) control; no glycosuria would trigger a decrease in hypoglycaemic therapy and 3+ an increase.[3] Initial comparison of the urine glucose with the blood glucose will detect patients with an increased renal threshold for glucose (associated with renal impairment) and those with a low threshold (renal glycosuria).

Cautions

After discontinuation, chlorpropamide and glibenclamide can produce hypoglycaemia for 48–72h, and up to 96h if there is renal or hepatic impairment. 1/3 of diabetics lose their adrenergic warning symptoms of hypoglycaemia within 20 years of developing diabetes; autonomic neuropathy may remove both the warning symptoms and the counter-regulatory mechanism of an epinephrine (adrenaline)-induced increase in blood glucose (Box 7.E). Malnourished patients with reduced hepatic glycogen stores will also have a reduced capacity to counteract hypoglycaemia.[4]

Box 7.E Treatment of hypoglycaemia

Hypoglycaemia should be treated with glucose 10–20g PO; this is contained in 3 sugar lumps, Lucozade 60ml or milk 200ml. If drowsy and swallowing unsafe, precede oral glucose with **glucagon** 1mg IV, IM or SC. Give 25–50ml of glucose 50% IV if no improvement within 10min.

Dose and use

Tolbutamide: starting dose 500mg b.d.; increase if necessary every 3 days to a maximum of 1g b.d.

Gliclazide: starting dose 40–80mg o.m. (with breakfast); increase if necessary every 3 days to a maximum of 160mg b.d. (maximum single dose 160mg).

Insulin: if the fasting blood glucose is >12mmol/L, the patient is symptomatic and already taking the maximal dose of an oral hypoglycaemic, prescribe **ultratard insulin** 10 units o.d. at 1800h and adjust the dose according to response. A *preprandial* sliding scale of short-acting (e.g. **Human Actrapid**) is occasionally necessary (Table 7.7).

Table 7.7 Preprandial sliding scale of insulin[a]

Preprandial blood glucose (mmol/L)	Short-acting insulin dose (units)
10–15	6
>15–18	8
>18–22	10
>22[b]	12

a. responses to insulin vary widely and sliding scales need to be individualized
b. patients with marked hyperglycaemia should have monitoring 2h after meals as well until the blood glucose is better controlled.

Supply

Tablets gliclazide 80mg scored, 20 = £2.34.
Tablets tolbutamide 500mg, 20 = 35p.
Gliclazide tablets are smaller than tolbutamide and easier to swallow, but are more expensive.

---

1 Glicksman AS and Rawson RW (1956) Diabetes and altered carbohydrate metabolism in patients with cancer. *Cancer.* **9**: 1127–1134.
2 Poulson J (1997) The management of diabetes in patients with advanced cancer. *Journal of Pain and Symptom Management.* **13**: 339–346.
3 Kovner VL (1998) Management of diabetes in advanced cancer: urine sugar tests. *Journal of Pain and Symptom Management.* **15**: 147–148.
4 Holroyde CP et al. (1975) Altered glucose metabolism in metastatic carcinoma. *Cancer Research.* **35**: 3710–3714.

*OCTREOTIDE   BNF 8.3.4.3

Class of drug: Synthetic hormone.

Indications: Symptoms associated with unresectable hormone-secreting tumours e.g. carcinoid, VIPomas, glucagonomas, gastrinomas, insulinomas, acromegaly and thyrotrophinomas; [†]bleeding oesophageal varices;[1] [†]pancreatic and enterocutaneous fistulas;[2] [†]prevention of complications after elective pancreatic surgery;[3] [†]intractable diarrhoea related to high output ileostomies, AIDS, radiation, chemotherapy or bone marrow transplant;[2,4] [†]inoperable bowel obstruction in patients with cancer.[5,6]

Pharmacology

Octreotide is a synthetic octapeptide analogue of somatostatin with a longer duration of action. Somatostatin is an inhibitory hormone found throughout the body. In the hypothalamus it inhibits the release of growth hormone, TSH, prolactin and ACTH. It inhibits the secretion of insulin, glucagon, gastrin and other peptides of the gastro-enteropancreatic system, reducing splanchnic blood flow, portal blood flow, bowel motility, gastric, pancreatic and small bowel secretion, and increases water and electrolyte absorption.[7] Octreotide has a direct anticancer effect on solid tumours of the gastro-intestinal tract and prolongs survival.[8,9] In hormone-secreting tumours, octreotide improves symptoms by inhibiting hormone secretion e.g.:

- 5HT in carcinoid (improving flushing and diarrhoea)
- VIP in VIPomas (improving diarrhoea)
- glucagon in glucagonomas (improving rash and diarrhoea).

In patients with cancer and inoperable bowel obstruction octreotide rapidly improves symptoms in about 75% of patients.[5,6] Doses of ≤1200µg daily were used but a beneficial effect is generally apparent with ≤600µg daily. At Sobell House, however, octreotide is rarely used because of its expense and a low success rate (≈ 20%) when used after standard UK palliative care regimens for bowel obstruction.[10]

At doses far below those necessary for an antisecretory effect (e.g. 1µg SC t.d.s.), octreotide protects the stomach from NSAID-related injury, probably via its ability to reduce NSAID-induced neutrophil adhesion to the microvasculature.[11] Somatostatin receptors have been identified on leucocytes and, in rats, octreotide has been shown to suppress inflammation.[12] Octreotide is also of value in chronic nonmalignant pancreatic pain caused by hypertension in the scarred pancreatic ducts.[13,14] Suppressing exocrine function by administering **pancreatin supplements** also reduces pain in 50–75% of patients with chronic pancreatitis.[15] The benefit reported with octreotide could therefore be secondary to its antisecretory action.[16] Octreotide is generally given as a bolus SC or by CSCI.[17] It can be given IV when a rapid effect is required. Octreotide has also been administered IT.[18] Newer longer acting depot preparations (e.g. **lanreotide**) for IM use are under investigation.[19]

Onset of action 30min.
Duration of action 8h.
Plasma halflife 2h.

Cautions

Insulinoma (may potentiate hypoglycaemia). In diabetes mellitus, insulin and oral hypoglycaemic requirements may be reduced.

Adverse effects

Bolus injection SC is painful (but less if the vial is warmed), dry mouth, flatulence (lowers oesophageal sphincter tone), anorexia, nausea, vomiting, bloating, abdominal pain, diarrhoea, steatorrhoea (>500µg daily), cholesterol gallstone formation (long-term treatment), post-prandial hyperglycaemia, hepatic dysfunction, lightheadedness.

Dose and use

Hormone-secreting tumours: **acromegaly** 100–200µg t.d.s.
carcinoid, VIPomas, glucagonomas initial dose 50–100µg t.d.s.; increased to 200µg t.d.s.; usual maximum dose 1500µg daily, rarely 6000µg daily.[20]

Intractable diarrhoea: starting dose 50–500µg daily; usual maximum dose 1500µg daily,[21] occasionally higher.[22]

Intestinal obstruction: starting dose 250–500µg daily; usual maximum dose 750µg daily, occasionally higher.

When given by CSCI octreotide is compatible with diamorphine, haloperidol, hyoscine butylbromide and midazolam. Precipitation may occur with cyclizine. Incompatible with dexamethasone (see Section 14).

Supply

Injection 50µg/ml, 1ml amp = £2.90; 100µg/ml, 1ml amp = £5.46; 200µg/ml, 5ml vial = £54.39 (14-day expiry once started); 500µg/ml, 1ml amp = £26.45.

1 Sung JJY et al. (1993) Octreotide infusion or emergency sclerotherapy for variceal haemorrhage. Lancet. 342: 637–641.

2 Harris AG (1992) Octreotide in the treatment of disorders of the gastrointestinal tract. Drug Investigation. 4: 1–54.

3 Bassi C et al. (1994) Prophylaxis of complications after pancreatic surgery: results of a multicenter trial in Italy. Digestion. 55 (suppl 1): 41–47.

4 Crouch MA et al. (1996) Octreotide acetate in refractory bone marrow transplant-associated diarrhoea. Annals of Pharmacotherapy. 30: 331–336.

5 Mercadante S et al. (1993) Octreotide in relieving gastrointestinal symptoms due to bowel obstruction. Palliative Medicine. 7: 295–299.

6 Riley J and Fallon MT (1994) Octreotide in terminal malignant obstruction of the gastrointestinal tract. European Journal of Palliative Care. 1: 23–25.

7 Lamberts SWJ et al. (1996) Octreotide. New England Journal of Medicine. 334: 246–254.

8 Cascinu S et al. (1995) A randomised trial of octreotide vs best supportive care only in advanced gastrointestinal cancer patients refractory to chemotherapy. British Journal of Cancer. 71: 97–101.

9 Pandha HS and Waxman J (1996) Octreotide in malignant intestinal obstruction. Anti-cancer Drugs. 7 (suppl 1): 5–10.

10 Twycross R (1997) Symptom Management in Advanced Cancer. Radcliffe Medical Press, Oxford.

11 Scheiman JM et al. (1997) Reduction of non-steroidal anti-inflammatory drug induced gastric injury and leucocyte endothelial adhesion by octreotide. Gut. 40: 720–725.

12 Karalis K et al. (1994) Somatostatin analogues suppress the inflammatory reaction in vivo. Journal of Clinical Investigations. 93: 2000–2006.

13 Donnelly PK et al. (1991) Somatostatin for chronic pancreatic pain. Journal of Pain and Symptom Management. 6: 349–350.

14 Okazaki K et al. (1988) Pressure of papillary zone and pancreatic main duct in patients with chronic pancreatitis in the early state. Scandinavian Journal of Gastroenterology. 23: 501–506.

15 Mossner J et al. (1989) Influence of treatment with pancreatic extracts on pancreatic enzyme secretion. Gut. 3: 1143–1149.

16 Lembcke B et al. (1987) Effect of the somatostatin analogue sandostatin on gastrointestinal, pancreatic and biliary function and hormone release in man. Digestion. 36: 108–124.

17 Mercadante S (1995) Tolerability of continuous subcutaneous octreotide used in combination with other drugs. Journal of Palliative Care. 11 (4): 14–16.

18 Chrubasik J (1985) Spinal infusion of opiates and somatostatin. Hygieneplan, Germany.

19 Scherübl H et al. (1994) Treatment of the carcinoid syndrome with a depot formulation of the somatostatin analogue lanreotide. European Journal of Cancer. 30A: 1591–1592.

20 Harris AG and Redfern JS (1995) Octreotide treatment of carcinoid syndrome: analysis of published dose-titration data. Alimentary Pharmacology and Therapeutics. 9: 387–394.

21 Cello JP et al. (1991) Effect of octreotide on refractory AIDS-associated diarrhoea: a prospective multicenter clinical trial. Annals of Internal Medicine. 115: 705–710.

22 Petrelli NJ et al. (1993) Bowel rest, intravenous hydration and continuous high-dose infusion of octreotide acetate for the treatment of chemotherapy-induced diarrhoea in patients with colorectal carcinoma. Cancer. 72: 1543–1546.

PROGESTOGENS

BNF 6.4.1.2 & 8.3.2

Class of drug: Sex hormones.

Indications: †Postcastration hot flushes (women and men), anticancer hormonal therapy. The licensed indications for **megestrol** are limited to breast and endometrial cancers, whereas the licence for **medroxyprogesterone** also includes renal cell cancer (Farlutal, Provera) and prostate cancer (Farlutal only).

Contra-indications: Hepatic impairment.

Pharmacology

There are two main groups of progestogens, **progesterone** and its analogues (dydrogesterone, hydroxyprogesterone, and medroxyprogesterone) and **testosterone** and its analogues (norethisterone and norgestrel). Progesterone analogues are less androgenic than the testosterone analogues; neither progesterone nor dydrogesterone causes virilization. Other synthetic derivatives are variably metabolized into testosterone and oestrogen; adverse effects vary with the preparation and the dose.

Hormonal manipulation has an important role in the treatment of metastatic cancers of the breast, prostate, and endometrium. Treatment is not curative but may induce remission in 15–30% of patients, occasionally for years. Tumour response and treatment toxicity need to be monitored and treatment changed if progression occurs or adverse effects exceed benefit.

Progestogens have been shown to stimulate appetite and weight gain in many patients, particularly those with breast cancer.[1] The impact is more long-lasting than with corticosteroids. Progestogens are relatively expensive, however, and should be used selectively. Doses of megestrol of up to 1600mg/day have been used and there is evidence of a dose-response effect;[2] elderly patients may respond to 80mg/day.

Plasma halflives of medroxyprogesterone and megestrol are similar, with mean values of ≥30h with wide variation from 13–105h.

Adverse effects

Urticaria, acne, weight gain, fluid retention, hypertension, nausea, constipation, fatigue, depression, insomnia. Alopecia, hirsutism, jaundice (all rare).

Dose and use

Appetite stimulation and weight gain: medroxyprogesterone 400mg o.m. *or* megestrol 80–160mg o.m. Consider doubling the dose if initial poor response.[3]
Hot flushes after surgical or chemical castration: medroxyprogesterone 5–20mg b.d.–q.d.s. *or* megestrol 40mg o.m.[4] The effect manifests after 2–4 weeks. (**Diethylstilbestrol** and **cyproterone**, which has weak progestogen activity, are alternatives.[5])

Supply

Tablets medroxyprogesterone acetate 100mg, 20 = £8.12; 200mg, 20 = £16.47; 250mg, 20 = £20.29; 400mg, 20 = £32.59; 500mg, 20 = £40.58.
Tablets megestrol acetate 40mg, 20 = £5.08; 160mg, 20 = £19.53.

1 Aisner J et al. (1990) Appetite stimulation and weight gain with megestrol acetate. *Seminars in Oncology.* **17** (6 suppl 9): 2–7.
2 Downer S et al. (1993) A double blind placebo controlled trial of medroxyprogesterone acetate (MPA) in cancer cachexia. *British Journal of Cancer.* **67**: 1102–1105.
3 Donnelly S and Walsh TD (1995) Low-dose megestrol acetate for appetite stimulation in advanced cancer. *Journal of Pain and Symptom Management.* **10**: 182–183.
4 Loprinzi CL et al. (1996) Megestrol acetate for the prevention of hot flushes. *New England Journal of Medicine.* **331**: 347–352.
5 Miller JI and Ahmann FR (1992) Treatment of castration-induced menopausal symptoms with low dose diethylstilbestrol in men with advanced prostate cancer. *Urology.* **40**: 499–502.

† unlicensed use.

STANOZOLOL   BNF 6.4.3

Class of drug: Anabolic steroid.

Indications: [†]Pruritus associated with obstructive jaundice when stenting of the common bile duct is contra-indicated and skin care alone is inadequate.

Pharmacology

The mechanism of action by which androgens relieve cholestatic pruritis is unknown. The effect was discovered serendipitously some 50 years ago when the co-incidental use of an androgen in a patient with primary biliary cirrhosis resulted in the amelioration of the associated pruritus.[1] In some patients the benefit is maintained even if the cholestasis is exacerbated by the androgen itself.[2] Androgens and oestrogens also relieve nonspecific pruritus in the elderly.[3]

Oral bio-availability no data.
Onset of action <7 days.
Duration of action 24–36h.
Plasma halflife 8h (slow metabolizer, 39h).

Adverse effects

Acne, hirsutism, amenorrhoea, oedema, cramp. Can enhance the effects of insulin and warfarin.

Dose and use

• 5–10mg o.d.; benefit noticed after about 1 week
• moisturizing the skin ('skin care') is a prerequisite for success.

Supply

Tablets 5mg, 56 = £26.26.

---

1 Ahrens EH *et al.* (1950) Primary biliary cirrhosis. *Medicine.* **29**: 299–364.
2 Lloyd-Thomas HGL and Sherlock S (1952) Testosterone therapy for the pruritus of obstructive jaundice. *British Medical Journal.* **ii**: 1289–1291.
3 Feldman S *et al.* (1942) Treatment of senile pruritus with androgens and estrogens. *Archives of Dermatology and Syphilology Chicago.* **46**: 112–127.

[†] unlicensed use.

8: Drugs used in
URINARY TRACT DISORDERS

Indoramin

Oxybutynin

Catheter patency solutions

INDORAMIN   BNF 7.4

Class of drug: Selective α_1-adrenoceptor antagonist.

Indications: Hesitancy of micturition, hypertension.

Contra-indications: Symptomatic postural hypotension, cardiac failure, concurrent use of MAOI.

Pharmacology
Indoramin is an α-adrenoceptor antagonist which acts selectively and competitively on post-synaptic α_1-adrenoceptors, causing a decrease in peripheral vascular resistance, relaxation of the bladder neck and contraction of the detrusor. Indoramin is used both in the treatment of essential hypertension and hesitancy of micturition associated with benign prostatic hypertrophy. Other selective α_1 antagonists are available, namely **prazosin, tamsulosin** and **terazosin**. All may cause severe hypotension, particularly with the first dose and in patients receiving diuretics or other antihypertensive medication. Low cost is the only advantage in using prazosin; this has to be balanced against ease of compliance with tamsulosin and terazosin (o.d. compared to b.d.). Indoramin is probably the safest in debilitated patients. Peak plasma concentrations are achieved in 1–4h, but it may take 4–8 weeks to obtain maximal urodynamic and symptomatic improvement. Muscarinic drugs and anticholinesterases are sometimes preferable to an α antagonist, e.g. **bethanechol** 10–25mg t.d.s.–q.d.s., **distigmine** 5mg o.d. If necessary, one of these may be used concurrently with indoramin.
Oral bio-availability 31%.
Onset of action 30–60min.
Duration of action 12–24h.
Plasma halflife 4–5h.

Cautions
If the patient is taking antihypertensives, the dose should be reduced and the blood pressure monitored. Baclofen also enhances the hypotensive effect.

Adverse effects
Sedation, dizziness, postural hypotension.

Dose and use
For hesitancy of micturition:
• starting dose 20mg b.d. (the first dose taken in bed at night); 20mg o.n. in the elderly
• increase dose if necessary by 20mg every 2 weeks to a maximum of 100mg/day.
Doses for hypertension tend to be higher, e.g. 25mg b.d. and increasing if necessary by 25–50mg every 2 weeks to a maximum of 200mg/day.

Supply
Tablets 20mg, 60 = £12.30.

OXYBUTYNIN BNF 7.4.2

Class of drug: Antimuscarinic.

Indications: Frequency of micturition not caused by infective cystitis, bladder spasms.

Contra-indications: Significant bladder outflow obstruction, intestinal atony, glaucoma, myasthenia gravis.

Pharmacology

Oxybutynin has an antispasmodic action on the detrusor muscle of the bladder and an anti-muscarinic (anticholinergic) effect on bladder innervation.[1] This helps to prevent bladder spasm and increase bladder capacity. The plasma halflife of oxybutynin increases in the elderly, generally allowing smaller doses to be given less frequently. An alternative drug may be more appropriate for some patients (Box 8.A).

Oral bio-availability 100%.
Onset of action 30–60min.
Duration of action 6–10h.
Plasma halflife 2–3h (4–5h in the elderly).

Box 8.A   Drugs for urinary frequency and bladder spasms

Antimuscarinics are the drugs of choice even though treatment may be limited by other antimuscarinic effects (see p.225):

- **oxybutynin** 2.5–5mg b.d.–q.d.s.; also has a topical anaesthetic effect on bladder mucosa[2]
- **amitriptyline** 25–50mg o.n.
- **propantheline** 15–30mg b.d.–t.d.s.

Sympathomimetics, e.g. **terbutaline** 5mg t.d.s.

Musculotropic drug, **flavoxate** 200mg t.d.s.

NSAIDs, e.g.:

- **flurbiprofen** 50–100mg b.d.
- **naproxen** 250–500mg b.d.

Topical analgesics, e.g. **phenazopyridine** 100–200mg t.d.s. (not available in the UK).

Vasopressin analogues, e.g. **desmopressin**, are of value in refractory nocturia (see p.141); hyponatraemia is a possible complication.

Adverse effects

Dry mouth, other antimuscarinic effects (see p.225), cognitive dysfunction and delirium in the elderly,[3] nausea, abdominal discomfort.

Dose and use
- starting dose 2.5–5mg b.d.
- increase if necessary to 5mg q.d.s.

Supply
Tablets 2.5mg, 20 = £2.45; 5mg, 20 = £4.97.
Suspension 2.5mg/5ml, 150ml = £4.78.

1 Andersson KE (1988) Current concepts in the treatment of disorders of micturition. *Drugs.* **35**: 477–494.
2 Robinson TG and Castleden CM (1994) Drugs in focus: 11. Oxybutynin hydrochloride. *Prescribers' Journal.* **34**: 27–30.
3 Donnellàn CA *et al.* (1997) Oxybutynin and cognitive dysfunction. *British Medical Journal.* **315**: 1363–1364.

CATHETER PATENCY SOLUTIONS   BNF 7.4.4

Deposit which forms on the surface of indwelling urinary catheters is composed chiefly of phosphate crystals. To minimize this a latex catheter should be changed at least every 6 weeks. If the catheter is to be left for longer periods a silicone catheter should be used together with the appropriate use of catheter maintenance solutions. Repeated blockage generally indicates that the catheter needs to be changed. In some patients blockage is caused by blood clots.

Supply and use
A range of prepacked 100ml solutions is available (see below). Bladder washouts do not cure infection; their main purpose is to reduce the frequency of catheter blockage.[1] There is no evidence that chlorhexidine has any advantage over sodium chloride, it may cause irritation or lead to the emergence of resistant bacterial strains.[2,3] Administer washouts daily; reduce to alternate days or change to sodium chloride once problem resolved.

Sodium chloride 0.9% recommended for flushing of debris and small blood clots, 100ml sachet = £2.00.

Chlorhexidine 0.02% antiseptic solution aimed at preventing or reducing bacterial growth, particularly *Escherichia coli* and *Klebsiella*; ineffective against most *Pseudomonas* species, 100ml sachet = £2.13.

Solution G (Suby G) 3.23% citric acid solution containing magnesium, reduces encrustation, 100ml sachet = £2.13.

The BNF also contains **Mandelic acid 1%** and **Solution R** solutions.

1 Getliffe KA (1996) Bladder instillations and bladder washouts in the management of catheterized patients. *Journal of Advanced Nursing.* **23**: 548–554.
2 Baillie L (1987) Chlorhexidine resistance among bacteria isolated from urine of catheterized patients. *Journal of Hospital Infection.* **10**: 83–86.
3 Davies AJ *et al.* (1987) Does instillation of chlorhexidine into the bladder of catheterized geriatric patients help reduce bacteria? *Journal of Hospital Infection.* **9**: 72–75.

9: Drugs affecting

NUTRITION AND BLOOD

Ascorbic acid (vitamin C)

Ferrous sulphate

Multivitamin preparations

Phytomenadione (vitamin K₁)

Potassium supplements

ASCORBIC ACID (VITAMIN C)   BNF 9.6.3

Class of drug: Vitamin.

Indications: [†]Decubitus ulcers, [†]furred tongue (topical), [†]urinary infection, scurvy.

Pharmacology

Ascorbic acid (vitamin C) is a powerful reducing agent. It is obtained from fresh fruit and vegetables, particularly blackcurrant and kiwifruit; it cannot be synthesized by the body. It is involved in the hydroxylation of proline to hydroxyproline, which is necessary for the formation of collagen. The failure of this accounts for most of the clinical effects found in deficiency (scurvy), e.g. keratosis of hair follicles with 'corkscrew hair', perifollicular haemorrhages, swollen spongy infected and bleeding gums, loose teeth, spontaneous bruising and haemorrhage, anaemia and failure of wound healing. Repeated infections are also common. In healthy adults, a dietary intake of 30–60mg/day is necessary; in scurvy, a rapid clinical response is seen with 100–200mg/day. Absorption occurs mainly from the proximal small intestine by a nonpassive saturable process. In health, body stores of ascorbic acid are about 1.5g, although larger stores may occur with intakes higher than 200mg daily. It is excreted as oxalic acid, unchanged ascorbic acid and small amounts of dehydro-ascorbic acid. Ascorbic acid is used to acidify urine in patients with alkaline urine and recurrent urinary infections.

A beneficial effect of megadose ascorbic acid therapy has been claimed for many conditions,[1] including the common cold, asthma, atherosclerosis, cancer, psychiatric disorders, increased susceptibility to infections related to abnormal leucocyte function, infertility, and osteogenesis imperfecta. Ascorbic acid has also been tried in the treatment of wound healing, pain in Paget's disease and opioid withdrawal. There are few controlled studies to substantiate these claims. High-dose vitamin C is not effective against advanced cancer.[2] Vitamin C alone or with β-carotene and vitamin E does not prevent the development of colorectal adenoma.[3] Ascorbic acid does, however, reduce the severity of a cold but not its incidence.[4] On the other hand, enthusiasm for high-dose ascorbic acid for HIV-positive people waned after many died from disease progression.[5] Although it has been postulated that ascorbic acid might help prevent ischaemic heart disease, in contrast to other anti-oxidant vitamins there is little demonstrable benefit in controlled studies.[6,7] Of more concern are data which indicate that a daily dose as small as 500mg has a pro-oxidant effect which could result in genetic mutation.[8]

Adverse effects

Excess ascorbic acid (>3g/day) may result in acidosis, diarrhoea, glycosuria, oxaluria and renal stones. Tolerance may be induced with prolonged use of large doses, resulting in symptoms of deficiency when intake is returned to normal.

Dose and use

- furred tongue, place 1/4 of 1g effervescent tablet on the tongue and allow it to dissolve; repeat up to q.d.s. for <1 week

---

[†] unlicensed use.

- acidification of urine, give 100–200mg b.d.; test urine with litmus paper until constant acid result is obtained
- enhancement of healing of decubitus ulcers, give 100mg b.d. for 4 weeks
- scurvy, 100mg b.d. for 4 weeks.

Supply
Tablets 50mg, 20 = 8p; 100mg, 20 = 23p; 200mg, 20 = 34p.
Tablets effervescent 1g, 20 = £2.28 (~~NHS~~).

---

1 Ovesen L (1984) Vitamin therapy in the absence of obvious deficiency: what is the evidence? *Drugs.* **27**: 148–170.
2 Moertel CG *et al.* (1985) High-dose vitamin C versus placebo in the treatment of patients with advanced cancer who have had no prior chemotherapy: a randomized double-blind comparison. *New England Journal of Medicine.* **312**: 137–141.
3 Greenberg ER *et al.* (1994) A clinical trial of antioxidant vitamins to prevent colorectal adenoma. *New England Journal of Medicine.* **331**: 141–147.
4 Hemila H (1994) Does vitamin C alleviate the symptoms of the common cold? – a review of current evidence *Scandinavian Journal of Infectious Diseases.* **26**: 1–6.
5 Abrams DI (1990) Alternative therapies in HIV infection. *AIDS.* **4**: 1179–1187.
6 Rimm EB (1993) Vitamin E consumption and the risk of coronary heart disease in men. *New England Journal of Medicine.* **328**: 1450–1456.
7 Stampfer MJ (1993) Vitamin E consumption and the risk of coronary disease in women. *New England Journal of Medicine.* **328**: 1444–1449.
8 Podmore ID *et al.* (1998) Vitamin C exhibits pro-oxidant properties. *Nature.* **392**: 559.

FERROUS SULPHATE   BNF 9.1.1

Class of drug: Elemental salt.

Indications: Iron deficiency anaemia.

Contra-indications: Anaemia of chronic disease (mimics true iron deficiency in terms of standard haematological parameters).

Pharmacology
Ferrous salts are better absorbed than ferric salts. Because there are only marginal differences in terms of efficiency of iron absorption, the choice of ferrous salt is based mainly on the incidence of adverse effects and cost. Adverse effects relate directly to the amount of elemental iron and an apparent improvement in tolerance on changing to another salt may be because of a lower elemental iron content (Table 9.1). M/r preparations are designed to reduce adverse effects by releasing iron gradually as the capsule or tablet passes along the bowel. However, these preparations are likely to carry most of the iron past the first part of the duodenum into parts of the bowel where iron absorption is poor. Such preparations have no therapeutic advantage and should not be used.

Table 9.1 Elemental ferrous iron content of different iron salts

Iron salt	Amount	Ferrous content
Ferrous fumarate	200mg	65mg
Ferrous sulphate, dried	200mg	65mg
Ferrous sulphate	300mg	60mg
Ferrous gluconate	300mg	35mg
Ferrous succinate	100mg	35mg

Some oral preparations contain ascorbic acid to aid absorption, or the iron is in the form of a chelate. These modifications have shown experimentally to produce a modest increase in absorption of iron. However, the therapeutic advantage is minimal and cost may be increased. There is no clinical justification for the inclusion of other therapeutically active ingredients, such as the B group of vitamins (except folic acid for pregnant women). In the treatment of iron deficiency, the haemoglobin concentration should rise by about 1g/dl per week. After the haemoglobin has risen to normal, treatment should be continued for a further 3 months in an attempt to replenish the iron stores. Epithelial tissue changes such as atrophic glossitis and koilonychia also improve but generally more slowly.

Adverse effects
Dyspepsia, nausea, epigastric pain, constipation, diarrhoea. Elderly patients are more likely to develop constipation, occasionally leading to faecal impaction; m/r preparations are more likely to cause diarrhoea (in patients with inflammatory bowel disease).

Dose and use
Ideally, the diagnosis of iron deficiency should be confirmed before iron supplements are prescribed (Table 9.2). For iron deficiency the daily dose of elemental ferrous iron should be 100–200mg PO:
• give as dried ferrous sulphate 200mg b.d.
• if adverse effects occur, reduce the dose or change to an alternative iron salt.

Table 9.2   Iron deficiency anaemia compared with anaemia of chronic disorders[1]

	Normal	Iron deficiency anaemia	Anaemia of chronic disorders
Morphology of blood	Normochromic normocytic	Hypochromic microcytic	Normochromic or hypochromic normocytic; rarely microcytic
Plasma iron (µmol/L)	20.6 ± 9	Low <7.2	Low <12.0
TIBC (µmol/L)	58.0 ± 4.5	High 71.6 ± 9	Low 44.8 ± 9
Plasma ferritin (µg/L)	100 ± 60	Low <10	Often high >200

Supply
Tablets **dried ferrous sulphate** 200mg, 20 = 11p.
Syrup **ferrous fumarate** 140mg/5ml, 200ml = £2.35.

1 Callender ST (1987) Normochromic, normocytic anaemias. In: Ledingham JGG, Warrell DA (eds) *Oxford Textbook of Medicine. (2nd edn) volume II.* Oxford Medical Publications, Oxford. pp 19.91–19.93.

MULTIVITAMIN PREPARATIONS   BNF 9.6.7

Indications: Vitamin deficiency, e.g. sore red tongue, angular stomatitis, painful neuropathy.

Dose and use
Use multivitamin capsules 1 b.d.–t.d.s.

Supply
Capsules **vitamins** (ascorbic acid 15mg, nicotinamide 7.5mg, riboflavine 500μg, thiamine 1mg, vitamin A 2500 units, vitamin D 300 units), 20 = 20p.

PHYTOMENADIONE (VITAMIN K₁) BNF 9.6.6

Indications: Vitamin K deficiency, reversal of anticoagulant effects of warfarin, †haemorrhage in patients with severe hepatic impairment in advanced cancer.

Pharmacology
Phytomenadione (vitamin K₁) is the active form of vitamin K. It is necessary for the production of blood clotting factors and proteins involved in bone calcification. Because vitamin K is fat-soluble, patients with fat malabsorption may become deficient, particularly in biliary obstruction or hepatic disease. Oral coumarin anticoagulants act by interfering with vitamin K metabolism in the liver and their effects are antagonized by giving exogenous vitamin K. Vitamin K is *not* indicated routinely in severe liver failure, nor even in moribund patients with manifestations of a bleeding diathesis (e.g. petechiae, purpura, multiple bruising, nose and gum bleeds) and it should not be used merely to prevent an imminent inevitable death. Its use is limited to conscious patients with a reasonable performance status for whom other supportive measures are deemed appropriate (e.g. blood transfusion).
Plasma halflife 1.5–3h.

Cautions and adverse effects
Konakion, a proprietary preparation of phytomenadione containing polyethoxylated castor oil, has been associated with anaphylaxis.

Dose and use
Partial reversal of warfarin anticoagulation: the recommendations of the British Society of Haematology should be followed (see BNF 2.8.2).
Correction of a bleeding tendency in liver failure: give **Konakion MM** 10mg by slow IV injection; repeat p.r.n.
Prevention of vitamin K deficiency in malabsorption: use an oral water-soluble preparation, i.e. **menadiol sodium phosphate** 10mg o.d.

Supply
Tablets **menadiol sodium phosphate** (= 10mg of menadiol phosphate), 100 = £9.28.
Injection **Konakion** 2mg/ml, 0.5ml amp = 24p. Konakion is for IM and slow IV use. *Must not be diluted, therefore should not be given by IV infusion.*
Colloidal injection **Konakion MM** 10mg/ml, 1ml amp = 45p. Konakion MM may be administered by slow IV injection or by IV infusion in 5% glucose; *not for IM injection.*

POTASSIUM SUPPLEMENTS BNF 9.2.1.1

Class of drug: Elemental salt.
Indications: Hypokalaemia (<3.5mmol/L).

Pharmacology
In palliative care, hypokalaemia is most common in patients receiving diuretics, particularly if also taking a corticosteroid and/or a NSAID. Hypokalaemia is also associated with chronic diarrhoea and persistent vomiting. Correction of hypokalaemia is important in patients taking digoxin or other anti-arrhythmic drugs because of the risk of an arrhythmia. Potassium supplements are seldom required with small doses of diuretics given to treat hypertension. When larger doses

of thiazide or loop diuretics are given to eliminate oedema, potassium-sparing diuretics (e.g. **amiloride**) rather than potassium supplements are recommended for the prevention of hypokalaemia. Dietary supplements can help maintain plasma potassium; 10mmol of potassium is contained in a large **banana** and in 250ml of **orange juice**.

Cautions
Smaller doses must be used if there is renal insufficiency (common in the elderly) so as to avoid switching from hypokalaemia to hyperkalaemia.

Adverse effects
Nausea and vomiting, often resulting in poor compliance. Liquid or effervescent preparations are distasteful.

Dose and use
Whenever possible orange juice and bananas should be used as a palatable source of potassium. To minimize nausea and vomiting, potassium supplements are best taken during or after a meal.
Prevention of hypokalaemia
• **amiloride** 5–10mg o.d. (see BNF 2.2.3)
• **potassium chloride** 2–4g daily (24–48mmol) = **Slow K** 3–6 tablets or **Sando-K** 2–4 tablets.
Treatment of hypokalaemia
The aim is to give 60-80mmol daily:
• **Kloref-S** 1 sachet t.d.s.–q.d.s. after meals
• **Sando-K** 2 tablets t.d.s.

Supply
Tablets m/r **Slow K** 600mg (8mmol K$^+$), 20 = 10p.
Tablets effervescent **Sando-K** 470mg (12mmol K$^+$), 20 = 34p.
Granules effervescent **Kloref-S** 1.5g (20mmol K$^+$), 30 sachets = £3.30.

10: Drugs used in
MUSCULOSKELETAL AND JOINT DISEASES

Depot corticosteroid injections

Hyaluronidase

Rubefacients and other topical preparations

Skeletal muscle relaxants
   Baclofen
   Dantrolene
   Quinine

DEPOT CORTICOSTEROID INJECTIONS   BNF 10.1.2.2

Indications: [†]Pain in superficial bones (e.g. rib, scapula, iliac crest), [†]pain caused by spinal metastases.

Contra-indications: Untreated local or systemic infection.

Pharmacology
Corticosteroids have an anti-inflammatory effect, i.e. they reduce the concentration of algesic substances present in inflammation which sensitize or stimulate nerve endings.[1] They also have a direct inhibitory effect on spontaneous activity in excitable damaged nerves.[2]

Cautions
May mask or alter presentation of infection in immunocompromised patients; such patients should not receive live vaccines and may need to take precautions if exposed to chickenpox. Depot preparations may result in symptomatic hyperglycaemia for several days in patients with diabetes mellitus and suppression of the hypothalamic-pituitary-adrenal axis for up to 4 weeks. Pneumothorax may follow injection of a rib. *See also p.137.*

Adverse effects
Occasionally, a patient develops lipodystrophy (local fat necrosis), resulting in indentation of the overlying skin. Antagonism of antihypertensive, antidiabetic and diuretic drugs. Enhanced effect of potassium-losing drugs. *See also pp 137–138.*

Dose and use
Intralesional injection[3]
- infiltrate the skin and SC tissues overlying the point of maximal bone tenderness with local anaesthetic
- with the tip of the needle pressing against the tender bone, inject **depot methylprednisolone** 80mg in 2ml.

In addition for rib lesions, reposition the needle under the rib and inject 5ml of **bupivacaine** 0.5% to anaesthetize the intercostal nerve. Complete or good relief occurs in more than 2/3 of patients. If of benefit, injections can be repeated if the pain returns but not more than every 2 weeks. **Triamcinolone hexacetonide (Lederspan)** may be used as an alternative.
Epidural injection[3, 4]
Depot methylprednisolone 80mg in 2ml or **triamcinolone hexacetonide** 40–80mg in 2–4ml. A single ED injection is given, or daily for 3 days, via an indwelling catheter. The effect of

---

[†] unlicensed use.

ED corticosteroids is unpredictable and may not peak until 1 week after injection; some patients obtain weeks of benefit from one injection. Further injections can be given at monthly or longer intervals. Depot corticosteroids cannot be injected through an epidural bacterial filter.

Supply
Injection **methylprednisolone acetate** 40mg/ml, 1ml vial = £2.70; 2ml vial = £4.87; 3ml vial = £7.05.
Injection **triamcinolone hexacetonide** 20mg/ml, 1ml vial = £2.48; 5ml vial = £9.65.

---

1 Pybus PK (1984) Osteoarthritis: a new neurological method of pain control. *Medical Hypothesis.* **14**: 413–422.
2 Twycross RG (1994) *Pain Relief in Advanced Cancer.* Churchill Livingstone, Edinburgh.
3 Rowell NP (1988) Intralesional methylprednisolone for rib metastases: an alternative to radiotherapy. *Palliative Medicine.* **2**: 153–155.
4 Devor M et al. (1985) Corticosteroids reduce neuroma hyperexcitability. In: Fields HL, Dubner R, Cervero F (eds) *Advances in pain research and therapy, vol 9.* Raven Press, New York. pp 451–455.

HYALURONIDASE   BNF 10.3

Class of drug: Enzyme.

Indications: To enhance absorption of SC infusions of fluid (hypodermoclysis), [†]inflammatory reactions caused by CSCI.

Contra-indications: Local infection or local malignancy.

Pharmacology
Hyaluronidase has a rapid temporary depolymerizing action on hyaluronic acid, a mucopolysaccharide component of the intercellular matrix, thereby rendering the tissues more permeable to injected or excess fluids. The natural process of repair to the intercellular matrix takes about 24h; repeat injections are therefore time-contingent (o.d. at most) and *not* related to the volume of fluid infused. *Hyaluronidase is not generally necessary when the daily SC infusion is ≤2L/24h.*[1]
Onset of action within minutes.
Duration of action about 24h.

Adverse effects
Occasional allergy.

Dose and use
Hyaluronidase is not used at Hayward House or Sobell House.
Hypodermoclysis: 1500 units dissolved in 1ml WFI or 0.9% sodium chloride and administered SC *before* starting an infusion of 500–1000ml: [1,2]
• prime the tubing attached to the butterfly needle with hyaluronidase 0.5ml
• position the butterfly needle SC
• inject remainder of hyaluronidase (0.5ml)
• commence infusion.
CSCI skin reaction: start with hyaluronidase 1500 units *as for hypodermoclysis* and repeat every 24h p.r.n.

Supply
Injection, 1500 unit amp = £6.91.

---

† unlicensed use.

1 Constans T et al. (1991) Hypodermoclysis in dehydrated elderly patients: local effects with and without hyaluronidase. *Journal of Palliative Care.* **7** (2): 10–12.
2 Stanley A et al. (1996) Workshop on Hyalase in hypodermoclysis.

RUBEFACIENTS AND OTHER TOPICAL PREPARATIONS   BNF 10.3.2

Indications: Muscle, tendon and joint pains (**rubefacients, topical NSAIDs**), severe skin reaction to an indwelling SC cannula and/or phlebitis (**kaolin poultices**).

Contra-indications: Inflamed or broken skin.

Pharmacology
Rubefacients act by counter-stimulation of the skin, thereby closing the pain 'gate' in the dorsal horn of the spinal cord.[1,2] Algipan Rub contains capsicin, glycol salicylate and methyl nicotinate. Kaolin poultices applied warm also act by counter-stimulation, substituting the pleasure of warmth for the stinging/burning of the skin reaction.

Topically applied salicylates and certain other NSAIDs can achieve high local SC concentrations and therapeutically effective concentrations within synovial fluid and peri-articular tissues similar to those seen after oral administration.[3-5] The benefit of topical ibuprofen has been demonstrated in a randomized controlled trial; a trial with piroxicam failed to show benefit.[6,7]
Onset of action immediate.
Duration of action 3–6h.

Cautions
Large quantities of topical NSAIDs have been associated with systemic effects, e.g. hypersensitivity, rash, asthma and renal impairment.[8]

Dose and use
Algipan Rub applied b.d.–q.d.s. according to results and patient preference.
Topical NSAIDs applied b.d.–q.d.s.
Kaolin poultices generally applied b.d.
The patient should be advised to wash hands after application.

Supply
Cream **Algipan Rub**, 80g = £3.15.
Cream **benzydamine 3%**, 100g = £7.00.
Gel **ibuprofen 5%**, 100g = £6.53.
Poultice **kaolin**, 4 × 100g pouches = £5.19.

1 Melzack R (1971) Phantom limb pain: implications for treatment of pathologic pain. *Anaesthesiology.* **35**: 409–419.
2 Anonymous (1976) The pain paradox. *Lancet.* **i**: 945–946.
3 Chlud K and Wagener HH (1987) Percutaneous nonsteroidal anti-inflammatory drug (NSAID) therapy with particular reference to pharmacokinetic factors. *EULAR Bulletin.* **2**: 40–43.
4 Mondino A et al. (1983) Kinetic studies of ibuprofen on humans: comparative study for the determination of blood concentration and metabolite following local and oral administration. *Med Welt.* **34**: 1052–1054.
5 Peters H et al. (1987) Percutaneous kinetics of ibuprofen (German). *Acta Rheumatologica.* **12**: 208–211.
6 Anonymous (1990) More topical NSAIDs: worth the rub? *Drug and Therapeutics Bulletin.* **28**: 27–28.
7 Kageyama T (1987) A double blind placebo controlled multicenter study of piroxicam 0.5% gel in osteoarthritis of the knee. *European Journal of Rheumatology and Inflammation.* **8**: 114–115.

8 O'Callaghan CA et al. (1994) Renal disease and use of topical NSAIDs. *British Medical Journal.*
308: 110–111.

SKELETAL MUSCLE RELAXANTS   BNF 10.2.2

Skeletal muscle relaxants are used to relieve painful chronic muscle spasm. Also used for
spasticity secondary to injury to the CNS, e.g. in paraplegia, poststroke, multiple sclerosis and,
occasionally, motor neurone disease. [†]**Baclofen** is sometimes used to relieve hiccup.

   Baclofen and **diazepam** act principally on spinal and supraspinal sites within the CNS;
dantrolene and **quinine** act upon muscle. The use of diazepam as a muscle relaxant is discussed
elsewhere (see pp 52 & 53).

BACLOFEN   BNF 10.2.2

Class of drug: Skeletal muscle relaxant.

Indications: Painful muscle spasm, spasticity secondary to CNS injury, [†]hiccup.

Contra-indications: Peptic ulcer.

Pharmacology

Baclofen is a chemical congener of the naturally occurring neurotransmitter, GABA (gamma-
aminobutyric acid). It acts on the GABA-receptor, inhibiting the release of excitatory amino acids,
glutamate and aspartate, principally at the spinal level.[1]
Bio-availability >90%.
Onset of action 3–4 days.
Duration of action 4–8h.
Plasma halflife 3.5h; 4.5h in the elderly.

Cautions

Withdrawal: serious adverse psychiatric reactions can occur with abrupt withdrawal (agitation,
delirium, delusions, hallucinations, paranoia and psychosis). Discontinue by gradual dose
reduction over 1–2 weeks, or longer if symptoms occur.[2]

History of peptic ulceration, severe psychiatric disorders, epilepsy, liver disease (monitor liver
function tests), renal impairment (reduce dose), respiratory impairment, diabetes mellitus, hesitancy of micturition (may precipitate urinary retention), patients who use spasticity to maintain
posture or to aid function. Drowsiness may affect skilled tasks/driving; effects of alcohol enhanced.

Adverse effects

Hypotonia and sedation (increase dose slowly particularly in the elderly), euphoria, insomnia,
depression, tremor, nystagmus, paraesthesia, convulsions, muscular pain and weakness, respiratory
or cardiovascular depression, hypotension, dry mouth, gastro-intestinal and urinary disturbances.
Rarely visual disorders, taste alterations, sweating, rash, blood glucose changes, altered liver
function tests, and a paradoxical increase in spasticity.

Dose and use

Starting doses are the same for muscle spasm, spasticity and hiccup:
- start with 5mg b.d.–t.d.s., preferably p.c., and increase if necessary by 5mg b.d.–t.d.s. every
  3 days
- effective doses for hiccup are often relatively low, e.g. 5–10mg t.d.s., although higher doses may
  be necessary

• for spasticity, the effective dose is generally ≤20mg t.d.s. (maximum 100mg daily)
• effective doses for muscle spasm fall somewhere in the middle.
With spasticity, if no improvement with maximum tolerated dose after 6 weeks, withdraw
gradually.

Supply
Tablets 10mg, 20 = £1.08.
Tablets scored (Lioresal) 10mg, 20 = £2.15.
Liquid sugar-free 5mg/5ml, 300ml = £7.46.

1 Kochak GM et al. (1985) The pharmacokinetics of baclofen derived from intestinal infusion. *Clinical Pharmacology and Therapeutics*. **38**: 251–257.
2 Anonymous (1997) Reminder: severe withdrawal reactions with baclofen. *Current Problems in Pharmacovigilance*. **23**: 3.

DANTROLENE   BNF 10.2.2

Class of drug: Skeletal muscle relaxant.
Indications: CNS spasticity.

Contra-indications: Hepatic impairment (may cause severe liver damage).

Pharmacology
Dantrolene acts directly on skeletal muscle reducing the amount of intracellular calcium available
for contraction. It produces fewer central adverse effects than baclofen and diazepam.
Bio-availability 35%.
Onset of action up to 1 week.
Duration of action variable.
Plasma halflife 9h.

Cautions
The dose of dantrolene must be built up slowly, not more than 25mg per week.

Adverse effects
Transient drowsiness, dizziness, muscle weakness, diarrhoea. Rarely severe hepatotoxicity
develops after 1–6 months in people over 30; fatalities have occurred only with doses over
200mg/day.[1,2]

Dose and use
• starting dose 25mg o.d.
• increased by 25mg *weekly*
• usual effective dose 75mg t.d.s.; maximum dose 100mg q.d.s.
Some centres increase the dose more rapidly because of the patient's limited prognosis.

Supply
Capsules 25mg, 20 = £3.42; 100mg, 20 = £11.97.

1 Utili R et al. (1977) Dantrolene-associated hepatic injury: incidence and character. *Gastroenterology*. **72**: 610–616.
2 Wilkinson SP et al. (1979) Hepatitis from dantrolene sodium. *Gut*. **20**: 33–36.

QUININE BNF 10.2.2

Class of drug: Antimalarial.

Indications: Nocturnal calf and foot cramps.

Pharmacology

Quinine reduces the amount of intracellular calcium available for muscle contraction. It reduces the frequency of cramps, thereby improving sleep, but does not always reduce cramp severity.[1,2] Maximum benefit takes up to 4 weeks. Smoking can block the effect of quinine.

Oral bio-availability 76–88%.

Onset of action <1h.

Duration of action 8h.

Plasma halflife 8–12h.

Cautions

Quinine is very toxic in overdosage and fatalities have occurred in children.

Adverse effects

Cinchonism (i.e. tinnitus, headache, hot flushed skin, nausea, abdominal pain, rashes, visual disturbances/temporary blindness, confusion), hypersensitivity reactions including angioedema, blood disorders including thrombocytopenia and DIC, acute renal failure, hypoglycaemia (unlikely with oral administration).

Dose and use

- quinine **sulphate** 200–300mg o.n.[1–4] *or*
- quinine **bisulphate** 300mg o.n.

Stop if no improvement in 4 weeks; interrupt treatment every few months to see if it is still needed.

Supply

Quinine base 100mg = quinine **sulphate** 121mg or quinine **bisulphate** 169mg. Thus, quinine bisulphate 300mg contains 177mg of quinine base, and quinine sulphate 300mg contains 248mg, whereas quinine sulphate 200mg contains 165mg; i.e. *quinine bisulphate 300mg is approximately equivalent to quinine sulphate 200mg.*

Tablets sulphate 200mg, 20 = 76p; 300mg, 20 = 82p.

Tablets bisulphate 300mg, 20 = 76p.

---

1 Connolly PS *et al.* (1992) The treatment of nocturnal leg cramps: a crossover trial of quinine vs. vitamin E. *Archives of Internal Medicine.* **152**: 1877–1880.

2 Jansen PHP *et al.* (1997) Randomised controlled trial of hydroquinine in muscle cramps. *Lancet.* **349**: 528–532.

3 Warburton A *et al.* (1987) A quinine a day keeps the leg cramps away? *British Journal of Clinical Pharmacology.* **23**: 459–465.

4 Man-Son-Hing M and Wells G (1995) Meta-analysis of efficacy of quinine for treatment of nocturnal leg cramps in elderly people. *British Medical Journal.* **310**: 13–17.

11: Drugs used in
EAR, NOSE AND THROAT DISORDERS

Mouthwashes

Artificial saliva

Pilocarpine

Drugs for oral inflammation and ulceration

Cerumenolytics

MOUTHWASHES   BNF 12.3.4

Mouthwashes cleanse and freshen the mouth, e.g. **compound mouthwash solution**. Compound **thymol glycerin** is generally not recommended because glycerin can have a rebound drying effect. Mouthwashes containing an oxidizing agent, such as **hydrogen peroxide** or **sodium perborate** froth when in contact with oral debris, and help to debride a heavily furred tongue; **sodium bicarbonate mouthwash** is probably equally effective. **Ascorbic acid (vitamin C)** effervescent tablets can be used for debriding the tongue (*see* p.153). They taste nice but are expensive; gentle brushing with a child's soft toothbrush is generally more effective. **Chlorhexidine** inhibits the formation of plaque on teeth and may be a useful adjunct to other measures for oral infection or when toothbrushing is not possible. **Povidone-iodine** is useful for mucosal infections but does not inhibit plaque. It should not be used for more than 2 weeks because a significant amount of iodine is absorbed.

Supply and use
Compound mouthwash solution tablets sodium benzoate BP, oil mentha BP, thymol BP, menthol BP, oil of cinnamon BP, saccharin BP, 100 = £1.95. Dissolve in 50–60ml water and rinse mouth p.r.n.
Tablets effervescent ascorbic acid, 10 = £1.14 (NHS). Place 1/4 of 1g tablet on the tongue and allow it to dissolve q.d.s.
Mouthwash chlorhexidine gluconate 0.2%, 300ml (original or mint) = £1.93, 600ml (mint) = £3.85. Rinse the mouth with 10ml for 1min b.d.
Mouthwash or gargle hexetidine 0.1%, 100ml = £1.13; 200ml = £1.78. Use 15ml undiluted b.d.–t.d.s.

ARTIFICIAL SALIVA   BNF 12.3.5

Artificial salivas help provide relief of dry mouth. They should be used only in conjunction with standard oral hygiene and mouth care. Patients should be encouraged to adopt strategies such as sucking boiled sweets and sipping ice-cooled drinks.[1] The proportion of patients prescribed an artificial saliva varies widely between palliative care services.

Ideally artificial saliva should be of a neutral pH and contain electrolytes (including fluoride) to correspond approximately to the composition of saliva. Proprietary artificial salivas available in the UK include:
* pastilles containing acacia, malic acid etc. (**Salivix**)
* porcine gastric mucin spray and lozenges (**Saliva Orthana**)
* carmellose-based sprays (**Glandosane, Luborant, Salivace, Saliveze**)
* hydroxyethylcellulose-based gel (**Oralbalance**); contains salivary peroxidase which enhances the production of hypothiocyanite, an antibacterial ion.

Luborant is licensed for any condition giving rise to a dry mouth; Saliva Orthana, Salivace, Saliveze, Glandosane, Oralbalance and Salivix pastilles are approved for dry mouth associated with radiotherapy or sicca syndrome. Saliva Orthana has a sorbitol base which is cooling to taste. Artificial salivas are generally used frequently, including before and during meals.

Supply and use

Pastilles sugar-free Salivix acacia, malic acid etc. 50 = £2.86. Use p.r.n.
Oral spray Saliva Orthana gastric mucin 3.5%, xylitol 2%, sodium fluoride 4.2mg/l, 50ml = £3.80; 450ml refill = £25.10. Apply 2–3 sprays p.r.n.
Lozenges Saliva Orthana mucin 65mg and xylitol 59mg in sorbitol, 45 = £2.75. Use p.r.n.
Oral spray e.g. **Luborant** sorbitol 1.8g and carmellose sodium 390mg in 60ml, 60ml unit = £3.96. Apply 2–3 sprays q.d.s. p.r.n.
Saliva replacement gel Oralbalance lactoperoxidase, glucose oxidase and xylitol in gel, 50g tube = £3.60. Apply p.r.n. Also available with mouthwash and toothpaste as a total package for dry mouth **(Biotene)**.

---

1 Twycross R (1997) *Symptom Management in Advanced Cancer* (2nd edn) Radcliffe Medical Press, Oxford.

PILOCARPINE   BNF 12.3.5

Class of drug: Parasympathomimetic.

Indications: Xerostomia (dry mouth) associated with hypofunction of salivary glands after radiation for head and neck cancer, [†]dry mouth from other causes.

Contra-indications: Intestinal obstruction, uncontrolled asthma and COPD, narrow-angle glaucoma.

Pharmacology

Pilocarpine is a parasympathomimetic (predominantly muscarinic) with mild β-adrenergic activity which stimulates secretion from exocrine glands, including salivary glands. Pilocarpine also increases the concentration of mucins in saliva which protect the oral mucosa from trauma and dryness. Up to 75% of patients with dry mouth are helped by pilocarpine. [1,2] Maximum therapeutic benefit may be seen only after 4–8 weeks of treatment. In a controlled study, half the patients preferred pilocarpine and half preferred **artificial saliva** (mainly because it was a spray and not a tablet).[2] Adverse effects were far more common in patients receiving pilocarpine (84% v 22%), with more than 1/4 of the patients withdrawing from the study in consequence.
Oral bio-availability 96%.
Onset of action 20min.
Duration of action 3–5h.
Plasma halflife 1h.

Adverse effects

Sweating, dizziness, rhinitis, urinary frequency, diarrhoea, nausea, vomiting, intestinal colic, blurred vision, excess salivation, increased bronchial secretions and increased airway resistance.[2]

Dose and use

• starting dose 5mg t.d.s. with or immediately p.c. (last dose with evening meal)
• if dose tolerated but response not sufficient increase dose after 1 week
• maximum dose 10mg t.d.s.
• discontinue if no improvement after 2 weeks.

---

† unlicensed use.

Supply
Tablets 5mg, 84 = £51.43.

1 Anonymous (1994) Oral pilocarpine for xerostomia. *Medical Letter.* **34**: 76.
2 Davies AN *et al.* (1998) A comparison of artificial saliva and pilocarpine in the management of xerostomia in patients with advanced cancer. *Palliative Medicine.* **12**: 105–111.

DRUGS FOR ORAL INFLAMMATION AND ULCERATION
BNF 12.3.1

The causes of ulceration of the oral mucosa include trauma (physical or chemical), recurrent aphthae, infections, cancer, skin disorders, nutritional deficiencies and drug therapy. It is important to determine the cause so that, if appropriate, specific as well as symptomatic treatment is given. For example, teeth and dentures should be checked, and ill-fitting dentures relined.

Mechanical protection
Carbenoxolone sodium gel or granules and **carmellose gelatin** paste relieve discomfort by adhering to the raw ulcer surface. The paste can be difficult to apply effectively.

Corticosteroids
Used primarily for aphthous ulcers (Box 11.A). Candidiasis is a recognized complication of oral corticosteroid treatment.

Box 11.A Treatment of aphthous ulcers

Aphthous ulcers are caused by auto-antibodies and opportunistic infection.

Suppression of immune system

Hydrocortisone 2.5mg lozenges 1 q.d.s. placed in contact with the ulcer.
Triamcinolone 0.1% paste (Adcortyl in Orabase); apply a thin layer b.d.–q.d.s. for 5 days.

Antibiotics and antiseptics

Chlorhexidine 0.2% mouthwash; rinse the mouth with 10ml for about 1min b.d.
Tetracycline suspension 250mg t.d.s. for 3 days; prepared by mixing the contents of a capsule with a small quantity of water; hold in the mouth for 3min and then spit out.

Immunomodulation
*†**Thalidomide** (an immunomodulator) 100mg o.d. or b.d. for 10 days is sometimes used in resistant cases of mouth ulceration in patients with AIDS. It is unlicensed because it causes severe congenital abnormalities (absent or shortened limbs) and irreversible peripheral neuropathy. *The use of thalidomide is best limited to centres with the necessary expertise.*

Local analgesics
Local analgesics have a definite but limited role in the management of painful oral ulceration, including postradiation and postchemotherapy mucositis. When applied topically their action is of relatively short duration; pain relief cannot be maintained continuously throughout the day. **Benzydamine** mouthwash or spray eases the discomfort associated with various causes of sore mouth, including postradiation mucositis. **Choline salicylate** dental gel provides similar relief, but excessive application or confinement under a denture irritates the mucosa and can itself cause ulceration.

---

* specialist use only. † unlicensed use.

Local anaesthetics

Lidocaine 5% ointment (or lozenges containing a local anaesthetic) can be applied to the ulcer or spread around the mouth by the tongue in cases of more generalized mucositis. †**Cocaine hydrochloride 2%** solution is of particular benefit in cases of severe mucositis. With all topical local anaesthetic preparations care must be taken not to produce anaesthesia of the pharynx before meals because it might lead to aspiration and choking.

Supply and use

Oral paste carmellose, pectin and gelatin, 30g = £1.72; 100g = £3.81. Apply a thin layer after meals p.r.n.

Powder carmellose, pectin and gelatin, 25g = £1.98. Sprinkle on the affected area.

Gel carbenoxolone 2% in adhesive base, 5g = £2.12. Apply p.c. and o.n.

Granules carbenoxolone 1% 20mg/sachet, 24 = £9.60. Dissolve contents of sachet in 30–50ml of warm water and rinse mouth p.c. and o.n.

Oral paste triamcinolone acetonide 0.1% in adhesive base, 10g = £1.27. Apply a thin layer to the ulcers b.d.–q.d.s.

Pellets (lozenges) hydrocortisone 2.5mg, 20 = £1.40. Dissolve 1 lozenge q.d.s. slowly in the mouth in contact with an ulcer for ⩽5 days; if necessary, continue treatment b.d. for 2–3 weeks.

Oral rinse benzydamine 0.15% 300ml = £4.10. Rinse or gargle 15ml every 1.5–3h p.r.n. for ⩽7 days. If the full strength mouthwash stings, dilute with an equal volume of water.

Spray benzydamine 0.15% 30ml unit = £3.57. 4–8 sprays to affected area every 1.5–3h.

Oral gel sugar-free choline salicylate 8.7%, **Bonjela** 15g = £1.53; **Dinnefords Teejel**, 10g = £1.02. Apply 1cm of gel with gentle massage q3h p.r.n. (maximum 6 applications daily).

†**Solution** cocaine hydrochloride 2% is prepared extemporaneously. 10ml (200mg) q4h p.r.n. is swished around the mouth for 2–3min and then spat out; swallowing cocaine 200mg would act as a powerful cerebral stimulant and could lead to agitation and hallucinations.

CERUMENOLYTICS   BNF 12.1.3

Indications: Impacted ear wax (cerumen).

Pharmacology

Ear wax is secreted to provide a protective film on the skin of the external auditory meatus. Keratin is a major constituent of ear wax. Disintegration is facilitated by keratin cell hydration and lysis. Keratolysis is optimal in aqueous solutions. In one study, **water** and **docusate 0.5%** (**Waxsol**) were more effective than **sodium bicarbonate 5% BP**[1] whereas, in a second study, sodium bicarbonate 5% and 10% acted more quickly than both water alone and **hydrogen peroxide** (1.5h compared with 3h and 18h at 37°C).[2] In contrast, organic-based OTC preparations had no effect or took ⩾1 week to bring about disintegration and should therefore not be used. One organic-based preparation, **Cerumol,** causes meatal irritation as does docusate in high concentrations, i.e. 5%.[1]

Dose and use

Ear wax should be removed only if it causes deafness or prevents examination of the ear drum. Wax may be removed by syringing with warm water. If necessary first soften with water or sodium bicarbonate 5% BP; tap water is more convenient and costs nothing. Aqueous preparations are truly cerumenolytic and 'liquefy' ear wax; use over several days may obviate the need for syringing. However, syringing is likely to be necessary to remove a firmly impacted plug of ear wax:

- lie the patient down with the affected ear uppermost
- instil a few drops of tap water 15–30min before syringing
- if syringing is unsuccessful, instil water or docusate 0.5% or sodium bicarbonate ear drops BP b.d. for 3 days, and then repeat syringing.

† unlicensed use.

Supply

Ear drops **tap water**, 1ml = 0p.
Ear drops **sodium bicarbonate 5%** from Thornton and Ross, 10ml = £1.10.
Ear drops **docusate 0.5%**, 10ml = 95p.

1   Bellini MJ et al. (1989) An evaluation of common cerumenolytic agents: an in-vitro study. *Clinical Otolaryngology.* **14**: 23–25.
2   Robinson AC and Hawke M (1989) The efficacy of cerumenolytics: everything old is new again. *Journal of Otolaryngology.* **18**: 263–267.

12: Drugs acting on the
SKIN

Emollients

Crotamiton

Barrier preparations

Surface cleansing agents and disinfectants

EMOLLIENTS   BNF 13.2

Indications: Dry or rough skin.

Pharmacology
Emollients soothe, smooth and hydrate the skin and are indicated for all causes of dry flaky skin. Some ingredients occasionally cause sensitization and this should be suspected if an eczematous reaction occurs. Benefit is relatively short-lasting and, depending on the condition of the under-lying skin, application may be necessary several times daily. Emollients are useful in dry eczematous disorders and, to a lesser extent, in psoriasis.

Dose and use
A simple preparation such as **aqueous cream** (containing emulsifying ointment 30%) is generally as effective as more complex proprietary formulations. **Diprobase cream** and **Oilatum** are paraffin-based; they are more convenient to use but more expensive. Apply up to q.d.s.; long-term treatment o.d.–b.d. is often advisable.

Supply
Cream **aqueous BP** 100g = 24p. *1% menthol* can be added to aqueous cream to enhance its antipruritic effect.
Cream **Diprobase** 50g = £1.61, 500g = £6.92.
Bath additive **Oilatum emollient** 250ml = £2.75; 500ml = £4.57.
Paraffin white soft (petroleum jelly) 100g = 32p.

CROTAMITON   BNF 13.3

Class of drug: Acaricide (antiscabetic) antipruritic.
Indications: Pruritus.

Contra-indications: Acute exudative dermatoses.

Pharmacology
There is no highly effective topical antipruritic preparation. **Aqueous cream** (see above) is the initial treatment of choice because of the common association in debilitated patients of pruritus with dry skin. **Calamine** which contains 0.5% phenol is as effective as **crotamiton** but is unsightly.

Cautions
Avoid contact with eyes and broken skin.

Dose and use
Apply to pruritic areas and gently rub in t.d.s.–q.d.s.

Supply
Cream 10%, 30g = £1.97; 100g = £3.38.
Lotion 10%, 100ml = £2.55.

BARRIER PREPARATIONS   BNF 13.2.2

Indications: Skin protection, napkin rash.

Pharmacology
Barrier preparations contain water-repellent substances which help to protect skin around stomas and, in patients with urinary or faecal incontinence, in the perineum and peri-anal areas. They are, however, no substitute for nursing care. Traditional formulations include **compound zinc ointments**. **Morhulin ointment** (38% zinc oxide in cod-liver oil, wool fat and paraffin) is the barrier preparation used at Sobell House. Some proprietary formulations include **dimeticone** or other water-repellent silicone.

Dose and use
Apply to the area in need of protection t.d.s.–q.d.s. after appropriate cleansing and gentle drying.

Supply
Ointment **Morhulin** 50g = £1.08; 350g = £5.06.

SURFACE CLEANSING AGENTS AND
DISINFECTANTS   BNF 13.11

Indications: Cleansing skin and wounds.

Pharmacology
Antiseptics are used less often than in the past because many of them have adverse effects (Table 12.1). **Sodium chloride solution 0.9%** (normal saline) is suitable for general cleansing of skin and wounds (or tap water if safe to drink). Useful disinfectants include **benzalkonium chloride, cetrimide** (also has detergent properties), **chlorhexidine** and **potassium permanganate solution** (1 in 10 000). **Povidone-iodine** is preferred to chlorinated solutions (e.g. dilute sodium hypochlorite solution) which are irritant. Astringent preparations, such as **potassium permanganate** solution are useful for oozing eczematous reactions. Because of a risk of carcinogenesis, **gentian violet** (**crystal violet**) and **Bonney's blue (brilliant green and crystal violet)** are available only on a named patient basis for marking skin before an operation.

Supply
Solution (sterile) **sodium chloride 0.9%**, 20 × 25ml amp = £6.20; 25 × 25ml sachet = £5.85.
Solution **chlorhexidine 0.05%**, 1 l = 77p.
Solution **povidone-iodine 10%**, 500ml = £1.83.
Spray **povidone-iodine 2.5%**, pressurized aerosol 150g = £2.92.
Spirit **industrial methylated BP**, 100ml = 19p.

---

1 Hatz RA *et al.* (1994) *Wound healing and wound management.* Springer-Verlag, London. p.128.

Table 12.1 Properties of antiseptics[1]

	Bactericidal (++) Bacteriostatic (+)	Fungicidal (++) Fungistatic (+)	Virucidal (++) Virustatic (+)	Other characteristics
Alcohols	++	++	+	Rapid onset of action at high concentrations; painful if skin broken
Phenol derivatives, e.g. hexachlorophane (Ster-Zac) chloroxylenol (Dettol)	++	++		Some absorption may occur
Iodine	++	++	++	Some iodine is absorbed; less effective in the presence of organic material; may cause contact dermatitis
Povidone-iodine	++	++	+	Some iodine is absorbed; has an inhibitory effect on wound healing
Chlorhexidene	++	+	+	Some iodine is absorbed; has an inhibitory effect on wound healing
Cationic compounds e.g. benzalkonium chloride, cetrimide cetylpyridinium (Merocet)	++	++		Adsorption at the surface; weak antibacterial action against Gram-negative bacteria
Quinoline derivatives e.g. dequalinium	+	+		
Heavy metals	+	+		Enzyme blocking; coagulatory action
Light metals	+			Astringent
Gentian (crystal) violet	+	+		Strong inhibition of wound healing *and risk of carcinogenesis*
Brilliant green	?	?		Strong inhibition of wound healing
Eosin	?	?		No inhibition of wound healing

13: Drugs used in
ANAESTHESIA

Glycopyrollate

*Ketamine

*Propofol

GLYCOPYROLLATE BNF 15.1.3

Class of drug: Quarternary ammonium antimuscarinic.

Indications: [†]Colic in patients with inoperable bowel obstruction, [†]death rattle, [†]sialorrhoea (drooling).

Pharmacology
Glycopyrollate is 2–5 times more potent than hyoscine hydrobromide as an antisecretory agent,[1] and may be effective in some patients who fail to respond to hyoscine. The optimal single dose is 200μg.[2] It does not cross the blood–brain barrier and is free of central effects; it causes less tachycardia than atropine.[3]
Onset of action 20–40min.
Duration of action 7h.
Plasma halflife 1.7h.

Dose and use
- stat dose 0.2–0.4mg SC
- followed by 0.6–1.2mg/24h CSCI.

When given by CSCI, glycopyrollate is compatible with cyclizine, diamorphine, haloperidol, levomepromazine (methotrimeprazine), midazolam, morphine (see p.183). Glycopyrrolate has also been used PO in the management of sialorrhoea in children with cerebral palsy and related neurodevelopmental disabilities and via a gastrostomy in an adult (0.6–1mg t.d.s.).[4,5]

Supply
Injection 200μg/ml, 1ml amp = 63p; 3ml amp = £1.06.

1 Mirakhur RK and Dundee JW (1980) A comparison of the effects of atropine and glyco-pyrollate on various end organs. *Journal of the Royal Society of Medicine.* **73**: 727–730.
2 Mirakhur RK et al. (1978) Evaluation of the anticholinergic actions of glycopyrronium bromide. *British Journal of Clinical Pharmacology.* **5**: 77–84.
3 Mirakhur RK et al. (1978) Atropine and glycopyrronium premedication. *Anaesthesia.* **33**: 906–912.
4 Blasco PA and Stansbury JCK (1996) Glycopyrrolate treatment of chronic drooling. *Archives of Pediatrics and Adolescent Medicine.* **150**: 932–935.
5 Lucas V and Amass C (1998) Use of enteral glycopyrrolate in the management of drooling. *Palliative Medicine.* **12**: 207.

*KETAMINE BNF 15.1.1

Class of drug: General anaesthetic.

Indications: [†]Neuropathic, inflammatory and ischaemic pain unresponsive to standard therapies.

Contra-indications: Raised intracranial pressure, epilepsy.

---

* specialist use only. 175

Pharmacology

Ketamine has analgesic properties in subanaesthetic doses.[1] Its principal site of analgesic action is in the dorsal horn of the spinal cord where it blocks the N-methyl D-aspartate (NMDA) receptor-channel complex (Figure 13.1). The NMDA-glutamate receptor is closely involved in the development of central (dorsal horn) sensitization. At normal resting membrane potentials, the channel is blocked by magnesium.[2] When the resting membrane potential is changed by prolonged excitation, the channel unblocks with a reduction in opioid-responsiveness and the development of allodynia and hyperalgesia. Ketamine has other actions which probably also contribute to its analgesic effect, including interactions with calcium and sodium channels, cholinergic transmission, noradrenergic and serotonergic re-uptake inhibition (intact descending inhibitory pathways are necessary for analgesia).[3] Ketamine also has κ and μ opioid-like actions. Ketamine may be less effective in neuropathic pain of long duration ($\geqslant$3 years).[4]

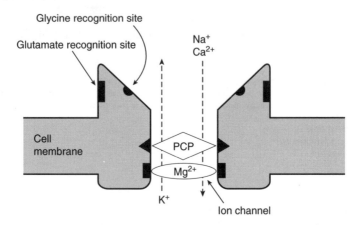

Figure 13.1   Simplified diagram of NMDA (excitatory) receptor-channel complex. The channel is blocked by Mg^{2+} when the membrane potential is at its resting level (voltage-dependent block) and by drugs which act at the phencyclidine (PCP) binding site in the glutamate-activated channel, e.g. MK 801 (use-dependent block).[5]

As an analgesic, ketamine is generally administered SC or PO;[6] it is also effective PR and can be administered spinally.[7] Oral ketamine undergoes extensive first-pass hepatic metabolism to norketamine which is about 1/3 as potent as ketamine; the maximum blood concentration of norketamine is greater after oral administration than after injection.[8] Less than 10% of ketamine is excreted unchanged, half in the faeces and half renally. Long-term use of ketamine leads to hepatic enzyme induction and enhanced ketamine metabolism. Ketamine is used less in centres where spinal analgesia is readily available and when methadone is used as the NMDA-receptor antagonist of choice; the receptor affinity of methadone and ketamine for the NMDA-receptor is approximately the same.[9]

Ketamine causes tachycardia and intracranial hypertension. Most patients experience vivid dreams, misperceptions, hallucinations and alterations in body image and mood after anaesthetic use, i.e. as the effects of a bolus dose wears off. These occur to a lesser extent with CSCI or regular PO use, and generally can be controlled by diazepam, midazolam or haloperidol.[10]

Bio-availability 93% IM; 20% PO.

Onset of action 15–30min SC; 30min PO.

Duration of action generally given by CSCI; 4–6h PO.

Plasma halflife 1–3h IM; 3h PO; 2.5h norketamine.

Cautions

Hypertension, cardiac failure, history of cerebrovascular accidents. Plasma concentration increased by diazepam.

Adverse effects

Occur in about 40% of patients when given by CSCI; less PO. Hypertension, tachycardia; psychoto-mimetic phenomena (dysphoria, vivid dreams, nightmares, hallucinations, altered body image), delirium, diplopia, nystagmus. Also erythema and pain at injection site.

Dose and use

Recommendations for the starting dose and route vary (Box 13.A). One PCU starts with 10–20mg PO q4h and titrates up to 50mg q4h; those cases which are responsive generally experience relief within this range (equivalent to 2–10mg SC q4h or 12–60mg/24h CSCI.[11] A starting dose of 25mg PO q.d.s. & p.r.n. is perhaps more typical (Box 13.A). With higher doses by CSCI, the dose of morphine should be reduced if the patient becomes drowsy. If a patient experiences dysphoria, hallucinations etc., the dose of ketamine should be reduced and a benzodiazepine prescribed (e.g. diazepam 5mg PO stat & o.n., midazolam 5mg SC stat and 5–10mg CSCI) or haloperidol (e.g. 2–5mg PO stat & o.n., 2–5mg SC stat and 2–5mg CSCI). Patients at home will generally be maintained on PO ketamine.

Box 13.A Dose recommendations for ketamine

SC[6]

- 10–25mg p.r.n.

CSCI[6,12]

Because ketamine is irritant, dilute with sodium chloride 0.9% to the largest volume possible (i.e. for a Graseby syringe driver, 18ml in a 30ml luerlock syringe given over 12–24h). Ketamine is compatible with dexamethasone (low-dose), diamorphine, haloperidol, levomepromazine (methotrimeprazine), metoclopramide, midazolam:

- starting dose 0.1–0.5mg/kg/h, typically 150–200mg/24h

- increase by 50–100mg/24h; maximum reported dose 2.4g/24h[13]

- inflammation at infusion site may be helped by hydrocortisone 1% cream or by adding dexamethasone 0.5–1mg to the infusion (dilute in 5–10ml sodium chloride 0.9% and then add ketamine).

PO[6,14]

Use direct from vial or dilute for convenience to 50mg/5ml (patient adds flavouring of choice to mask the bitter taste):

- starting dose 25mg q.d.s. & p.r.n. (equivalent to 5mg SC)

- increase dose in steps of 10–25mg; maximum reported dose 200mg q.d.s.[15]

- give a smaller dose more frequently if psychotomimetic phenomena or drowsiness occurs which does not respond to a reduction in opioid.

Supply

Injection 10mg/ml, 20ml vial = £3.52; 50mg/ml, 10ml vial = £7.31; 100mg/ml, 10ml vial = £13.42. *Available only in hospitals; in the community obtained on a* **named patient and named pharmacy basis** *by arrangement with the manufacturer* (Box 13.B).

Box 13.B Prescribing ketamine in the community

The UK product licence for ketamine is for use as an anaesthetic agent only and supply is restricted to use in hospital under the supervision of an anaesthetist. In the community, therefore, a named patient supply has to be obtained.

Requesting the patient's GP to prescribe ketamine
Before a patient returns home, the GP should be contacted by a doctor to ascertain whether he/she is willing to prescribe ketamine. The process for obtaining a named patient and named pharmacy supply is outlined, and detailed written information sent preferably by fax (Box 13.C).

Obtaining a supply
The GP has to ring the manufacturer, Parke Davis, on 01703 620500 and ask for a *named patient request form*. This will be faxed through (Box 13.D). The GP needs to know the address of the patient's community pharmacist where the supply will be sent and how much to request calculated on a weekly basis (the solution has a shelf-life of 1 week). One 100mg vial of ketamine makes 100ml of 50mg/5ml ketamine oral solution. For example:

Mr Colin White is prescribed ketamine 50mg q.d.s. & p.r.n.
= 5ml q.d.s. & p.r.n., i.e. 20ml × 7 = 140ml + 50ml (10 p.r.n. doses).

This amounts to a total of 190ml oral solution 50mg/5ml, so 2 vials will be needed each week. The GP initiates the supply and the community pharmacist can then order further supplies directly from the manufacturer.

Prescription writing
Advise the GP to prescribe for 1 month at a time:

Ketamine oral solution 50mg/5ml
50mg q.d.s. & p.r.n.
Supply: 28 days

Continuity of supply
When going home patients should receive a 7-day supply of medication. If there is a delay in obtaining the community ketamine supply, the hospital manufacturing department will need to dispense a further supply on an outpatient prescription.

The hospital/palliative care pharmacist should contact the patient's community pharmacist and supply written information regarding the formulation and practical aspects of supplying oral ketamine solution to the patient (Boxes 13.D & 13.E).

---

1 Fallon MT and Welsh J (1996) The role of ketamine in pain control. *European Journal of Palliative Care.* **3**: 143–146.
2 Mayer ML *et al.* (1984) Voltage-dependent block for Mg^{2+} of NMDA responses in spinal cord neurones. *Nature.* **309**: 261–263.
3 Meller ST (1996) Ketamine: relief from chronic pain through actions at the NMDA receptor. *Pain.* **68**: 435–436.
4 Mathisen LC *et al.* (1995) Effect of ketamine, an NMDA receptor inhibitor, in acute and chronic orofacial pain. *Pain.* **61**: 215–220.
5 Richens A (1991) The basis of the treatment of epilepsy: neuropharmacology. In: Dam M (ed) *A practical approach to epilepsy.* Pergamon Press, Oxford. pp 75–85.

Box 13.C   Ketamine in the community: letter to the patient's GP

Hayward House
Hucknall Road
Nottingham NG5 1PB

Date:

Dear Dr

┌───┐
│   │
│   Attach patient identification label here │
│   │
│   │
└───┘

Thank you for agreeing to prescribe ketamine for this patient. The manufacturer, Parke Davis, may be contacted either by telephone (01703 620500) or by fax (01703 628010). On request, they will fax a 'named patient request form' to you. This has to be completed and returned to Parke Davis before a supply of ketamine can be sent to the designated community pharmacist.

I enclose a copy of the entry in the Palliative Care Formulary on the use of ketamine for pain relief. Please follow the advice in Box 13.B about the best way to prescribe oral ketamine. If you require any further information/references, please do not hesitate to contact me.

Yours sincerely

Senior House Officer/Specialist Registrar in Palliative Medicine

Encs

Box 13.D Ketamine in the community: example of a request for named patient medication

Request for named patient medication

In response to your request for **ketamine**
we require the completion of this form which should be returned to:

Parke Davis   *Tel: 01703 620500*   *Fax: 01703 628010*

Product: *Ketamine injection*
Strength and form: *100mg/ml 10ml vials*
Quantity required: *2 vials each week for 4 weeks*
Use: *Neuropathic pain*   Unlicensed   (Yes) / No
                                                            Licensed   Yes / (No)

Patient: *Mr C White*

First supply   (Yes) / No   Continuation of supply   Yes / No

Clinician (block capitals):   *GP's details*
Position:
Address:

Address for dispatch (if different):   *Patient's designated pharmacy*

Signature (prescriber):
Date:

---

6 Luczak J et al. (1995) A role of ketamine, an NMDA receptor antagonist, in the management of pain. *Progress in Palliative Care.* **3**: 127–134.
7 Lin TC et al. (1998) Long-term epidural ketamine, morphine and bupivacaine attenuate reflex sympathetic dystrophy neuralgia. *Canadian Journal of Anaesthesia.* **45**: 175–177.
8 Clements JA et al. (1982) Bio-availability of pharmacokinetics and analgesic activity of ketamine in humans. *Journal of Pharmaceutical Sciences.* **71**: 539–542.
9 Hughes A et al. (1997) Hayward House, Nottingham. Personal communication.
10 Gorman AL et al. (1997) The d- and l- isomers of methadone bind to the non-competitive site on the N-methyl-D-aspartate (NMDA) receptor in rat forebrain and spinal cord. *Neuroscience Letters.* **223**: 5–8.
11 Hall E (1997) Personal communication.
12 Oshima E et al. (1990) Continuous subcutaneous injection of ketamine for cancer pain. *Canadian Journal of Anaesthetics.* **37**: 385–386.
13 Clark JL and Kalan GE (1995) Effective treatment of severe cancer pain of the head using low-dose ketamine in an opioid-tolerant patient. *Journal of Pain and Symptom Management.* **10** 310–314.
14 Broadley KE et al. (1996) Ketamine injection used orally. *Palliative Medicine.* **10**: 247–250.
15 Mercadante S (1996) Ketamine in cancer pain: an update. *Palliative Medicine.* **10**: 225–230.

Box13.E   Ketamine in the community: letter to the pharmacist

Hayward House
Hucknall Road
Nottingham NG5 1PB

Date:

Dear Colleague

Attach patient identification label here

The above patient, who obtains medication from you, has started ketamine oral solution for pain relief. I enclose a copy of the entry in the Palliative Care Formulary on the use of ketamine for pain relief.

Manufacture
We generally use ketamine 100mg/ml 10ml vials because this is the cheapest concentration. Initially we tried raspberry syrup BP for dilution and gave a 1 week expiry when kept refrigerated. However, many patients found this formulation too sweet, so now we use purified water as the diluent and suggest that patients add their own flavouring, e.g. fruit cordial, to disguise the bitter taste.

Formula
To prepare ketamine oral solution 50mg/5ml, use ketamine injection 100mg/1ml.

	Example:
Ketamine injection 100mg/1ml	*10ml*
Purified water to 100ml	*to 100ml*
	i.e. 100ml of 50mg/5ml oral solution

We suggest storage in a refrigerator and an expiry date of 1 week.

Supply
The patient's GP arranges the initial supply of ketamine injection from the manufacturer, Parke Davis, on a named patient basis. This will be delivered directly to you as the patient's designated pharmacy. Thereafter you can request the supply weekly/fortnightly/monthly as convenient, directly from Parke Davis on 01703 620500 (tel) or 01703 628010 (fax). AAH are the distributors and delivery is usually on the following day.

Prescriptions
We have suggested that the GP writes a prescription for 'ketamine oral solution 50mg in 5ml', stating a dose and requesting a 1 month supply. If the prescription is endorsed 'short expiry', then payment will be made by the Prescription Pricing Authority for all four dilutions/dispensings.

Please contact me if you require any further information.

Yours sincerely

Palliative Care Pharmacist

Encs

*PROPOFOL   BNF 15.1

Class of drug: General anaesthetic.

Indications: [†]Used on rare occasions at some centres for agitated terminal delirium unresponsive to usual therapies.

Pharmacology

Propofol is an ultrafast-acting anaesthetic agent. Propofol is rapidly metabolized, mainly in the liver, to inactive conjugates and its corresponding quinol; these are excreted in the urine.The incidence of untoward haemodynamic changes is low. Propofol reduces cerebral blood flow, intracranial pressure and cerebral metabolism. The reduction in intracranial pressure is greater if the baseline pressure is raised. Propofol also has an anti-emetic effect as evidenced by a reduced incidence of postoperative vomiting compared with other anaesthetic agents,[1] and by a reduction in nausea and vomiting during the first 24h after chemotherapy when given in subhypnotic doses.[2,3]
Bio-availability 100%.
Onset of action 0.5min.
Duration of action 5min.
Plasma halflife 40min.

Cautions

There is a risk of convulsions in epileptic patients.

Adverse effects

Bradycardia, myoclonus.

Dose and use

Propofol is not used at Hayward House or Sobell House.
Propofol should not be used unless other measures have failed to relieve a patient's distress such as a combination of SC haloperidol/levomepromazine (methotrimeprazine) with SC midazolam, or SC phenobarbital (see p.81).[4,5] Propofol is given IV as a 1% solution (10mg/ml) in doses ranging from 5–70mg/h (0.5–7ml) using a computer-controlled volumetric infusion pump. 10mg/h (1ml) is a typical starting dose with 10mg/h increments every 15min until a satisfactory level of sedation is achieved. Any change in rate has an effect in 5–10min. If it is necessary to increase the level of sedation quickly, boluses of 20–50mg can be given by increasing the rate to 1ml/min for 2–5min. If the patient is too sedated, the infusion should be turned off for 2–3min and then restarted at a lower rate. It is important to replenish the infusion quickly when a container empties, otherwise the sedation will wear off after a few minutes.[2]

Supply

Injection 10mg/ml, 20ml amp = £3.88, 50ml vial = £9.70.

1 Korttila K (1993) Recovery from propofol: does it really make a difference? *Journal of Clinical Anesthesia.* **5**: 443–446.

2 Borgeat A et al. (1992) Propofol and chemotherapy emesis. *Canadian Journal of Anaesthesia.* **39**: 578–579.

3 Borgeat A et al. (1994) Adjuvant propofol enables better control of nausea and emesis secondary to chemotherapy for breast cancer. *Canadian Journal of Anaesthesia.* **41**: 1117–1119.

4 Mercadante S et al. (1995) Propofol in terminal care. *Journal of Pain and Symptom Management.* **10**: 639–642.

5 Moyle J (1995) The use of propofol in palliative medicine. *Journal of Pain and Symptom Management.* **10**: 643–646.

14:
SYRINGE DRIVERS

Indications

Rate setting

Drug compatibility

Setting up a syringe driver

Checks in use

Infusion site problems

Drug compatibility charts

Subcutaneous, epidural and intrathecal syringe driver prescription charts

Indications
The syringe driver is a small portable battery-driven pump used to deliver medication SC, ED or IT via a syringe, generally over 24h. Indications for use include:
* persistent nausea and vomiting
* intestinal obstruction
* when ED or IT route is used for drug administration
* poor absorption of oral drugs (rare)
* swallowing difficulties
* comatose patient.

Before setting up a syringe driver, its use should be discussed with the patient and the family. Explanation is needed about what a syringe driver is, how it works, why it is planned to use one, together with comments about its advantages and possible disadvantages (Box 14.A). It is important that the syringe driver is not seen just as the last resort but as an effective method of relieving certain symptoms by injection. It is equally important to appreciate that the syringe driver is merely a convenient alternative route of administration and is not step 4 on the analgesic ladder.

Box 14.A Advantages and disadvantages of a syringe driver

Advantages

Increased comfort for the patient because there is less need for repeated injections.

Control of multiple symptoms with a combination of drugs.

Round-the-clock comfort because plasma drug concentrations are maintained without peaks and troughs.

Independence and mobility maintained because the device is lightweight and can be worn in a holster either under or over clothes.

Generally needs to be reloaded only o.d.

Disadvantages

Fear that it is a last resort.

Training necessary for staff.

Possible inflammation and pain at the infusion site leading to decreased drug absorption (diazepam and chlorpromazine are too irritant to administer by CSCI).

Occasional technical problems with ED/IT infusions, e.g. a leaking connection causing a resurgence of symptoms and a risk of infection.

Lack of flexibility with o.d. prescription.

Rate setting

Graseby Medical manufacture two portable syringe drivers:

- **MS16A** with an **hourly** rate (mm/h) syringe driver and a **blue** front panel
- **MS26** with a **daily** rate (mm/24h) syringe driver and a **green** front panel.

The rate settings are mm per unit time and not ml; this allows any brand of syringe to be used (Box 14.B). There are several published reports about 'infusion confusion'[1,2] and a Department of Health Hazard 94(12) has been issued. Errors have arisen from confusion between the two different ways of determining the rate of drug delivery (hourly v daily). Staff training is essential in order to highlight the differences and the potentially fatal hazards.[1,2] Graseby Medical offer staff training, including a videofilm, a manual and instruction by their local representatives.

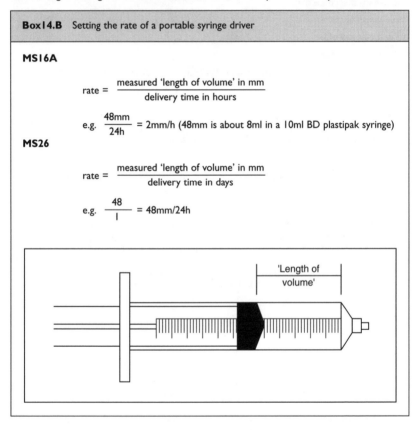

Box14.B Setting the rate of a portable syringe driver

MS16A

$$rate = \frac{\text{measured 'length of volume' in mm}}{\text{delivery time in hours}}$$

e.g. $\dfrac{48mm}{24h}$ = 2mm/h (48mm is about 8ml in a 10ml BD plastipak syringe)

MS26

$$rate = \frac{\text{measured 'length of volume' in mm}}{\text{delivery time in days}}$$

e.g. $\dfrac{48}{1}$ = 48mm/24h

'Length of volume'

Drug compatibility

The prescription should be checked to ascertain whether the drug combination is compatible (see pp 189 & 191). Many combinations have been successfully used in clinical practice without supporting laboratory data. Where this is the case, regular monitoring of the contents of the syringe and the tubing will detect evidence of physical incompatibility (e.g. precipitation, colour change). It is helpful to record details for future reference of those combinations where problems arise (see **red cards** inside the back cover). Laboratory data about the drugs to be mixed help in deciding whether to attempt to mix them (Table 14.1 & Figure 14.1). As a general rule, drugs with similar pH are more likely to be compatible than those with widely differing pH. Concentrations of the individual drugs also influence compatibility.

Saline is recommended as the diluent for **granisetron, ketamine, ketorolac, octreotide** and **ondansetron.** For other drugs the recommended diluent is **water for injections (WFI)** because there is less chance of precipitation. As a general rule, dilute the drug contents by at least 100% (if necessary using a 20ml or 30ml syringe) because this helps to reduce inflammation at the infusion site. Information about drug compatibility is summarized in the two charts (see pp 189 & 191).

Table 14.1 The pH values of drugs delivered by syringe drivers[a]

Drug	pH	Drug	pH
Bupivacaine	4–6.5	Hyoscine butylbromide	3.7–5.5
Clonidine	4–4.5	Hyoscine hydrobromide	5–7
Cyclizine lactate	3.3–3.7[b]	Ketamine	3.5–5.5
Dexamethasone	7–8.5	Ketorolac	6.9–7.9
Diamorphine	2.5–6	Levomepromazine	4.5
Diclofenac	7.8–9	Methadone	3–6.5
Droperidol	3–3.8	Metoclopramide	4.5–6.5
Glycopyrrolate	2–3	Midazolam	3
Granisetron	4.7–7.3	Morphine	2.5–6
Haloperidol	3–3.8	Octreotide	3.9–4.5
Hyaluronidase	6.4–7.4	Ondansetron	3.3–4
Hydromorphone	4–5.5	Tropisetron	4.5–5.2

a. manufacturers' information
b. above pH 6.8 cyclizine base precipitates;[1] if diluted with saline, cyclizine hydrochloride precipitates out.[3]

Setting up a syringe driver[4]
The diagram of a portable syringe driver illustrates its main features (Figure 14.2).

1 *Insert the battery:* the alarm will sound (press the start/test button to silence). An alkaline 9V battery should last for about 50 full syringes; the light stops flashing 24h before it runs out.

2 *Fix the syringe onto the syringe driver:*
• fit a flange of the syringe into the slot provided on the syringe driver
• secure the syringe firmly with the rubber strap
• press the white button on the actuator assembly and slide along the lead screw until firmly against the syringe plunger
• connect the syringe to the butterfly tubing
• press the start/test button to operate; the indicator light will flash every second in the MS16A and every 25 seconds in the MS26
• place the syringe driver in the plastic holder and place in the holster or appropriate cover to protect the contents from light.
If the alarm subsequently sounds, check to identify fault, e.g. empty syringe, kinked tubing, blocked needle/tubing, jammed plunger.

3 *Subcutaneous siting:* an 18 gauge butterfly needle should be inserted at a 30–45° angle into subcutaneous tissue, avoiding oedematous sites, skin folds and breast tissue. Usual sites are the anterior chest wall or anterior/lateral aspects of upper arms. Sometimes the anterior abdominal wall or anterior aspects of the thighs is used. The tubing should be secured with a dressing (e.g. **Tegaderm**) incorporating a loop to avoid pulling on the needle.

Checks in use
The use of a dedicated chart for SC, ED and IT routes not only serves as a prescription chart and record of administration but also re-inforces training on the use of syringe drivers. Checks q4h on the rate, condition of infusion site and measurement of remaining volume should be documented. The calculation to determine whether the driver is running to time is based on the preceding 4h period. The comments/action section is completed, for example, if the infusion needs to be resited and hence reprimed. If so, record the time, the new site and the new syringe volume (priming a new line uses about 0.5ml). Other comments might include details of evidence of incompatibility or if the syringe driver was found disconnected or tubing split etc.

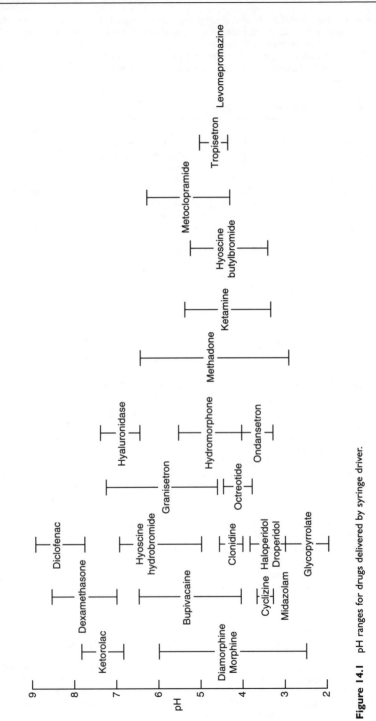

Figure 14.1 pH ranges for drugs delivered by syringe driver.

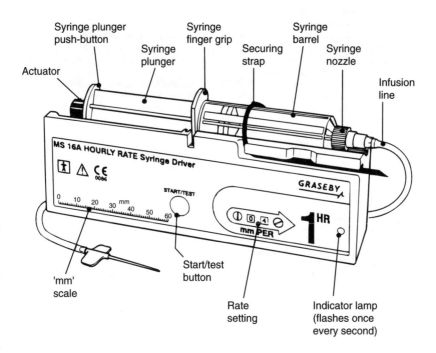

Figure 14.2   The Graseby Medical MS16A hourly rate syringe driver.

Infusion site problems

Irritation at the injection site is most commonly found with **cyclizine** or **levomepromazine** (**methotrimeprazine**).[4] Occasionally patients may be allergic to the nickel needles. Sites may last up to a week, depending on the drugs used. The site should be changed if painful or inflamed. If frequent resiting is necessary (i.e. every 24–48h), consider the following strategies:

- using a larger syringe to enable a more dilute mixture to be used, thereby decreasing the final drug concentrations
- changing to a q12h regimen, thereby permitting further dilution of the drugs
- changing an irritant drug to a less irritant alternative (e.g. cyclizine → hyoscine butylbromide)
- adding hyaluronidase 1500 units to the syringe (see p.160)
- adding hydrocortisone 50–100mg or dexamethasone 0.5–1mg to the syringe
- using a plastic (teflon) cannula instead of a butterfly needle (have a tendency to kink)[5]
- placing the needle IM rather than SC.

1 Carlisle D et al. (1996) Infusion Confusion. *Nursing Times*. **92** (48): 48–49.
2 Cousins DH and Upton DR (1995) Make infusion pumps safer to use. *Pharmacy in Practice*. October, 401–406.
3 Fawcett JP et al. (1994) Compatibility of cyclizine lactate and haloperidol lactate. *American Journal of Hospital Pharmacists*. **51** (18): 2292–2294.
4 Latham J (1987) Syringe Drivers in Pain Control. *The Professional Nurse*. **April**, 207–209.
5 Ventafridda V et al. (1986) The importance of continuous subcutaneous morphine administration for cancer pain control. *The Pain Clinic*. **1**: 47–55.

Drug compatibility charts

Main sources for compatibility charts

1 Thorp SA Collection of inhouse data. Hayward House, City Hospital, Nottingham.
2 French SA Collection of inhouse data. Pharmacy Department, City Hospital, Nottingham.
3 Dickman A (December 1997) The syringe driver in palliative care. Data from Countess Mountbatten House, Southampton.
4 Grassby PF (April 1995 and July 1997) UK Stability Database. Welsh Pharmaceutical Services, St. Mary's Pharmaceutical Unit, Corbett Road, Penarth, South Glamorgan.
5 Trissel LA (1996) Handbook on Injectable Drugs. (9th edn) American Society of Health-System Pharmacists.

Other sources for compatibility charts

1 Bradley K (1996) Swap data on drug compatibilities. *Pharmacy in Practice.* **6** (3): 69–72.
2 Allwood MC (1984) **Diamorphine** mixed with **anti-emetic** drugs in plastic syringes. *British Journal of Pharmaceutical Practice.* **6** (3): 88–90.
3 Allwood MC (1991) The stability of **diamorphine** alone and in combination with **anti-emetics** in plastic syringes. *Palliative Medicine.* **5**: 330–333.
4 Allwood MC et al. (1994) Stability of injections containing **diamorphine** and **midazolam** in plastic syringes. *International Journal of Pharmacy Practice.* **3**: 57–59.
5 Collins AJ et al. (1986) Stability of **diamorphine** hydrochloride with **haloperidol** in prefilled syringes for continuous subcutaneous administration. *Journal of Pharmacy and Pharmacology.* **38**: 51.
6 Fawcett JP et al. (1994) Compatibility of **cyclizine** lactate and **haloperidol** lactate. *American Journal of Hospital Pharmacists.* **51** (18): 2292–2294.
7 Grassby PF and Hutchings L (1997) Drug combinations in syringe drivers: the compatibility and stability of **diamorphine** with **cyclizine** and **haloperidol.** *Palliative Medicine.* **11**: 217–224.
8 Hutchinson HT et al. (1981) Continuous subcutaneous **analgesics** and **anti-emetics** in domiciliary terminal care. *Lancet.* **2**: 1279.
9 Kyaterekera N et al. (1997) Stability of **octreotide** in the presence of **diamorphine** hydrochloride. *Journal of Pharmacy and Pharmacology.* **49** (suppl 4): 63.
10 Mehta AC (1996) Admixtures' storage is extended. *Pharmacy in Practice.* **6**: 113–118.
11 Regnard C et al. (1986) **Anti-emetic/diamorphine** mixture compatibility in infusion pumps. *British Journal of Pharmaceutical Practice.* August: 218–220.

SUBCUTANEOUS SYRINGE DRIVER CHECKLIST

If fast (>30 minutes)

1 Check the rate setting is correct.

2 Change entire syringe driver for a new one and send for servicing.

3 Inform doctor if patient's clinical condition gives cause for concern.

If slow (>30 minutes)

1 Check the rate setting is correct.

2 Check syringe driver light is flashing.

3 Check that syringe is inserted correctly into the Graseby pump.

4 Check battery using meter – change if voltage is low.

5 Ascertain if syringe driver has been stopped and then restarted for any reason.

6 Check contents of syringe and line – is there any evidence of crystallization?

7 Check site of subcutaneous needle – is this red/hard/lumpy/sore? Change if necessary. Consider further dilution of drugs to minimize irritation.

8 Inform a doctor if patient's clinical condition warrants this i.e.: symptoms not relieved and patient needs p.r.n. drugs prescribing or has needed repeated p.r.n. doses.

At next four-hourly check

1 See steps 1–8.

2 If continuing to run through too slowly change entire driver and send for servicing.

Setting up a new driver

Always check:

1 The battery voltage using meter.

2 The rate set.

NAME:

HOSPITAL NO:

DRUGS	DOSE	Measurement in syringe at start		CHECKS IN USE					
				Time	Rate set	Site	mm left	Slow/fast/on time	Signature
Date		Start time	Rate set						
Route		Site	Syringe size						
Duration		Nurses signature							
Drs signature		Comments/Action							

DRUGS	DOSE	Measurement in syringe at start		CHECKS IN USE					
				Time	Rate set	Site	mm left	Slow/fast/on time	Signature
Date		Start time	Rate set						
Route		Site	Syringe size						
Duration		Nurses signature							
Drs signature		Comments/Action							

DRUGS	DOSE	Measurement in syringe at start		CHECKS IN USE					
				Time	Rate set	Site	mm left	Slow/fast/on time	Signature
Date		Start time	Rate set						
Route		Site	Syringe size						
Duration		Nurses signature							
Drs signature		Comments/Action							

Twelve hourly drivers run at **4mm** per hour. **Twenty-four** hourly drivers run at **2mm** per hour.

Nottingham City Hospital NHS Trust
HAYWARD HOUSE
Macmillan Specialist Palliative Care Unit

EPIDURAL Syringe Driver Prescription Chart

Affix addressograph label here:

Name: DOB: Ward:

Hospital No: Sex: Consultant:

Address:

Instructions for setting up EPIDURAL syringe drivers

1 Always use a **luerlock** syringe.

2 All epidurals should be administered using a BD Plastipak luerlock syringe. The appropriate volume that measures 48mm is ≈ 14ml. **Saline** should always be used as a diluent.

3 Set appropriate rate:

Graseby MS16A delivers in **millimetres per hour**.
Set at **02** to run at 2mm/h over **24** hours.
Set at **04** to run at 4mm/h over **12** hours.

Graseby MS26A delivers in **millimetres per 24 hours**.
Set at **48** to run at 2mm/h over **24** hours.
Set at **96** to run at 4mm/h over **12** hours.

4 Checks in use:

Check the contents of the syringe and tubing and the rate set.
Also measure the volume remaining every **four** hours. If **not** running on time – refer to check list.

Examine the exit site if visible. *If red/inflamed – inform doctor – need for antibiotics?*

Each prescription must be rewritten **daily**.

The dose of diamorphine must be written in words and figures i.e.: 15mg (fifteen) for clarity.

If syringe driver is to be stopped indicate clearly on prescription sheet.

When changing an epidural drug combination, consider changing the external line and priming it with the new combination as well, otherwise it may take up to 12 hours to detect any benefits of the new combination (generally make up two syringes – one for priming and one for infusion). The doctor will decide whether this is necessary according to the patient's pain.

EPIDURAL/INTRATHECAL CHECKLIST

If fast (>30 minutes)

1 Check the rate setting is correct.

2 Change entire syringe driver for a new one and send for servicing.

3 Inform doctor if patient's clinical condition gives cause for concern.

If slow (>30 minutes)

1 Check the rate setting is correct.

2 Check syringe driver light is flashing.

3 Check that syringe is inserted correctly into the Graseby pump.

4 Check battery using meter – change if voltage is low.

5 Ascertain if syringe driver has been stopped and then restarted for any reason.

6 Check contents of syringe and line – is there any evidence of crystallization?

7 Check the exit site – is this red/inflamed? If so, inform doctor – patient may need antibiotics.

8 Inform a doctor if patient's clinical condition warrants this i.e.: symptoms not relieved and patient needs p.r.n. drugs prescribing or has needed repeated p.r.n. doses.

At next four-hourly check

1 See steps 1–8.

2 If continuing to run through too slowly change entire driver and send for servicing.

Setting up a new driver

Always check:

1 The battery voltage using meter.

2 The rate set.

EPIDURAL INFORMATION

Drugs given by the spinal route must be preservative-free. A combination of diamorphine and bupivacaine is most commonly used with clonidine occasionally added.

Doses:

Bupivacaine: 0.25%, 0.5% and 0.75%; dose according to advice from an anaesthetist.

Diamorphine: starting dose generally 10–60mg (often one-tenth of previous 24-hour oral morphine dose).

Clonidine: 150–300 micrograms per 24 hours.

Dose increments should be small:

Bupivacaine usually 1–2ml.

Diamorphine usually 2.5–5mg.

p.r.n. doses of oral morphine should be calculated as one-sixth of the equivalent 24-hour oral morphine dose.

e.g. diamorphine 10mg epidurally daily = morphine 100mg PO daily.

p.r.n. dose = morphine 15mg PO (diamorphine 5mg SC).

Note: laxative doses may need to be reduced when opioids are given via the spinal route.

NAME:

HOSPITAL NO:

DRUGS		DOSE	Measurement in syringe at start		CHECKS IN USE				
					Time	Rate set	Site	mm left	Slow/fast/on time	Signature
			Start time	Rate set						
			Site	Syringe size						
Date			Nurses signature							
Route										
Duration			Comments/Action							
Drs signature										

DRUGS		DOSE	Measurement in syringe at start		CHECKS IN USE				
					Time	Rate set	Site	mm left	Slow/fast/on time	Signature
			Start time	Rate set						
			Site	Syringe size						
Date			Nurses signature							
Route										
Duration			Comments/Action							
Drs signature										

DRUGS		DOSE	Measurement in syringe at start		CHECKS IN USE				
					Time	Rate set	Site	mm left	Slow/fast/on time	Signature
			Start time	Rate set						
			Site	Syringe size						
Date			Nurses signature							
Route										
Duration			Comments/Action							
Drs signature										

Twelve hourly drivers run at **4mm** per hour. **Twenty-four** hourly drivers run at **2mm** per hour.

Nottingham City Hospital NHS Trust
HAYWARD HOUSE
Macmillan Specialist Palliative Care Unit

INTRATHECAL Syringe Driver Prescription Chart

Affix addressograph label here:

Name:　　　　　　　　DOB:　　　　　　　Ward:

Hospital No:　　　　　　Sex:　　　　　　　Consultant:

Address:

Instructions for setting up INTRATHECAL syringe drivers

1　Always use a **luerlock** syringe.

2　All epidurals should be administered using a BD Plastipak luerlock syringe. The appropriate volume that measures 48mm is ≈ 14ml. **Saline** should always be used as a diluent.

3　Set appropriate rate:

　Graseby MS16A delivers in **millimetres per hour**.
　Set at **02** to run at 2mm/h over **24** hours.
　Set at **04** to run at 4mm/over **12** hours.

　Graseby MS26A delivers in **millimetres per 24 hours**.
　Set at **48** to run at 2mm/h over **24** hours.
　Set at **96** to run at 4mm/h over **12** hours.

4　Checks in use:

　Check the contents of the syringe and tubing and the rate set.
　Also measure the volume remaining every **four** hours. If **not** running on time – refer to check list.

　Examine the exit site if visible. *If red/inflamed – inform doctor – need for antibiotics?*

Each prescription must be rewritten **daily**.

The dose of diamorphine must be written in words and figures i.e.: 15mg (fifteen) for clarity.

If syringe driver is to be stopped indicate clearly on prescription sheet.

When changing an intrathecal drug combination, consider changing the external line and priming it with the new combination as well, otherwise it may take up to 12 hours to detect any benefits of the new combination (generally make up two syringes – one for priming and one for infusion). The doctor will decide whether this is necessary according to the patient's pain.

EPIDURAL/INTRATHECAL CHECKLIST

If fast (>30 minutes)

1   Check the rate setting is correct.

2   Change entire syringe driver for a new one and send for servicing.

3   Inform doctor if patient's clinical condition gives cause for concern.

If slow (>30 minutes)

1   Check the rate setting is correct.

2   Check syringe driver light is flashing.

3   Check that syringe is inserted correctly into the Graseby pump.

4   Check battery using meter – change if voltage is low.

5   Ascertain if syringe driver has been stopped and then restarted for any reason.

6   Check contents of syringe and line – is there any evidence of crystallization?

7   Check the exit site – is this red/inflamed? If so, inform doctor – patient may need antibiotics.

8   Inform a doctor if patient's clinical condition warrants this i.e.: symptoms not relieved and patient needs p.r.n. drugs prescribing or has needed repeated p.r.n. doses.

At next four-hourly check

1   See steps 1–8.

2   If continuing to run through too slowly change entire driver and send for servicing.

Setting up a new driver

Always check:

1   The battery voltage using meter.

2   The rate set.

INTRATHECAL INFORMATION

Drugs given by the spinal route must be preservative-free. A combination of diamorphine and bupivacaine is most commonly used with clonidine occasionally added.

Doses:

Bupivacaine: 0.25% (only this strength is used); dose according to advice from an anaesthetist.

Diamorphine: starting dose can be as low as 0.5–1mg, but generally 5–20mg (often one-hundredth of previous 24-hour oral morphine dose).

Clonidine: 15–30 micrograms per 24 hours.

Dose increments should be small:

Bupivacaine usually 1ml.

Diamorphine usually 0.5–1mg, depending on total dose administered.

Clonidine usually 15 micrograms.

p.r.n. doses of oral morphine should be calculated as one-sixth of the equivalent 24-hour oral morphine dose.

e.g. diamorphine 5mg intrathecally daily = morphine 500mg PO daily.

p.r.n. dose = morphine 80mg PO (diamorphine 25mg SC).

Note: laxative doses may need to be reduced when opioids are given via the spinal route.

NAME:

HOSPITAL NO:

DRUGS	DOSE	Measurement in syringe at start		CHECKS IN USE					
				Time	Rate set	Site	mm left	Slow/fast/on time	Signature
Date		Start time	Rate set						
Route		Site	Syringe size						
Duration		Nurses signature							
Drs signature		Comments/Action							

DRUGS	DOSE	Measurement in syringe at start		CHECKS IN USE					
				Time	Rate set	Site	mm left	Slow/fast/on time	Signature
Date		Start time	Rate set						
Route		Site	Syringe size						
Duration		Nurses signature							
Drs signature		Comments/Action							

DRUGS	DOSE	Measurement in syringe at start		CHECKS IN USE					
				Time	Rate set	Site	mm left	Slow/fast/on time	Signature
Date		Start time	Rate set						
Route		Site	Syringe size						
Duration		Nurses signature							
Drs signature		Comments/Action							

Twelve hourly drivers run at **4mm** per hour. **Twenty-four** hourly drivers run at **2mm** per hour.

Appendix 1: Anaphylactic shock

Anaphylactic shock is rare in palliative care and is generally associated with **antibiotics, aspirin, and other NSAIDs**. It is:
- specific to a given drug or chemically-related class of drugs
- more likely after parenteral administration
- more frequent in patients with systemic lupus erythematosus or with aspirin-induced asthma.

A possible case of anaphylactic shock has been recorded in a woman with known peanut allergy who received an arachis (peanut) oil enema.[1]

Clinical manifestations of anaphylactic shock typically develop *within seconds or minutes* of taking the causal drug due to the release of large amounts of histamine:

flushing	tingling of the extremities
palpitations	urticaria
weakness	angioedema
dizziness	bronchoconstriction
hypotension	agitation.

Anaphylaxis requires urgent treatment with epinephrine (adrenaline) backed up by an antihistamine and hydrocortisone (Box A1.A). Because their impact is not immediate, corticosteroids are only of secondary value.

Box A1.A Treatment of anaphylactic shock[2,3]

Epinephrine (adrenaline) 1 in 1000, 0.5–1ml (0.5–1mg) IM:

- if the patient is unconscious, double the dose

- repeat every 10min until pulse and blood pressure are satisfactory.

Administer oxygen.

Chlorphenamine (chlorpheniramine) 10–20mg IV over 1min is a useful adjunct.

Hydrocortisone 100–300mg IV to prevent further deterioration.

Chlorphenamine (chlorpheniramine) 4–8mg PO q.d.s. should be given for 24–48h to prevent relapse.

---

1 Pharmax (1998) Data on file.
2 Szczeklik A (1986) Analgesics, allergy and asthma. *Drugs.* **32** (suppl 4): 148–163.
3 Anonymous (1998) *British National Formulary.* British Medical Association and the Royal Pharmaceutical Society of Great Britain, London, No. 35 (March), pp 145–147.

Appendix 2: Synopsis of pharmacokinetic data

Table A2.1 contains selected pharmacokinetic data for most of the drugs featured in the PCF. The plasma halflives given in the table sometimes differ from those in the main text. This is because, for most drugs, several values have been published and here a single value has been chosen.[1] It is important to remember that interindividual variability of pharmacokinetic parameters is generally considerable. For example, the typical range for the total clearance of various drugs is 4- to 5-fold. Further, bio-availability may vary according to formulation.

Key for Table A2.1:

a. A = acid; Aa = amino acid; Alc = alcohol; Amf = ampholyte; B = base; B_4 = base with quaternary ammonium group; Gly = glycoside; Pep = peptide; S = steroid; Sa = substituted amide.

b. the pH at which the drug is 50% ionized.

c. the fraction of the drug eliminated by nonrenal pathways in normal individuals; 1 – [fraction] gives an estimate of how much of the drug is excreted unchanged in the urine.

d. pharmacologically active metabolite(s).

e. metabolite(s) with possible pharmacological activity.

f. apparent volume of distribution at steady state.

g. after oral administration.

1 Holford NHG (ed) (1998) *Clinical pharmacokinetics: drug data handbook.* (3rd edn) Adis International, Auckland.

Table A2.1 Pharmacokinetic drug data

	Nature[a]	pKa[b]	Oral bio-availability (%)	Clearance (L/h)	Plasma halflife (h)	Volume of distribution (L)	Protein binding (%)	Nonrenal elimination[c]	Comments
Acetylcysteine			9	58 #/8 ##	2 #/5.5 ##	42 #/35 ## f		0.7 #	# Reduced acetylcysteine ### Total acetylcysteine
Amiloride [e]	B	8.7	50	≈31 g	≈9.6	≈350 g	95	0.25 e	
Amitriptyline [d]	B	9.4	48	51	19	1085 f		1.0 d	
Aspirin [d]	A	3.5	68	39	0.25 #	10.5	≈70	1.0 #	# Active metabolite (salicylate) t½ 2–30h
Atropine	B	9.25		70	2.2	231	50	0.45	
Baclofen [e]	A	3.9/9.6	60–90		3.5		30	0.15 e	
Beclometasone	S				15				
Betamethasone	S		72	11	6.5	126	6.4	0.95	
Bromocriptine [e]	Pep	4.9	6	56	3	≈238	90	1.0 e	# High first-pass metabolism
Budesonide	S		10 #	84	2.7	308	88		
Bumetanide [e]	A		90	12	1.75	16.8	96	0.35 e	
Bupivacaine	B	8.1		35	2.7	70 f	96	0.95	
Buprenorphine	B	8.49/10.03	30 #	70	2.5	140	≈96	1.0	# Sublingual
Carbamazepine [d]	Sa		>70	1.1/4.5 g	36/16 #	84 g	75	1.0 d	# Single-dose/long-term treatment
Cetirizine				3	7–10	35	93	0.4	
Chlorpropamide [d]	A	4.8	>90	0.13 g	40	≈10.5 g	90	0.2 d	
Chlordiazepoxide [d]	B	4.8	>86	1	20	28	96	1.0 d	
Chlorphenamine [d]	B	9.2		7.2	20	238	72	0.8 d	
Chlorpromazine [d]	B	9.3	32 #	38 ##	30	1470 ##	98	1.0 d	# After PO administration ### After IM administration
Cimetidine	B	6.8	70 #	36	2	91	20	0.3	# IM >90%
Cisapride			40–50		10	168	98	1.0	
Clonidine [e]	B	8.25	90	0.16–0.6 #	6.2–12.8 #	241.5	20	0.4 e	# Dose-dependent
Clodronate disodium				6	2 #			≈0.1	# Terminal elimination phase t½ 13h

Table A2.1 Continued

	Nature[a]	pKa[b]	Oral bio-availability (%)	Clearance (L/h)	Plasma halflife (h)	Volume of distribution (L)	Protein binding (%)	Nonrenal elimination[c]	Comments
Clomipramine[d]	B			45	20	1162	98	1.0[d]	
Clonazepam	Amf	1.5/10.5	98	≈6[g]	25	210[g]	85	1.0	
Codeine[d]	B	7.95	55	98[#]	2.8	378[#]	≈7	1.0[d]	# After PO administration, corrected for bio-availability
Dantrolene[d]	A	7.5			≈9			0.95[d]	
Desipramine[d]	B	10.2	51	130[g]	22	1568[g]	80	1.0[d]	
Demeclocycline	Amf	3.3/7.2/9.4	80		12	126	≈70		
Dexamethasone	S			14.7	3	52.5	77	1.0	
Dextropropoxyphene	B	6.3		66	2.7	189	78	≈1.0	
Diazepam[d]	B	3.3	100	1.8	40[#]	140	98	1.0	# Active metabolite t½ 30–200h
Diclofenac[e]	A		60	15.6	1.5	10.5	>99	1.0[e]	
Diflunisal	A		100	0.35–0.49[#]	5–20[#]	7.7	99	0.95	# Dose-dependent
Digoxin	Gly		70	4.5	40	420	27	0.3	Recommended therapeutic plasma concentration 0.8–2µg/L
Diltiazem	B	7.7	41	60	5.1	315	98	1.0	
Diphenhydramine[e]	B	8.3	42	47	5	280	98.5	0.9[e]	
Diphenoxylate	B	7.07			2.5	322			
Dosulepin (dothiepin)			30	146	25	4900			
Ethinylestradiol	S		40	23	13	203	97		
Fentanyl[e]	B			47	3	≈210	83	0.95[e]	
Flecainide[d]	B	8.43	95	42.8[#]	12[#]/19.5[###]	588[#]	52	0.7[d]	Recommended therapeutic plasma concentration <800µg/L # Healthy volunteers ## Arrhythmia patients

Table A2.1 Continued

	Nature^a	pKa^b	Oral bio-availability (%)	Clearance (L/h)	Plasma half-life (h)	Volume of distribution (L)	Protein binding (%)	Nonrenal elimination^c	Comments
Fluconazole			90		30	56	11	0.3	
Fludrocortisone					0.5		75		
Flunitrazepam^e	B	1.84	85	8 g	29	259 g		1.0 e	
Fluoxetine				40 (10) #	48 (96) #	1400(2940) #	94	0.97	# Multiple dose data in parenthesis
Flurbiprofen	A		>85	1.3 g	3.5	7 g	>99	0.9	
Fluvoxamine			77		20	1400		0.95	
Furosemide(frusemide)	A	3.9	65	8	1	21	97	0.35	
Gabapentin			60	7.5	5–7	49	0		
Glibenclamide^d	A	5.3		5.5	1.5–10 #	10.5	>99	1.0 d	# Divergent values reported
Gliclazide		5.8		0.8	12	21	90	1.0	
Glyceryl trinitrate				≈1260	0.05	≈210			Wide interindividual variability
Granisetron				14.7	11	231		0.9	
Haloperidol	B	8.3	65	46	20	1400	90	1.0	# Dose- and assay-dependent ## Lipoproteins
Heparin	A		0	2.5 #	1.5 #	4.9	95 ##	0.8	
Hydrocortisone	S			21–30 #	1.3–1.9 #	21–35 #	75–95 #		# Dose-dependent
Hyoscine hydrobromide	B	7.55	23	45	2.5	140		0.45	
Hyoscine butylbromide	B₄				14		11 #		# Albumin
Ibuprofen	A	4.4/5.2	>80 #	3.5 g	2.5	9.8 g	99	1.0	# Dose-dependent
Imipramine^d	B	9.5	27	58	18	1470	89	1.0 d	# Wide interindividual variability
Indoramin	B	7.8		66	5–15 #	518	90	0.95	# Divergent values reported
Insulin	Pep			10–40 #	0.25–2 #		≈5	0.4	
Ipratopium	B				≈3.5			0.3	
Isosorbide-5-mononitrate			93	7.6	4.4	49	0	0.8	
Itraconazole			40		30 #		>99		# At steady state

Table A2.1 Continued

	Nature[a]	pKa[b]	Oral bio-availability (%)	Clearance (L/h)	Plasma halflife (h)	Volume of distribution (L)	Protein binding (%)	Nonrenal elimination[c]	Comments
Ketamine[e]		7.5	20#	60	3	140	12	1.0[e]	# IM
Ketoconazole		2.9/6.5	80	2	8	17.5	99	1.0	
Ketorolac		3.49			5.6		99		
Lamotrigine			98	1.9	30	80.5	55	0.9	
Lansoprazole					2			1.0	
Levodopa[d]	Aa	2.3/8.7	35		1.4			1.0[d]	
Lidocaine	B	7.86		40	3.9	210	60	0.95	Recommended therapeutic plasma concentration 2–5mg/L
Lithium			>85	1.6	27	56		1.02	Therapeutic plasma concentration 0.4–1.2 mmol/L
Lofepramine[d]	B			686[g]	2.2		>99	1.0	Active metabolite desipramine
Loperamide[e]		8.7	<10		10		97	1.0[e]	
Lorazepam	Amf	1.3/11.5	93	3[g]	20	105[g]	90	1.0	
Medroxyprogesterone[e]	S			≈76#	≈36	≈42#	94	0.55[e]	# After PO and IM administration
Metformin			50	26–42#	1.5–4.5#	70–280#	<5	0.01	# Divergent values reported; terminal elimination phase t½ ≈ 10h
Methadone	B	8.25	92	7.5	29	280	80	0.6	
Methylprednisolone	S	4.6	82	15	3	49		1.0	
Metoclopramide			85	38/23#	4/7#	210	30	0.7	# Possibly dose-dependent
Metronidazole[d]	B?	2.62	100#	3	8	49	<20	0.85[d]	# Rectal 70%
Mexiletine[e]#		8.75	85	27	10	350	70	0.8[e]	# Recommended therapeutic plasma concentration 0.8–2mg/L
Miconazole[e]		6.65	27	46	23	1400	99	1.0[e]	
Midazolam	B	6.1	35	20	3.0	84	95	1.0	

Table A2.1 Continued

	Nature[a]	pKa[b]	Oral bio-availability (%)	Clearance (L/h)	Plasma half-life (h)	Volume of distribution (L)	Protein binding (%)	Nonrenal elimination[c]	Comments
Misoprostol[d]					1.5 #		85		# Active metabolite. Parent drug undetectable in plasma after oral dose
Morphine[e]	Amf	9.85/7.87	20–33	72	2.5 #	245	35	0.9 [e]	# Active metabolite (morphine-6-glucuronide) $t_{1/2}$ ≤7.5h in renal failure
Naloxone[e]	B	7.94	2	104	1.5	210	20	=1.0 [e]	
Naltrexone	A		5–60 #	94	2.7	994	99	1.0	# Dose-dependent
Naproxen		4.15	99	0.3	14	7	97	0.9	
Nifedipine			50	42	1.8	98	99	1.0	
Nimesulide					4.8		99		
Nitrazepam	Amf	3.4/10.8	78	4	30	175	85	1.0	
Nordiazepam[d] (desmethyldiazepam)	Amf	11.65/3.35	50	1.5	80	175	97	1.0 [d]	Active metabolite of diazepam
Nortriptyline[d]	B	9.73	51	40	28	1470	93	1.0 [d]	
Octreotide	Pep		<5	11.4	1.5	23.8	95		
Omeprazole	Amf	3.97/8.8	67	35	0.5	24.5	95	0.9	
Ondansetron			60	29	3	161	70–76	1.0	
Orphenadrine	B	8.4			18		20		
Oxazepam	Amf	11.51/1.56	>90	8 [g]	7	70 [g]	>95	1.0	
Pamidronate disodium					27				
Paracetamol[d]	A	9.5	70–90	19.3	2.5	65.8	low #	1.0 [d]	# At therapeutic doses
Paroxetine			50		24		95	0.98	
Phenobarbital	A	7.2	100	0.3	100	49	50	0.7	Recommended therapeutic plasma concentration 10–35 mg/L

Table A2.1 Continued

	Nature[a]	pK_a[b]	Oral bioavailability (%)	Clearance (L/h)	Plasma halflife (h)	Volume of distribution (L)	Protein binding (%)	Nonrenal elimination[c]	Comments
Phenytoin	A	8.33	98	#	9–40	56	90	1.0	Recommended therapeutic plasma concentration 10–20 mg/L # Dose-dependent # Concentration-dependent
Prednisolone	B		80	6.3–15 #	3.6	28–91 #	65–91 #	1.0	
Pethidine[d]	B	6.3	54	38	6.9	280	70	0.9[d]	
Prochlorperazine	B	3.73/8.1			≈23				
Promethazine	B	9.1	25	68	12	910[f]			
Propanetheline[e]	B4		≈30	79	1.8				
Propofol	B	9.45		104	0.05:0.5:4 #	280[f]	93	0.85[e]	# Tri-exponential
Propranolol[d]	B			63	4	196		1.0	
Quinine	B	4.3/8.4		5.5	14	112	90	1.0[d]	
Ranitidine[d]	B	2.7	50	35	2	105	15	0.8	
Salbutamol	B	9.3	10.3		≈5			0.3[d]	
Salmeterol					67		95–98		
Sertraline					26	>1400	99	1.0	
Sodium cromoglicate	A	2.0			0.1		7.0	0.6	
Spironolactone[d]	S		70		19 #		98 #	1.0[d]	# Active metabolite (canrenone)
Sulindac[d]	A	4.5	>88		7 #		96	1.0 #	# Active sulfide metabolite $t_{1/2}$ 18h
Temazepam	B	1.31	>80	4[g]	13	70[g]	97	1.0	
Tenoxicam				0.13	72	14	99	1.0	
Terazosin			82	3.3	12	21	90	0.9	
Terbutaline	Amf	10.1/11.2 /8.8		13	15	112[f]	25	0.45	
Terfenadine[d]					20		97	1.0[d]	

Table A2.1 Continued

Nature[a]	pKa[b]	Oral bioavailability (%)	Clearance (L/h)	Plasma halflife (h)	Volume of distribution (L)	Protein binding (%)	Nonrenal elimination[c]	Comments
Theophylline[d] — Amf	8.6/3.5	96	3	8	35	50	0.9[d]	Recommended therapeutic plasma concentration 10–20 mg/L
Thioridazine[d]			0.1	≈20	≈14	99 #	1.0[d]	#Concentration-dependent
Thyroxine			3	150	45.5	>99	0.75	
Tinidazole — A	5.43	>90	≈1[g]	13		12		
Tolbutamide				7	10.5[g]	95 #	0.7[d]	#Concentration-dependent
Tramadol[d]		34	26	6	231	4	0.03	
Tranexamic acid — A	4.3/10.6		6.7	10			1.0	
Triamcinolone — S		100	45–70 #	1.4	98–147 #			#Dose-dependent
Trimethoprim — B	7.2	41	4.5[g]	11	91[g]	45	0.45	
Trimipramine[e] — B			67	23	2170	95	1.0[e]	
Tropisetron		52–66 #	60/12 ##	8/35	546	59–71 #	0.9	#Dose-dependent ## Two hydroxylation phenotypes
Valproic acid[d] — A	4.95	100	0.5	13	10.5	90		Recommended therapeutic plasma concentration 50–100mg/L
Venlafaxine — A	5.0			4/10 #	525/400 #	27		#Parent drug/active metabolite
Vigabatrin			5.6	7	56	<1	0	
Warfarin[d] — A	5.0	100	0.2/0.15 #[g]	35/50 #	10.5[g]	99	1.0[d]	#S/R enantiomers
Zolpidem		70	18.2	2	37.8	90	1.0	
Zopiclone		80	14.8	4.9	98	45	1.0	

a. A = acid; Aa = amino acid; Alc = alcohol; Amf = ampholyte; B = base; B_4 = base with quaternary ammonium group; Gly = glycoside; Pep = peptide; S = steroid; Sa = substituted amide.

b. the pH at which the drug is 50% ionized.

c. the fraction of the drug eliminated by nonrenal pathways in normal individuals; 1 – [fraction] gives an estimate of how much of the drug is excreted unchanged in the urine.

d. pharmacologically active metabolite(s).

e. metabolite(s) with possible pharmacological activity.

f. apparent volume of distribution at steady state.

g. after oral administration.

Appendix 3: Polypharmacy and cytochrome P450

Polypharmacy (i.e. using more than one drug concurrently) introduces the possibility of clinically important drug interactions. In the past, concern about interactions focused mainly on changes in drug absorption, protein binding in the blood and renal excretion. There was also recognition of important metabolic interactions such as the serotonin syndrome observed with pethidine and MAOIs (see p.62). Studies over the last 20 years, however, have demonstrated that most of the potentially serious drug interactions involve hepatic biotransformation pathways catalyzed by the cytochrome P450 mixed-function oxidase group of enzymes. These are the major drug metabolizing enzymes involved in intramolecular biotransformation processes, principally *oxidation* and *reduction*.

The name cytochrome P450 is derived from the spectrometer characteristics of the group of enzymes; maximum absorbance is produced at or near 450nm. Cytochrome P450 enzymes exist in virtually all tissues but their highest concentration is in the liver. The cytochrome P450 group of enzymes comprises at least 12 families (>40% identical gene content) with some 30 active subfamilies (>55% identical gene content) (Figure A3.1). Cytochrome P450 enzymes are identified by the root symbol CYP, followed by:
- a number representing the enzyme family
- a capital letter designating the subfamily
- a number which represents the individual enzyme.

The mammalian P450 families can be functionally divided into two major classes; those involved in the synthesis of steroids and bile acids and those which primarily metabolize foreign substances (xenobiotics). Enzymes of the CYP1, CYP2 and CYP3 families are responsible for many drug biotransformations and account for 70% of the total P450 content of the liver (Figure A3.2).

Drugs responsible for interactions act either as *inhibitors* or *inducers* and have been nicknamed *accomplice* drugs. The drugs affected by enzyme inhibition or induction are the enzyme substrates and have been nicknamed *bullets* if made more active and *blanks* if made less active.

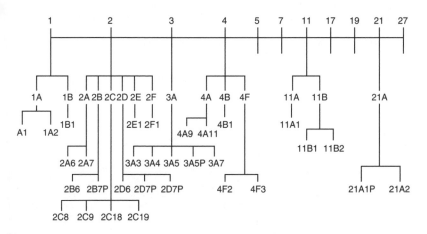

Figure A3.1 Cytochrome P450 enzyme tree.[1]

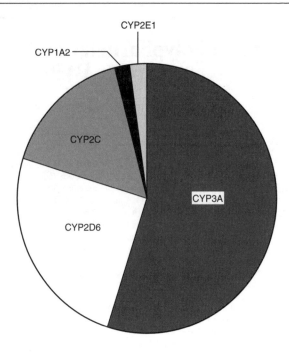

Figure A3.2 Proportion of drugs metabolized by different cytochrome P450 iso-enzymes. CYP2C includes all the 2C subfamily of enzymes.[1]

Inhibition

Inhibition of drug biotransformation begins within a few hours of the administration of the inhibitor drug, leading to an increase in the substrate drug plasma concentration, drug response and toxicity (*except prodrugs* which will have a corresponding reduced effect). The mechanism of enzymatic inhibition is either competitive or noncompetitive. In competitive inhibition, the accomplice drug (e.g. **cimetidine**, **ketoconazole** and **macrolide antibiotics**) binds to the P450 enzyme and prevents the metabolism of the substrate drug. The extent of inhibition of one drug by another depends on their relative affinities for the P450 enzyme. In noncompetitive inhibition the enzyme is destroyed or inactivated by the accomplice drug or its metabolites (e.g. **chloramphenicol** and **spironolactone**). The occurrence of serious cardiac arrhythmias seen with concurrent administration of the accomplice drug **ketoconazole** and the bullet drug **terfenadine** is an example of a noncompetitive inhibitory drug interaction involving CYP3A3/4[2] (Box A3.A).

Box A3.A   Ketoconazole-induced terfenadine cardiotoxicity[3]

A 39 year-old woman began a course of **terfenadine** and, 8 days later, started **ketoconazole**. Two days later she developed syncopal symptoms, prolongation of her QT interval on the ECG and Torsades de Pointes. Plasma assay showed high concentrations of terfenadine and reduced concentrations of its main metabolite suggesting inhibition of metabolism. It was concluded that ketoconazole-induced inhibition of terfenadine metabolism caused the cardiotoxicity.

A food–drug interaction has been highlighted involving **grapefruit juice** and substrates of CYP3A3/4 iso-enzymes such as **felodipine, nifedipine, ciclosporin** and **terfenadine.**[4] Grapefruit juice contains several bioflavonoids (naringenin, kaempferol and quercetin) which noncompetitively inhibit oxidation reactions in the CYP3A3/4 enzymes in the gastro-intestinal wall.[5] The effect is variable because the flavonoids in grapefruit products vary up to 6-fold;[6] it is maximal when grapefruit juice is ingested 30–60min before the drug. In contrast, orange juice does not contain these bioflavonoids and does not inhibit drug metabolism. Box A3.B gives examples of enhanced drug effects resulting from enzyme inhibition. Figures A3.3–A3.9 at the end of this appendix give numerous examples of cytochrome P450 enzyme inhibitors which may increase the plasma concentrations of various substrate drugs.[7]

Box A3.B   Examples of drug interactions → increased effect

Cimetidine reduces **diazepam** clearance → increased effect.[8]

Ciprofloxacin reduces **theophylline** clearance by 18–113% → increased effect.[9]

Diltiazem prolongs the halflife of **propranolol** and **metoprolol** → increased effect.[10]

Erythromycin increases **cisapride** concentration → possible cardiac effects.

Fluvoxamine increases **warfarin** concentration by 65% → increased effect.[11]

Ketoconazole increases **terfenadine** concentration → possible life-threatening cardiac arrhythmias.[12]

Mexiletine reduces clearance of **amitriptyline** → increased effect.

SSRIs reduce clearance of **tricyclic antidepressants** → increased plasma concentrations by 50–350% → increased effect.[13-15]

Induction

Induction of the rate of drug biotransformation results in a decrease in the parent drug plasma concentrations and either decreased pharmacological effect or increased toxicity if active metabolites are formed. The onset and offset of enzyme induction is gradual because:
- onset depends on drug-induced synthesis of new enzyme
- offset depends upon elimination of the enzyme-inducing drug and the decay of the increased enzyme stores.

Several molecular mechanisms for enzyme induction have been characterized, including increased DNA transcription (the most common), increased RNA processing and mRNA stabilization.

Accomplice drugs like **rifampicin, dexamethasone, griseofulvin** and anti-epileptics such as **carbamazepine, phenobarbital** and **phenytoin** induce members of the CYP3A subfamily. Rifampicin is the most potent inducer of cytochrome CYP3A in clinical use. Some estrogens are metabolized by CYP3A3/4 and induction by **rifampicin** has caused oral contraceptive failure. In fact, any enzyme inducer can potentially result in oral contraceptive failure. Box A3.C gives examples of decreased drug effects as a result of enzyme induction. Figures A3.3–A3.9 give numerous examples of cytochrome P450 enzyme inducers which may decrease the plasma

---

Box A3.C   Examples of drug interactions → decreased effect

Carbamazepine and **phenytoin** increase midazolam metabolism → decreased effect.[16]

Phenytoin increases **carbamazepine** metabolism → possible therapeutic failure.

Quinidine inhibits biotransformation of **codeine** to morphine → decreased analgesic effect.[17]

Rifampicin increases **phenytoin** clearance (halflife halved) → decreased effect.[18]

---

concentrations of various substrate drugs. **Carbamazepine** can potentially decrease the effect of many other drugs by decreasing their plasma concentrations, or it can expedite the biotransformation of a drug to an active metabolite. For example, **carbamazepine** increases **diazepam** metabolism but, in this case, there may be no detectable clinical effect because of active metabolites.

General polymorphism

Genetic differences in the amount of drug metabolized by an enzymatic pathway has resulted in the classification of individuals into slow (poor) metabolizers and rapid (extensive) metabolizers.[1,19] Recent data suggest that, for some pathways, there may also be ultra-rapid metabolizers. Inevitably, even within the general population of rapid metabolizers, there is a normal distribution ranging from well below-average to well above-average. However, the slow metabolizers (and ultra-rapid ones) form a discontinuous genetically distinct group – they are not merely one end of a spectrum. Slow metabolizer status is generally linked to only one enzyme in any one individual, and is inherited as an autosomal recessive trait (Table A3.1).

Nongenetic circumstances in which drug metabolism may become relatively slower include liver damage (with an associated disease in cytochrome P450 enzyme activity) and old age. In general, age-related decreases in liver mass, hepatic enzyme activity and hepatic blood flow result in a decrease in the overall metabolic capacity of the liver in the elderly. This is of particular importance in relation to drugs which have a high 'hepatic extraction ratio', e.g. amitriptyline, lidocaine, propranolol, verapamil.

Table A3.1 Genetic polymorphism and slow metabolizer status[1]

Pathway	Drugs affected	Population affected
N-acetylation	Caffeine Dapsone Hydralazine Isoniazid Procainamide	North European 60–70% American whites and blacks 50% Asians 5–10%
CYP2D6 (debrisoquine hydroxylase)	β-blockers Codeine Debrisoquine Flecainide Oxycodone Phenothiazines SSRIs (some) Tricyclic antidepressants (some)	Whites 5–10% Asians 1%
CYP2C19	Diazepam PPIs S-mephenytoin	Whites 3–5% Asians 20%

1 Riddick DS (1997) Drug biotransformation. In: Kalant H, Roschlau W (eds) *Principles of Medical Pharmacology. (6th edn)* Oxford University Press, New York.
2 Honig PK et al. (1993) Terfenadine-ketoconazole interaction: pharmacokinetic and electrocardiographic consequences. *Journal of the American Medical Association.* **269**: 1513–1518.
3 Monaham BP et al. (1990) Torsades de Pointes occurring in association with terfenadine. *Journal of the American Medical Association.* **264**: 2788–2790.
4 Benton R et al. (1996) Grapefruit juice alters terfenadine pharmacokinetics, resulting in prolongation of repolarization on the electrocardiogram. *Clinical Pharmacology and Therapeutics.* **59**: 383–388.

5 Gibaldi M (1992) Drug interactions. Part II. *Annals of Pharmacotherapy.* **26**: 829–834.

6 Tailor S et al. (1996) Peripheral oedema due to nifedipine-itraconazole interaction: a case report. *Archives of Dermatology.* **132**: 350–352.

7 Aeschlimann JR and Tyler LS (1996) Drug interactions associated with cytochrome P-450 enzymes. *Journal of Pharmaceutical Care in Pain and Symptom Control.* **4** (4): 35–54.

8 Klotz U et al. (1980) Delayed clearance of diazepam due to cimetidine. *New England Journal of Medicine.* **302**: 1012ff.

9 Nix DE et al. (1987) Effect of multiple dose oral ciprofloxacin on the pharmacokinetics of theophylline and indocyanine green. *Journal of Antimicrobial Chemotherapy.* **19**: 263ff.

10 Tateishi T et al. (1989) Effect of diltiazem on the pharmacokinetics of propranolol, metoprolol and atenolol. *European Journal of Clinical Pharmacology.* **36**: 67ff.

11 Tatro DS (1995) Fluvoxamine drug interactions. *Drug Newsletter.* **14**: 20ff.

12 Eller MG et al. (1991) Pharmacokinetic interaction between terfenadine and ketoconazole. *Clinical Pharmacology and Therapeutics.* **49**: 130.

13 Vandel S et al. (1992) Tricyclic antidepressant plasma levels after fluoxetine addition. *Neuropsychobiology.* **25**: 202–207.

14 Finley PR (1994) Selective serotonin reuptake inhibitors: Pharmacologic profiles and potential therapeutic distinctions. *Annals of Pharmacotherapy.* **28**: 1359–1369.

15 Pollock BG (1994) Recent developments in drug metabolism of relevance to psychiatrist. *Harvard Review of Psychiatry.* **2**: 204–213.

16 Backman JT et al. (1996) Concentrations and effect of oral midazolam were greatly reduced in patients treated with carbamazepine or phenytoin. *Epilepsia.* **37**: 253–257.

17 Sindrup HS et al. (1992) The effect of quinidine on the analgesic effect of codeine. *European Journal of Clinical Pharmacology.* **42**: 587–591.

18 Kay L et al. (1985) Influence of rifampicin and isoniazid on the kinetics of phenytoin. *British Journal of Clinical Pharmacology.* **20**: 323–326.

19 Meyer UA (1991) *Pharmacogenetics.* **1**: 66–67.

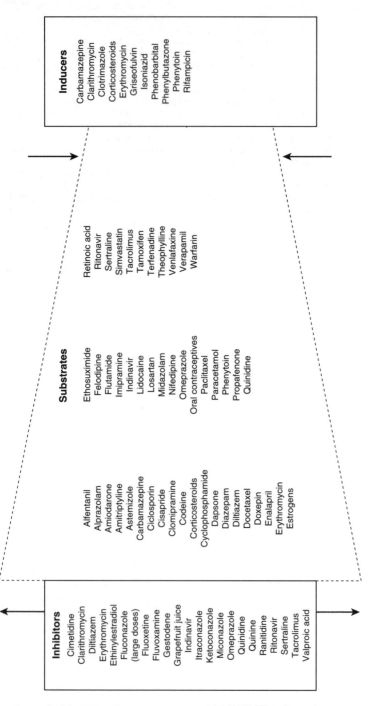

Inducers

Carbamazepine
Clarithromycin
Clotrimazole
Corticosteroids
Erythromycin
Griseofulvin
Isoniazid
Phenobarbital
Phenylbutazone
Phenytoin
Rifampicin

Substrates

Ethosuximide
Felodipine
Flutamide
Imipramine
Indinavir
Lidocaine
Losartan
Midazolam
Nifedipine
Omeprazole
Oral contraceptives
Paclitaxel
Paracetamol
Phenytoin
Propafenone
Quinidine

Retinoic acid
Ritonavir
Sertraline
Simvastatin
Tacrolimus
Tamoxifen
Terfenadine
Theophylline
Venlafaxine
Verapamil
Warfarin

Inhibitors

Cimetidine
Clarithromycin
Diltiazem
Erythromycin
Ethinylestradiol
Fluconazole
(large doses)
Fluoxetine
Fluvoxamine
Gestodene
Grapefruit juice
Indinavir
Itraconazole
Ketoconazole
Miconazole
Omeprazole
Quinidine
Quinine
Ranitidine
Ritonavir
Sertraline
Tacrolimus
Valproic acid

Alfentanil
Alprazolam
Amiodarone
Amitriptyline
Astemizole
Carbamazepine
Ciclosporin
Cisapride
Clomipramine
Codeine
Corticosteroids
Cyclophosphamide
Dapsone
Diazepam
Diltiazem
Docetaxel
Doxepin
Enalapril
Erythromycin
Estrogens

Figure A3.3   Selected list of CYP3A3/4 inhibitors and inducers and substrates.[7]

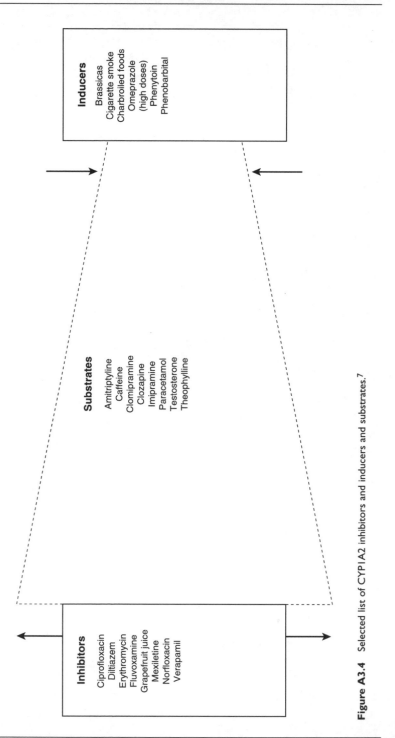

Inducers

Brassicas
Cigarette smoke
Charbroiled foods
Omeprazole
(high doses)
Phenytoin
Phenobarbital

Substrates

Amitriptyline
Caffeine
Clomipramine
Clozapine
Imipramine
Paracetamol
Testosterone
Theophylline

Inhibitors

Ciprofloxacin
Diltiazem
Erythromycin
Fluvoxamine
Grapefruit juice
Mexiletine
Norfloxacin
Verapamil

Figure A3.4 Selected list of CYP1A2 inhibitors and inducers and substrates.[7]

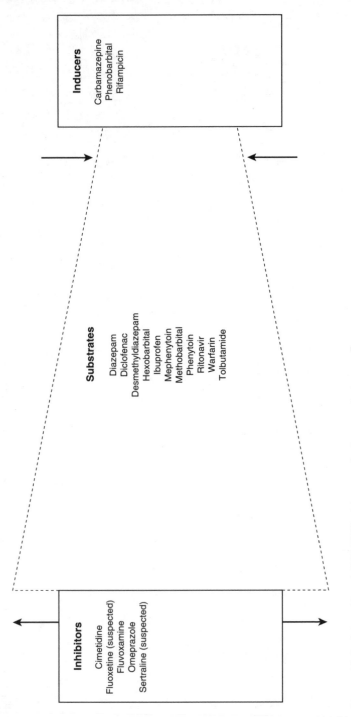

Figure A3.5 Selected list of CYP2C9/10 inhibitors and inducers and substrates.[7]

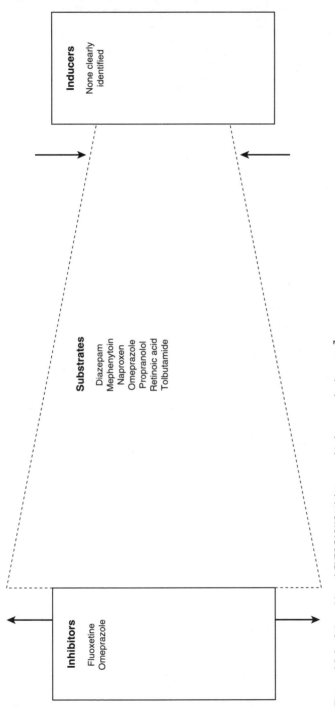

Figure A3.6 Selected list of CYP2C18/19 inhibitors and inducers and substrates.[7]

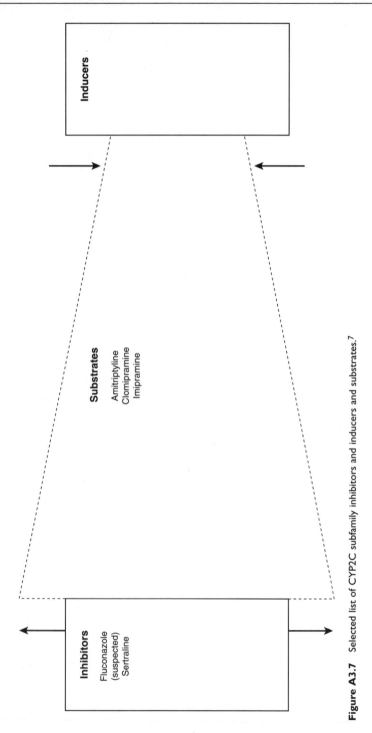

Figure A3.7 Selected list of CYP2C subfamily inhibitors and inducers and substrates.[7]

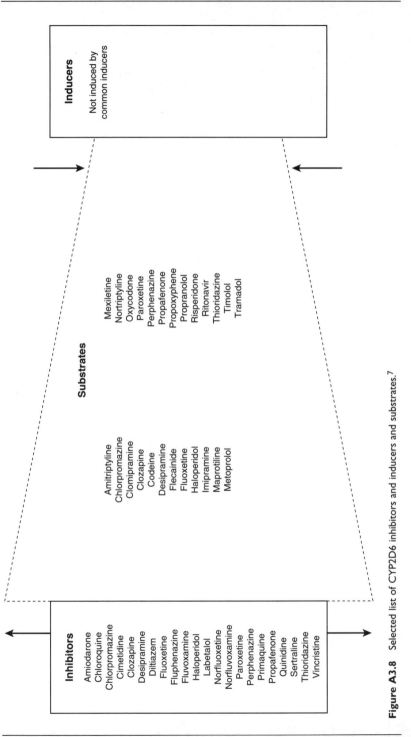

Inducers

Not induced by
common inducers

Substrates

Amitriptyline
Chlorpromazine
Clomipramine
Clozapine
Codeine
Desipramine
Flecainide
Fluoxetine
Haloperidol
Imipramine
Maprotiline
Metoprolol

Mexiletine
Nortriptyline
Oxycodone
Paroxetine
Perphenazine
Propafenone
Propoxyphene
Propranolol
Risperidone
Ritonavir
Thioridazine
Timolol
Tramadol

Inhibitors

Amiodarone
Chloroquine
Chlorpromazine
Cimetidine
Clozapine
Desipramine
Diltiazem
Fluoxetine
Fluphenazine
Fluvoxamine
Haloperidol
Labetalol
Norfluoxetine
Norfluvoxamine
Paroxetine
Perphenazine
Primaquine
Propafenone
Quinidine
Sertraline
Thioridazine
Vincristine

Figure A3.8   Selected list of CYP2D6 inhibitors and inducers and substrates.[7]

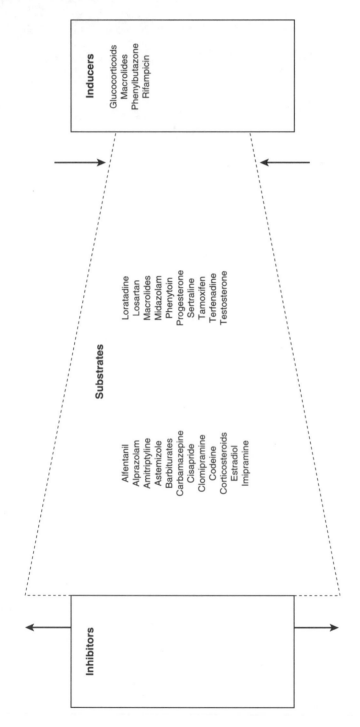

Figure A3.9 Selected list of CYP3A4 inhibitors and inducers and substrates.[7]

Appendix 4: Antimuscarinic effects

'Dry as a bone,
blind as a bat,
red as a beet,
hot as a hare,
mad as a hatter.'

Several drugs used in palliative care have antimuscarinic (anticholinergic) properties (Table A4.1). Antimuscarinic effects may be a limiting factor in symptom management (Table A4.2). The concurrent use of two antimuscarinics should generally be avoided.

Table A4.1 Antimuscarinic drugs used in palliative care

Antihistamines
  chlorphenamine
    (chlorpheniramine)
  cyclizine
  dimenhydrinate
  promethazine
	Belladonna alkaloids
	  atropine
	  hyoscine

	Glycopyrrolate

Antiparkinsonians
  orphenadrine
  procyclidine
	Phenothiazines
	  chlorpromazine
	  levomepromazine
	    (methotrimeprazine)
	  prochlorperazine
	  thioridazine

Antispasmodics
  mebeverine
  oxybutynin
  propantheline
	Tricyclic antidepressants

Table A4.2 Antimuscarinic (anticholinergic) effects

Visual Mydriasis Loss of accommodation }	blurred vision	*Gastro-intestinal* Dry mouth Heartburn Constipation	
Cardiovascular Palpitations Extrasystoles Arrhythmias }	also related to norepinephrine (noradrenaline) potentiation and a quinidine-like action	*Urinary tract* Hesitancy of micturition Retention of urine	

Appendix 5: Drug-induced movement disorders

Drug-induced movement disorders encompass:
• extrapyramidal effects:
  parkinsonism
  acute dystonia
  acute akathisia
  tardive dyskinesia
• malignant neuroleptic (antipsychotic) syndrome.

The features of the various syndromes are listed in Table A5.1 (see p.228). Extrapyramidal effects are caused mostly by drugs which block dopamine receptors in the CNS; this includes all antipsychotics and metoclopramide.[1] Other drugs have also been implicated, including antidepressants and ondansetron[2–4] (Table A5.2).

High potency antipsychotics possess a greater affinity for dopamine receptors and a lower affinity for muscarinic (cholinergic) receptors than low potency antipsychotics. They therefore cause a greater imbalance between dopamine and acetylcholine, and are more likely to cause extrapyramidal effects. Thus haloperidol is high risk but, for example, levomepromazine (methotrimeprazine) is low risk. More extrapyramidal effects occur at higher doses of any potentially causal drug. There is probably also a genetic factor. To explain the mechanism by which antidepressants and ondansetron cause extrapyramidal effects, a 'four neurone model' has been proposed which includes 5HT- and GABA-receptors.[5]

Table A5.2 Drugs which may cause extrapyramidal effects[3,6]

Palliative care	General
Antipsychotics	Diltiazem
haloperidol	Fenfluramine
phenothiazines	5-Hydroxytryptophan
Metoclopramide	Lithium
Ondansetron	Methyldopa
Antidepressants [a]	Methysergide
tricyclics	Reserpine
SSRIs	
Carbamazepine	

a. all classes of antidepressants have been implicated except RIMAs.

Parkinsonism

Parkinsonism develops in up to 40% of patients treated long-term with antipsychotic drugs. It develops at any stage after starting treatment, although generally not before the second week. It is most common in those over 60. Although normally symmetrical, there may be asymmetry in the early stages.

Regular rhythmic tremors of the hands, head, mouth or tongue with a frequency of 8–12cps may be induced by a wide range of drugs (Table A5.3). These must not be confused with drug-induced parkinsonism. Drug-induced tremor is generally absent at rest but intensifies when the affected part is used or held in a sustained position, e.g. hands outstretched, mouth held open. In contrast, the tremor of drug-induced parkinsonism is typically lower in frequency, worse

Table A5.1 Movement disorders associated with D_2-receptor antagonists[7]

Parkinsonism	Acute dystonias	Acute akathisia	Tardive dyskinesia	Neuroleptic malignant syndrome
Coarse resting tremor of limbs, head, mouth and/or tongue	One or more of Abnormal positioning of head and neck (retrocollis, torticollis)	One or more of Fidgety movements or swinging of legs	Exposure to neuroleptic medication for ⩾3 months (1 month if over 60)	Severe muscle rigidity Pyrexia +
Muscular rigidity (cogwheel or leadpipe)	Spasms of jaw muscles (trismus, gaping, grimacing)	Rocking from foot to foot when standing	Involuntary movement of tongue, jaw, trunk or limbs: choreiform	Two or more of Tremor Sweating Mutism
Bradykinesia (notably of face)	Tongue dysfunction (dysarthria, protrusion)	Pacing to relieve restlessness	(rapid, jerky, nonrepetitive) athetoid	Dysphagia Incontinence
Sialorrhoea (drooling)	Dysphagia	Inability to sit or stand still for several minutes	(slow, sinuous, continual) rhythmic	Drowsiness Tachycardia
Shuffling gait	Laryngo-pharyngeal spasm		(stereotypic)	Elevated/labile blood pressure Leucocytosis
	Dysphonia			Evidence of muscle injury (myoglobinuria, raised plasma creatine kinase concentration)
	Eyes deviated up, down, or sideways ('oculogyric crisis')			
	Abnormal positioning of limbs or trunk			

at rest, suppressed during intentional movements, and is typically associated with rigidity and bradykinesia (Table A5.1).

Treatment
- prescribe an antimuscarinic antiparkinsonian drug:
  benzatropine 1–2mg IV/IM → 2mg PO o.d.–b.d. or
  procyclidine 5–10mg IV/IM → 2.5–5mg PO t.d.s. or
  orphenadrine 50mg PO b.d.–t.d.s. (see p.82)
- if possible, reduce or stop causal drug.

Table A5.3 Drug-induced (nonparkinsonian) tremor[8]

Anticonvulsants
  sodium valproate
	Methylxanthines
	  caffeine
	  aminophylline
	  theophylline

Antidepressants
  SSRIs
  tricyclics	

β-adrenoceptors
  salbutamol
  salmeterol
	Antipsychotics
	  butyrophenones
	  phenothiazines

Lithium	Psychostimulants
	  dexamfetamine
	  methylphenidate

Acute dystonia

Acute dystonias occur in <10% of patients treated with antipsychotics. They develop abruptly within days of starting treatment, and are accompanied by anxiety (Table A5.1). They are most common in young adults.

Treatment
- **benzatropine** 1–2mg or **procyclidine** 5–10mg IV/IM for immediate relief. Benefit is seen within 10min; peak effect within 30min. If necessary, repeat after 30min
- continue treatment with a standard oral antimuscarinic antiparkinsonian drug e.g. **orphenadrine** 50mg b.d.–t.d.s. (see p.82)
- some centres use **diphenhydramine** 25–50mg IV/IM, followed by 25–50mg PO b.d.–q.d.s.
- if possible, reduce or stop causal drug
- if caused by metoclopramide, substitute **domperidone**.

Acute akathisia

Akathisia is a form of motor restlessness in which the subject is compelled to pace up and down or to change the body position frequently (Table A5.1). It is most common in the 16–50 age range. It occurs in up to 20% of patients receiving antipsychotics. It can develop within days of starting treatment. If the drug is continued, it may progress to parkinsonism. Haloperidol and prochlorperazine carry the highest risk.[9] It is uncommon for metoclopramide to cause akathisia. Concurrent administration of morphine or sodium valproate may be additional risk factors.[6]

Treatment
- if possible, reduce or stop causal drug
- switch to a neuroleptic with more antimuscarinic activity
- prescribe an antimuscarinic antiparkinsonian drug (as for acute dystonia)
- if only partial response, add **diazepam** 5mg nocte
- alternatively, prescribe a *lipophilic* β-adrenoceptor antagonist, i.e. **propranolol** 10–40mg b.d. or **metoprolol** 50–100mg b.d.
- in resistant cases, discontinue causal drug.

Akathisia responds less well to antiparkinsonian drugs than drug-induced parkinsonism and dystonias. Propranolol, a highly *lipophilic* nonselective β-receptor antagonist, and metoprolol, a lipophilic β_1-receptor antagonist, are equally effective. In contrast, atenolol, a *hydrophilic* β_1-receptor antagonist, has no effect.

Tardive dyskinesia

Tardive (late) dyskinesia is caused by the long-term administration of drugs which block dopamine receptors, particularly D_2-receptors. It occurs in 20% of patients receiving a neuroleptic for more than 3 months. Women, the elderly and those on high doses, e.g. chlorpromazine 300mg/day, are most commonly affected. Tardive dyskinesia typically manifests as involuntary stereotyped chewing movements of the tongue and orofacial muscles. The involuntary movements are made worse by anxiety and reduced by drowsiness and during sleep. Tardive dyskinesia seldom causes subjective distress, unless associated with akathisia. This is seen in 25% of cases. Early diagnosis is aided by the request to *'open your mouth and stick out your tongue'.* Inability to protrude the tongue for more than a few seconds and worm-like movements of the tongue indicate early tardive dyskinesia.

In younger patients, tardive dyskinesia may present as abnormal posturing of the limbs and tonic contractions of the neck and trunk muscles causing torticollis, lordosis or scoliosis. In younger patients, tardive dyskinesia may occur if neuroleptic treatment is stopped abruptly, but not if tailed off gradually.

Treatment

* withdrawal of the causal agent leads to resolution in 30% in 3 months and a further 40% in 5 years; sometimes irreversible particularly in the elderly
* often responds poorly to drug therapy; *antimuscarinic antiparkinsonian drugs may exacerbate*
* **tetrabenazine** depletes presynaptic biogenic amine stores and blocks postsynaptic dopamine receptors. Best not used in depressed patients. Start with 12.5mg t.d.s. → 25mg t.d.s.; increase the dose slowly to avoid troublesome hypotension
* **reserpine** depletes presynaptic biogenic amine stores. May be used in place of tetrabenazine; causes similar adverse effects
* **levodopa** may produce long-term benefit after causing initial deterioration
* GABA antagonists **baclofen**, **sodium valproate**, **diazepam** and **clonazepam** have all been tried with inconsistent results
* increasing the dose of the causal drug; paradoxically, this may help but should be considered only in desperation.

Neuroleptic (antipsychotic) malignant syndrome

Neuroleptic malignant syndrome occurs in 1–2% of patients receiving an antipsychotic, particularly in young adults; 2/3 of cases occur <1 week after starting treatment.[10] It is more likely to occur in patients also receiving lithium. The essential features of neuroleptic malignant syndrome are fever and muscle rigidity associated with some of the following: tremor, sweating, mutism, dysphagia, incontinence, drowsiness, tachycardia, elevated or labile blood pressure. Leucocytosis and evidence of muscle injury, i.e. myoglobinuria and raised plasma creatine kinase concentration, are laboratory features. It is possible that this syndrome is seen with other drugs; a case report suggests that it may occur with IV ondansetron.[11]

Treatment

* discontinue the causal drug
* prescribe a muscle relaxant.

In severe cases, **bromocriptine** (a dopamine-receptor agonist) has been used. Death occurs in <20% of cases, most commonly as a result of respiratory failure.

---

1 Tonda ME and Guthrie SK (1994) Treatment of acute neuroleptic-induced movement disorders. *Pharmacotherapy.* **14**: 543–560.

2 Zubenko GS *et al.* (1987) Antidepressant-related akathisia. *Journal of Clinical Psychopharmacology.* **7**: 254–257.

3 Arya DK (1994) Extra-pyramidal symptoms with selective serotonin reuptake inhibitors. *British Journal of Psychiatry.* **165**: 728–733.

4 Mathews HG and Tancil CG (1996) Extrapyramidal reaction caused by ondansetron. *Annals of Pharmacotherapy.* **30**: 196.

5 Hamilton MS and Opler LA (1992) Akathisia, suicidality, and fluoxetine. *Journal of Clinical Psychiatry.* **53**: 401–406.

6 Anonymous (1994) Drug-induced extrapyramidal reactions. *Current Problems in Pharmacovigilance.* **20**: 15–16.

7 American Psychiatric Association (1994) Neuroleptic-induced movement disorders. In: *Diagnostic and Statistical Manual of Mental Disorders. (4th edn) (DSM-IV).* American Psychiatric Association, New York. pp 736–751.

8 American Psychiatric Association (1994) Medication-induced postural tremor. In: *Diagnostic and Statistical Manual of Mental Disorders. (4th edn) (DSM-IV).* American Psychiatric Association, New York. pp 749–751.

9 Gattera JA et al. (1994) A retrospective study of risk factors of akathisia in terminally ill patients. *Journal of Pain and Symptom Management.* **9**: 454–461.

10 Launer M (1996) Selected side-effects: 17. Dopamine-receptor antagonists and movement disorders. *Prescribers' Journal.* **36**: 37–41.

11 Goswami DC (1996) Adverse reaction of ondansetron. *Journal of Anaesthesia and Clinical Pharmacology.* **12**: 59–60.

Appendix 6: Discoloured urine

There are many causes of discoloured urine (Table A6.1). If the urine is red, it is often assumed to be haematuria.

Table A6.1 Common causes of discoloured urine

Red/pink
Beetroot
Dantron (in co-danthramer and co-danthrusate)
Doxorubicin
Nefopam
Phenolphthalein (in alkaline urine) present in several proprietary laxatives (e.g. Agarol)
Rhubarb

Blue
Methylene blue; present in some proprietary urinary antiseptic mixtures, e.g. Urised (USA)
Pseudomonas aeruginosa (pyocyanin) – in alkaline urine

Dark
Metronidazole

Appendix 7: Using licensed drugs for unlicensed purposes

In palliative care the treatment of many symptoms involves the use of drugs for unlicensed indications or by unlicensed routes. Throughout the PCF the symbol[†] is used to draw attention to such use. It is important to understand that the licensing process for drugs *regulates the activities of pharmaceutical companies and not a doctor's prescribing practice*. Indeed, exemptions are specifically incorporated into the Medicines Act (1968) which preserve a doctor's clinical freedom. Further, drugs prescribed outside the licence can be dispensed by pharmacists and administered by nurses or midwives.[1]

The licensing process

A marketing licence is necessary in the UK for a product for which therapeutic claims are made. After receiving satisfactory evidence of quality, safety and efficacy, the Licensing Authority (working through the Medicines Control Agency) grants a licence, called the Marketing Authorisation. This allows a pharmaceutical company to market and supply a product for the specific indications listed in its Data Sheet or Summary of Product Characteristics. (Alternatively, since 1995, drugs can be licensed through the European Union). Restrictions are imposed by the Licensing Authority if evidence of safety and efficacy is unavailable in particular patient groups, e.g. children. Once a product is marketed, further clinical trials and experience may reveal other indications. For these to become licensed, however, additional evidence would need to be submitted. The considerable expense of this, perhaps coupled with a small market for the new indication, often means that a revised application is not made.

Prescribing outside the licence

In the UK, a doctor may legally:
- prescribe unlicensed medicines
- in a named patient, use unlicensed products specially prepared, imported or supplied
- supply another doctor with an unlicensed medicine
- with appropriate safeguards, use unlicensed drugs in clinical trials
- use or advise the use of licensed medicines for indications or in doses or by routes of administration outside the licensed recommendations
- override the warnings and precautions given in the licence.

The responsibility for the consequences of these actions lies with the doctor.[2] In addition to clinical trials such prescriptions may be justified:
- when prescribing generic formulations (for which indications are not described)
- with established drugs for proven but unlicensed indications
- with drugs for conditions for which there are no other treatments (even in the absence of strong evidence)
- when using drugs in individuals not covered by licensed indications, e.g. children.

Prescription of a drug (whether licensed use/route or not) requires a doctor to balance both the potential good and the potential harm which might ensue in the light of published evidence. Doctors have a duty in common law to act responsibly and with reasonable care and skill in a manner consistent with the practice of professional colleagues of similar standing. Thus, when prescribing outside the terms of a licence, doctors must be fully informed about the actions and uses of the drug and be assured of the quality of the particular product. It is possible to draw a hierarchy of degrees of reasonableness relating to the use of unlicensed drugs (Figure A7.1). The more dangerous the medicine and the more flimsy the evidence the more difficult it is to justify its prescription.

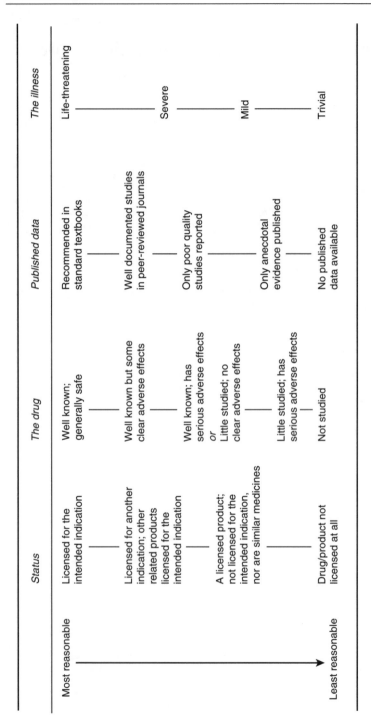

Figure A7.1 Factors influencing the reasonableness of prescribing decisions.[3]

It has been recommended that when prescribing a drug outside its licence, a doctor should:[1-4]
- record in the patient's notes the reasons for the decision to prescribe outside the licensed indications
- where possible explain the position to the patient (and family as appropriate) in sufficient detail to allow them to give informed consent (the Patient Information Leaflet obviously does not contain information about unlicensed indications)
- inform other professionals, e.g. pharmacist, nurses, general practitioner, involved in the care of the patient to avoid misunderstandings.

In palliative care, however, the use of drugs for unlicensed uses or by unlicensed routes is so widespread that such an approach is impractical. Indeed the harm done (e.g. by creating unnecessary anxiety and increasing noncompliance) is likely to exceed any benefits in most cases. Even so, in certain situations, it will be appropriate to explain the experimental nature of the treatment and to secure appropriate consent. There is clearly a grey area here and each doctor must decide how explicit he/she ought to be.

1 Anonymous (1992) Prescribing unlicensed drugs or using drugs for unlicensed indications. *Drug and Therapeutics Bulletin*. **30**: 97–99.
2 Tomkins CM (1988) Drugs without a product licence. *Journal of the Medical Defence Union*. Spring: 7.
3 Ferner RE (1996) Prescribing licensed medicines for unlicensed indications. *Prescribers' Journal*. **36**: 73–78.
4 Cohen PJ (1997) Off-label use of prescription drugs: legal, clinical and policy considerations. *European Journal of Anaesthesiology*. **14**: 231–235.

Appendix 8: Special orders and named patient supplies

The following companies manufacture special order products, e.g. liquid preparations of diuretics or analgesics in strengths appropriate for use in adults. Details of products and prices are supplied on request, and a prompt service is offered.

BCM Specials
Boots Contracting Manufacturing
1 Thane Road West
Nottingham NG2 3AA
Tel: 0500 925 935
Fax: 0115 959 1098

Martindale Pharmaceuticals Ltd
Bampton Road
Harold Hill
Romford RM3 8UG
Tel: 01708 386 660
Fax: 01708 384 866

Rosemont Pharmaceuticals Ltd
Rosemont House
Yorkdale Industrial Park
Braithwaite Street
Leeds LS11 9XE
Tel: 0113 244 1999
Fax: 0113 246 0738

Companies which will obtain information and organize the supply of drugs licensed in other countries include:

IDIS (International Drug Information Service) Ltd World Medicines
Millbank House
171 Ewell Road
Surbiton KT6 6AX
Tel: 0181 410 0700
Fax: 0181 410 0800

John Bell and Croyden
54 Wigmore Street
London W1H 0AU
Tel: 0171 935 5555
Fax: 0171 935 9605

Appendix 9: Nebulized drugs

Nebulizers are used in asthma and COPD for both acute exacerbations and long-term pro-phylaxis.[1] Other uses include the pulmonary delivery of antimicrobial drugs for cystic fibrosis, bronchiectasis and AIDS-related pneumonia. Nebulizers are also used in palliative care. The aim is to deliver a therapeutic dose of a drug as an aerosol in particles small enough to be inspired within 5–10min. A nebulizer is preferable to a hand-held inhaler when:
- a large drug dose is needed
- co-ordinated breathing is difficult
- if hand-held inhalers are ineffective
- if a drug is unavailable in an inhaler.

Commonly used nebulizers are:
Jet: the aerosol is generated by a flow of gas from, for example, an electrical compressor or an oxygen cylinder. At least 50% of the aerosol produced at the recommended driving gas flow should be particles small enough to inhale (British standard BS7711).
Ultrasonic: the aerosol is generated by ultrasonic vibrations of a piezo-electric crystal.
Aerosol output (the mass of particles in aerosol form produced/min) is not necessarily the same as drug output (the mass of drug produced/min as an aerosol). Ideally, the drug output of a nebulizer should be known for each of the different drugs given. Various factors affect the drug output and deposition:
- gas flow rate (generally air at 6–8 L/min but oxygen if treating acute asthma)
- chamber design
- volume (commonly 2–2.5ml, up to 4ml)
- residual volume (commonly 0.5ml)
- physical properties of the drug in solution
- breathing pattern of the patient.

The choice of nebulizer can be crucial, particularly when trying to produce an aerosol small enough to deliver a drug to the alveoli. Ideally, a nebulizer should be prescribed in co-operation with the local nebulizer service which can generally provide an assessment, information and education service for staff, patients and their families. Information should include:
- a description of the equipment and its use
- drugs used, doses and frequencies
- equipment maintenance/cleaning
- action to take if treatment becomes less effective
- action to take and emergency telephone number to use if equipment breaks down.

Written information should also be given to patients (Box A9.A). Patients should be instructed to take steady normal breaths (interspersed with occasional deep ones) and nebulization time should be less than 10min or 'to dryness'. Because there is always a residual volume, 'dryness' should be taken as 1min after spluttering starts. In general, whereas a mask can be used for bronchodilators, a mouthpiece should be used for other drugs to limit environmental contam-ination and/or contact with the patient's eyes. A mask may be preferable, however, in patients who are acutely ill, fatigued or very young, regardless of the nature of the drug.

Nebulizers in palliative care
Nebulizers are used to ease cough and breathlessness in advanced cancer (Tables A9.1 & A9.2); they should be reviewed after 2 days to check efficacy. When using **lidocaine** or **bupivacaine** for a dry cough (but not for breathlessness), pretreat with **salbutamol** because of the risk of bronchospasm. After treatment with a local anaesthetic, patients should be advised not to eat or drink for 1h because the reduced gag/cough reflex increases the risk of aspiration. Comparative pharmacokinetic data for inhaled **corticosteroids** are given in Table A9.3 (see also p.43).

Box A9.A Advice about using a nebulizer at home

To help your breathing, your doctor has prescribed a drug to be used with a nebulizer. The nebulizer converts the drug into a fine mist which you inhale.

The apparatus
Your nebulizer system consists of the following parts:

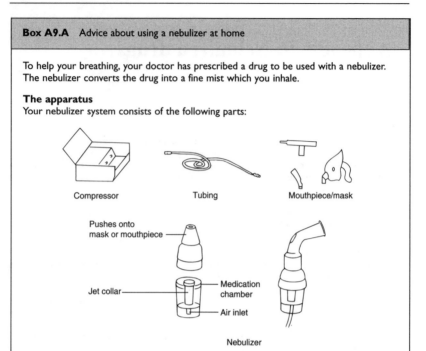

Compressor   Tubing   Mouthpiece/mask

Pushes onto mask or mouthpiece

Jet collar   Medication chamber

Air inlet

Nebulizer

The compressor is the portable pump which pumps air along the tubing into the nebulizer.

The nebulizer is a small chamber for the liquid medicine, through which air is blown to make a mist.

The nebulizer has a screw-on top onto which the mask or mouthpiece is attached.

How to use your nebulizer
Place the medication in the nebulizer, replace the screw-on top and turn the compressor on. Inhale by mouthpiece or mask while breathing at a normal rate. Stop 1 minute after the nebulizer contents start spluttering or after a maximum of 10 minutes.

General advice
If you have a cough, the nebulizer may help you to expectorate, so have some tissues nearby.

You may wish to use the nebulizer before attempting an activity which makes you feel out of breath.

If the effects of the nebulizer wear off or you have any questions or concerns about it, please speak to your doctor or nurse.

Cleaning
Wash the mouthpiece/mask and nebulizer in warm water and detergent, then rinse and dry well. Ideally this should be done after every use, but *once a day as a minimum*. Attach the tube and run the nebulizer empty for a few moments after cleaning it to make sure the equipment is dry. Once a week, unplug and wipe the compressor and tubing with a damp cloth.

Table A9.1 Nebulized drugs and cancer-related cough or breathlessness[2]

Class of drug	Indications	Scientific evidence	Comments
Normal saline	Loosening of tenacious secretions	None	Probably underused in this setting; may also help breathlessness
Mucolytic agents (e.g. hypertonic saline, acetylcysteine)	To thin viscous sputum	Conflicting evidence	May result in copious liquid sputum which the patient may still not be able to cough up
Corticosteroids (e.g. budesonide)	Stridor, lymphangitis, radiation pneumonitis, cough after the insertion of a stent	None	Very limited clinical experience only; may not be more beneficial than use of inhaler or oral routes
Local anaesthetics (e.g. lidocaine, bupivacaine)	Cough, particularly if caused by lymphangitis carcinomatosa	Conflicting evidence for both dyspnoea [3,4] and cough[5]	Risk of bronchospasm; reduces gag reflex
Opioids (e.g. morphine, diamorphine, fentanyl)	Breathlessness associated with diffuse lung disease	Anecdotal evidence supportive,[6] but controlled trials indicate that no better than saline[7,8]	Not recommended; risk of bronchospasm
Bronchodilators (e.g. salbutamol)	Treatment of reversible airway obstruction	Extrapolated from patients with asthma and COPD	Use only if trial of therapy demonstrates real benefit

Table A9.2   Recommended uses of nebulized drugs in palliative care

Indication	Drug	Initial regimen	Dose titration	Comments
Tenacious secretions	Saline 0.9%	5ml q6h	Up to q2h	
Reversible airway obstruction	Salbutamol	2.5mg q4h–q6h	Up to 5mg q4h	Risk of sensitivity to cardiac stimulant effects
	Terbutaline	5mg q4h–q6h	Up to 10mg q4h	
Cough	*†Lidocaine 2%	5ml p.r.n.	Up to q6h	Risk of bronchospasm; fast for 1h after nebulization
	*†Bupivacaine 0.25%	5ml p.r.n.	Up to q8h	

Table A9.3   Pharmacokinetic details of inhaled corticosteroids[9]

	Anti-inflammatory activity[a]	Affinity for lung tissue[b]	Human lung GR complex halflife (h)	Systemic bio-availability (%)		Plasma halflife (h)
				Inhaled	Oral	
Beclometasone	3.5	0.4	?	20	<20	15
Budesonide	1	9.4	5.1	25	11	2.8
Fluticasone	?	18.0	10.5	20	<1	3.1
Triamcinolone	5.3	3.6	3.9	21	22	1.5

a. thymic involution assay
b. compared to dexamethasone.

1 BTS and others (1997) Current best practice for nebuliser treatment. Thorax. **52** (suppl 2).
2 Ahmedzai S and Davis C (1997) Nebulised drugs in palliative care. Thorax. **52** (suppl 2): S75–S77.
3 Winning AJ et al. (1988) Ventilation and breathlessness on maximal exercise in patients with interstitial lung disease after local anaesthetic aerosol inhalation. Clinical Science. **74**: 275–281.
4 Wilcock A et al. (1994) Safety and efficacy of nebulized lignocaine in patients with cancer and breathlessness. Palliative Medicine. **8**: 35–38.
5 Howard P et al. (1997) Lignocaine aerosol and persistent cough. British Journal of Diseases of the Chest. **71**: 19–24.
6 Young IH et al. (1989) Effect of low dose nebulized morphine on exercise endurance in patients with chronic lung disease. Thorax. **44**: 387–390.
7 Davis CL et al. (1993) The pharmacokinetics of nebulized morphine. Proceedings of International Association for the Study of Pain. IASP Publications, Seattle. pp 379 (abstract 995).
8 Noseda A et al. (1997) Disabling dyspnoea in patients with advanced disease: lack of effect of nebulized morphine. European Respiratory Journal. **10**: 1079–1083.
9 Demoly P and Chung KF (1998) Pharmacology of corticosteroids. Respiratory Medicine. **92**: 385–394.

* specialist use only. † unlicensed use.

Index

Note: Drugs are indexed under their recommended International Nonproprietary Names. The British Approved Name appears in brackets following the rINN. Principal page references appear in bold.

Palliative Care Formulary

Report on syringe driver compatibility/incompatibility

- Compatibility

- Incompatibility

Please report any combination of drugs which have been used successfully and do not appear on the charts

Please report any combination of drugs which has caused problems (i.e. crystallization/discolouration)

Please send to: Dr Andrew Wilcock
Hayward House
City Hospital
Hucknall Road
Nottingham NG5 1PB

Reporting Unit

Name and professional address _____

_____

_____

Telephone _____   Fax _____

Signature _____   Date _____

Drug combination (give dose details)	Total volume	Diluent	Administration rate	Comments
Example: Diamorphine 60mg + Haloperidol 5mg + Midazolam 30mg	13.5ml	WFI	24 hours	Ran on time. No site problems. No visible evidence of incompatibility

Incompatible

Drug combination (give dose details)	Total volume	Diluent	Administration rate	Comments
Example: Diamorphine 30mg + Haloperidol 10mg + Hyoscine butylbromide 200mg	13.5ml	WFI	Set to run for 24 hours	Crystals found in line after 20 hours